Health Care System Transformation for Nursing and Health Care Leaders

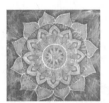

Anne Boykin, PhD, MN, founding dean of the Christine E. Lynn College of Nursing, Florida Atlantic University, is currently professor emeritus (retired). She is recognized internationally and nationally as an authority on caring science, and has coauthored and edited several books including *Nursing as Caring: A Model for Transforming Practice* (1993, 2001) and *Living a Caring-Based Program* (1994). She is a contributing author for many book titles and has authored more than 20 journal articles. Dr. Boykin is the past president of the International Association for Human Caring, and has served as a member of several boards at the international, national, state, and local levels, including the American Association of Colleges of Nursing, National League for Nursing, Southern Education Board Council on Collegiate Education for Nursing, and the Florida Association of Colleges of Nursing. She now serves as a consultant on nursing, nursing theory, and transforming health care environments, and works with a growing list of hospitals and hospital chains locally and nationally.

Savina Schoenhofer, PhD, MEd, MN, is professor (part-time) at the University of Mississippi Medical Center School of Nursing. Earlier academic appointments include those at Florida Atlantic University, Alcorn State University, Texas Tech University, and Wichita State University. As the collaborating author with Anne Boykin, Dr. Schoenhofer has published *Nursing as Caring: A Model for Transforming Practice,* and has written chapters in numerous other books and authored multiple journal articles in *Nursing Science Quarterly, Advances in Nursing Science, International Journal for Human Caring,* and others. She is noted as an authority on caring science and was named "Living Legend" in 2003 by the International Association for Human Caring, in recognition of her nursing scholarship.

Kathleen Valentine, PhD, RN, MS, is associate professor and associate dean for clinical affairs and community engagement at the School of Nursing at MGH Institute of Health Professions. At the time of writing this book, she was the director of the Louis and Anne Green Memory and Wellness Center and the Diabetes Education and Research Center at the Christine E. Lynn College of Nursing, Florida Atlantic University. Formerly, she was associate dean, College of Nursing, Florida State University, and department chair, University of Wisconsin, with clinical positions as practice director, Clinical Practice Model Resources Center, Grand Rapids, MI, and director, Health Care Delivery, Kaiser Permanente, Oakland, CA, among others. She has been awarded 18 research/practice grants, seven of them in the amount of six and seven figures. She has authored 15 journal articles, and presents nationally and internationally. She received her doctorate from Cornell University, specializing in human service program evaluation. She has worked on health system transformation as a specialty.

Health Care System Transformation for Nursing and Health Care Leaders

Implementing a Culture of Caring

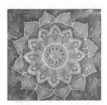

Anne Boykin, PhD, MN
Savina Schoenhofer, PhD, MEd, MN
Kathleen Valentine, PhD, RN, MS

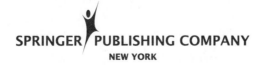
SPRINGER PUBLISHING COMPANY
NEW YORK

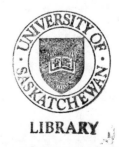

Springer Publishing Company, LLC
11 West 42nd Street
New York, NY 10036
www.springerpub.com

Acquisitions Editor: Joseph Morita
Composition: Newgen Imaging

ISBN: 978-0-8261-9643-9
e-book ISBN: 978-0-8261-9644-6

13 14 15 16 17 / 5 4 3 2 1

The author and the publisher of this Work have made every effort to use sources believed to be reliable to provide information that is accurate and compatible with the standards generally accepted at the time of publication. The author and publisher shall not be liable for any special, consequential, or exemplary damages resulting, in whole or in part, from the readers' use of, or reliance on, the information contained in this book. The publisher has no responsibility for the persistence or accuracy of URLs for external or third-party Internet websites referred to in this publication and does not guarantee that any content on such websites is, or will remain, accurate or appropriate.

Library of Congress Cataloging-in-Publication Data
Boykin, Anne, author.
  Health care system transformation for nursing and health care leaders : implementing a culture of caring / Anne Boykin, Savina Schoenhofer, Kathleen Valentine.
      p. ; cm.
  Includes bibliographical references and index.
  ISBN 978-0-8261-9643-9 — ISBN 978-0-8261-9644-6 (e-book)
  I. Schoenhofer, Savina O'Bryan, author. II. Valentine, Kathleen Louise, author. III. Title.
  [DNLM: 1. Models, Nursing. 2. Nursing Theory. 3. Nurse Administrators—psychology. 4. Nursing Care. WY 86]
  RT41
  610.73--dc23   2013017306

Special discounts on bulk quantities of our books are available to corporations, professional associations, pharmaceutical companies, health care organizations, and other qualifying groups. If you are interested in a custom book, including chapters from more than one of our titles, we can provide that service as well.

For details, please contact:
Special Sales Department, Springer Publishing Company, LLC
11 West 42nd Street, 15th Floor, New York, NY 10036–8002
Phone: 877-687-7476 or 212-431-4370; Fax: 212-941-7842
E-mail: sales@springerpub.com

Printed in the United States of America by Bradford & Bigelow.

We dedicate this book to all health care providers,
especially those in leadership roles,
who commit themselves
to humanize and transform systems of care.

To my husband, Steve Staudenmeyer, whose love, support, caring, and
*encouragement allow me to live my passion for nursing.—**Anne Boykin***

For Gwen, Carrie, and Emma, my love and gratitude.
*—**Savina Schoenhofer***

To my husband George DePuy and the extended circle of family,
friends, and colleagues who help me to grow in caring.
*With love, always.—**Kathleen Valentine***

Contents

Foreword

We are deepening our understanding of the operation of a complex world and the structures and processes that demonstrate its interactions. The introduction in the United States of concepts associated with complex adaptive systems has radically changed our understanding of human dynamics and the organizations and structures that support and advance them. Traditional industrial and linear notions of structure, culture, and leadership have essentially been eclipsed by the deeper richness of the levels of understanding of how people live, relate, interact, and work in highly complex systems.

As a result of this deeper understanding gleaned from the translation of complex adaptive systems into human organizations and relationships, much conflict and confusion with traditional structures and approaches to aligning, understanding, and applying developed processes to human dynamics have emerged in our traditional organizational constructs. The architecture, structure of work, characteristics of interaction, management and leadership capacities, and relational dynamics that developed over the full course of the 20th century have become less relevant and viable, and increasingly lacking in effectiveness. The more linear two-dimensional, vertical, hierarchical models and mechanisms of structuring work and relationships that were developed throughout the 20th century have become nonrelevant in a 21st-century social context.

The growing digital reality that increasingly defines and influences contemporary human experience has substantially changed the rules of the game with regard to human dynamics, interaction, and work. In the industrial age, models of work were fixed, finite, functional, and institutional. Twenty-first–century work and workplaces are characterized by structures and processes that are more fluid, flexible, focused, portable, and mobile. The portability and mobility of human life, relationships, interactions, and dynamics have altered our understanding of the operation of systems structures, processes, relationships, and leadership. This deepening understanding of the complexity that characterizes life at both the universal and subatomic levels has redefined the parameters within which human interaction unfolds and progresses.

Our understanding of complex adaptive systems leads us to raise questions about our ability to predict and adapt these forces for good use and their implications and actions in human dynamics and on human organization and work. Our awareness is now informed by such wide-ranging complexity characteristics as follows:

- The continuous interaction of large numbers of intersecting elements
- No one element ever understanding the operation of the entire system
- The depth in degree of rich interaction between elements and "agents" of the system
- Continuously open, transforming, altering, changing conditions and circumstances
- Unending operation and confluence of positive and negative feedback loops
- Continuous demand for disequilibrium in the environment
- Agents can influence others and are simultaneously being influenced by others
- Systems and organizational behavior are continuously emergent
- Patterns of synergy and effectiveness can be unknowable and unpredictable
- Big systems' changes emerge and generate from small causative drivers
- Systems interact with their environment in dynamic and nonlinear ways
- Effective systems operate best on the edges of chaos and stability
- All systems succeed as a function of their interaction with their own history

All of these characteristics, elements, and forces are acting constantly and consistently and are reflected in human experience and call us as leaders to a deeper understanding of their actions and operations as we more clearly develop mechanisms for engaging environmental dynamism, transformation, change, innovation, and leadership. Whatever approaches are undertaken by organizational leaders must now reflect the clear and abiding understanding of the normative action of these universal forces operating as both the backdrop of human action and the context that gives such action impetus, clarity, understanding, and veracity.

Societal and professional leaders must now make, as a part of their work obligations, the translation of these emerging realities into mechanisms, toolsets, and frames of reference that guide those we lead. This leadership must be expressed in ways that help those we lead reflect on their own responses and patterns of behavior and have a deeper understanding of the forces that can both enable or disable their best efforts. This is especially true as health professionals are challenged with fundamentally transforming the health care system that clearly represents the same many characteristics of complexity, and demands our deepening understanding of health care professionals' actions and influences on the relevance and effectiveness of the health system. In addition to the growing translation of the attributes of complexity to health care are the political and economic challenges codified in the Patient Protection and Affordable Care Act of 2010 (PPACA), which represents a substantive recalibration from a volume-based economic and delivery model for American health care to one that is grounded in a value-based, effectiveness-delineated health script attempting to advance the nation's health and provide a level of universal access.

Traditional and historic industrial-grounded approaches to transforming American health care simply can't succeed. Much of the historic industrial and linear thinking and models are no longer relevant, neither to the times nor the demand. Furthermore, the firmly entrenched digital infrastructure of social and human experience with all of its implications now demands entirely fresh thinking, innovations, and models disciplined by experimentation and testing in a wide variety of social and systems approaches.

Clearly, it is leaders who must understand this sea change within the health system in the broader social culture. Leaders must suspend attachment to traditional grounding in their leadership learning and experience and become increasingly available to approaches that may at first appear counterintuitive and even uncomfortable. Traditional attachment to historic transactional and even transformational models developed within an industrial/postindustrial paradigm must be suspended in a way that increases availability to a richer level of understanding of complexity leadership and its application to the challenges of the time.

This textbook serves as both a challenge and a bridge to nursing and health care leaders as they grapple with the need for changing structures, approaches, and skills necessary to support sustainable health transformation. Practice frequently changes; principle rarely does. The foundational and sustainable principles in caring so central to the nurse's role do not themselves change, yet, the expression of caring and its applications are necessarily constantly refined and altered to reflect the contemporary character of their expression. With all of the necessary incorporation, translation, and application of complex adaptive systems to health care, there is a strong need for a principle-based, theoretically grounded set of tools for transforming the culture of care in contemporary health care systems. There is a crying need for translational and practical strategies for living the shift to value-grounded caring throughout the health care system. While our understanding of systems and applications may be more deeply evolving, along with it comes a greater demand for intentional reflection and articulation of the living of caring values that sustains the focus on essential human relatedness and the need for refining and developing the enterprise in a way that demonstrates value for caring by translating it within a complex adaptive frame. Engaging stakeholders in the essential partnerships for caring creates both the urge and the obligation to align the contemporary complex culture with the principles and patterns of human caring that will both hominize it and sustain it. To do so creates a culture responsive to the environmental demands and shifts of the time, the converging forces of a complex adaptive milieu, and a community of careers guided by principles and practices that reflect the unique health needs of individuals and the collective sustainable health requisites of the human community.

The authors' approach to creating a transforming culture through use of foundations laid in the theoretical development of Nursing as Caring offers a solid foundation upon which to recalibrate and reconfigure toward a caring organizational health system. The use of the Dance of Caring Persons, grounded in value-based principles, serves as an effective vehicle for guiding and refining organizational and human systems in a way that grounds the further work of transforming health care systems in sustaining values of caring. While many of the beliefs, elements, and attitudes in the Dance of Caring Persons will need continuous further refinement as they are translated into complex adaptive systems, the fact that the approach requires the engagement of all organizational constituencies in the process of care transformation ensures continuing relevance and adaptation.

The increasing recognition and intentional articulation of the core values of respect for persons and sincere appreciation for the community of contribution of all participants in the health care systems' effectiveness are essential. This work will need collaboration from patients, families, nurses, physicians, and other health professionals, as well as administrators and managers in conjunction with the systems and models within which they operate as an essential construct for a sustaining transformation. Grounding that transformation in values and principles of caring ensures that the system and approaches will be open and responsive and that the essential elements of care will remain at the core of the collective conversation of service transformation. How systems respond to environmental changes and economic and resource challenges associated with human action, and how personal and collective human caring responses are calibrated, are addressed and will help maintain the caring-centric focus of both human design and response. In this way the authors and those who respond to their work will demonstrate the fundamental and essential core of our human existence and sustenance—the continuing capacity to love and care for each other.

Tim Porter-O'Grady, DM, EdD, APRN, FAAN, FACCWS
Senior Partner, Tim Porter-O'Grady Associates, Inc., Atlanta, GA
Associate Professor, Leadership Scholar, College of Nursing
and Health Innovation, Arizona State University, Phoenix, AZ
Clinical Professor, Leadership Scholar, College of Nursing
The Ohio State University, Columbus, OH

Preface

This book offers a perspective that health care systems are human systems as portrayed in the Dance of Caring Persons. It provides a values-based, theoretically grounded guide for transforming the culture of health care systems. It provides detailed, practical strategies for living the value of caring in the workplace using the Dance of Caring Persons as the framework for transformation. The Dance of Caring Persons emerged in the context of the nursing theory, Nursing as Caring. Although the theory of Nursing as Caring offers a theoretical framework for the study and practice of nursing, the Dance of Caring Persons is a value-based model designed to guide the organization and functioning of human systems, including health care systems, thus transforming the cultural environment. At its most basic level, the Dance of Caring Persons expresses certain fundamental beliefs and attitudes: Each person in the health care system lives caring meaningfully in unique and valuable ways; and the contributions of each person to the whole of the enterprise have a prized place in the enterprise.

The book addresses all stakeholders in the health care system—patients and families, nurses, physicians and other primary and adjunctive professional care providers, ancillary service providers, and administrators and managers. It also addresses all aspects of the system—organizational model, delivery of health care, human resource functions, and outcomes of all aspects of the system. Although broad in the scope of addressing all components of health care systems, there is a focus on specific caring-based strategies for transforming the culture of health care systems.

The book is organized into three sections. Embedded in each chapter are provocative questions intended to engage the reader and stimulate thinking. In addition to the traditional references, at the end of the book the reader will find a list of related resources. Section I includes three foundational chapters that offer a context and framework for the later chapters that address specific strategies relevant to aspects of the health care system. The first chapter emphasizes the inevitable need for transformation in health care systems compelled by health care reform through the Affordable Care Act. For persons not steeped in the issues confronting health care systems in the 21st century, this chapter provides a valuable overview of those issues, and an understanding of the value of bringing a caring perspective to the transformation of health care systems. Persons who are deeply aware of the world of health care and the significant challenges affecting that world may choose to begin with another chapter, depending on their background and interests. Chapters 2 and 3 establish the necessary foundation and framework for the remaining chapters. Chapter 2 provides a substantive understanding of the Dance of Caring Persons model that grounds the design and implementation of specific strategies; Chapter 3 focuses on the relationship of cultural aspects of a health care system to the experience of those within the system and ultimately to the success of the organization. These chapters are essential to understanding concepts in subsequent chapters.

Section II addresses strategies to prepare people and processes in all functions for whole system transformation. Chapter 4 focuses on "getting ready," by discussing ways in which leaders at all levels of the organization propel the desire for change into commitment for action. It addresses specific strategies for planning and designing for transformational change, and for engaging the leadership team in preparing for implementation. Chapter 5, focusing on "getting set," describes the functional timetable for specific actions for transforming the culture. Both of these chapters provide important, detailed guidance on the "how to" of transformation for leaders in health care and for students preparing to be leaders.

Section III offers practical strategies for living caring values throughout all aspects of the organization and infusing all functions of the health care system with the core values central to the Dance of Caring Persons. Successive chapters address practical strategies for transforming the organizational mission (Chapter 6); leadership structures and processes (Chapter 7); communication (Chapter 8); and outcomes (Chapter 9). Although there is a logical flow of ideas in these chapters, they do not necessarily have to be read in sequential order. For example, if the organization is focusing on transforming the mission of the institution, it would make sense to begin with reading Chapter 6, although Chapters 2 and 3 would provide valuable insight and support for transforming the organizational mission.

In keeping with the inclusive and dialogic character of the Dance of Caring Persons model, responses from health professionals representing a broad range of participants in health care are included in each chapter. The method of achieving dialogue in the book varies from formal written responses to chapter content, to transcriptions of small group conversations about the chapter topic and its contents. Also included are "questions to consider," exemplars, and suggested resources to assist with the implementation of suggested strategies. We offer this book for your consideration because of our fundamental belief in the value of caring and its ability to transform the health care system, and the practical value of the Dance of Caring Persons model as an overarching framework.

Anne Boykin, PhD, MN
Savina Schoenhofer, PhD, MEd, MN
Kathleen Valentine, PhD, RN, MS

Acknowledgments

We thank those who contributed to this book, those who influenced our understanding of caring and health care systems, and those aspiring to transform health care systems, all for whom we hope this book will be of value.

Introduction

Health Care System Transformation for Nursing and Health Care Leaders: Implementing a Culture of Caring describes a new approach to transforming our health care system based upon a model grounded in caring as an essential human value. Using the Dance of Caring Persons framework (originally developed as the nursing philosophical framework, Nursing as Caring) for transforming health care system culture, the book provides a values-based, theoretically grounded guide for transforming organizational culture with detailed, practical strategies for living the value of caring in the health care system workplace.

SO WHY IS TRANSFORMATION NEEDED IN HEALTH CARE?

The U.S. health care system has struggled for decades against seemingly intractable problems: safety problems, including more than 100,000 unexpected hospital deaths annually (Committee on Quality of Health Care in America, Institute of Medicine, 2000); incomplete and unequal access to care; perverse payment incentives that fail to reward good outcomes; fragmented, uncoordinated, and highly variable care processes that result in significant waste; a disconnect between quality and price; rising costs; inadequate consumer engagement and empowerment; and the absence of productivity and efficiency gains common in other industries.

Beyond life expectancy and other macro variables, even small, seemingly "controllable" variables often score poorly when measuring the performance of the U. S. health care system. For example, in 2003 McGlynn and colleagues showed that typical patients received only just over half of the recommended care. Later the study was repeated with children (Mangione-Smith et al., 2007) and showed that they received even less of the recommended care at just under half. These problems have resulted in various reform proposals including significant, and often emotional, dialogue during each of the 2008 and 2012 presidential political campaigns. Most proposals have focused on providing greater access to care, with intermittent focus on controlling the costs of care. Although understandable, this approach ignores the fundamental problem: Health care value (defined here as health outcomes relative to input costs) simply must increase.

Yet despite these valid concerns, health care is not just another "product or service." It is intensely personal, often consumed at the most vulnerable times of our lives, and highly dependent upon the values, desires, and beliefs of both those treating and those being treated. Unlike other industries, price transparency is noticeably absent—consumers often lack the knowledge to "know" what they need and frequently bear only a small fraction, if any, of the actual costs of the services provided, and physician and other provider intermediaries who "choose" for consumers have potentially conflicting incentives. These conditions are far different than the "perfect markets" described by economists in college texts.

So what to do given these circumstances? Enter Boykin and colleagues, who propose a radically different perspective on health care transformation. In contrast to the bottom-line, productivity, and benchmark-driven approaches exclusively used so often within health care, the authors recognize that health care is the "ultimate team sport" by explicitly defining that each person in the health care system lives caring meaningfully in unique and valuable ways and that the contributions of each person to the whole of the enterprise are meaningful and valuable and have a place in the enterprise. At Mission Health, we agree with this concept and explicitly refer to all staff—whether at the bedside, in billing, housekeeping, administration, or otherwise—as "caregivers."

The book approaches the opportunity for transformation in different ways, from formal written responses to chapter content, to transcriptions of small group conversations about the chapter topic and its contents. The approach is very practical, with each chapter including "questions to consider" relevant to the particular chapter topic, exemplars, and suggested resources to assist with implementation of strategies suggested. The Resources section provides invaluable information that can be used to support practical implementation of the model. This book explicitly questions how the organization might address traditional "myths" that have contributed to our dysfunctional system today, including the following:

- Hierarchy trumps collaboration
- Most legitimate outcomes are financial
- Change must come from the top
- Caring is a luxury
- Finance and caring are opposite poles
- Professional disciplinary accountability will ensure positive system accountability
- External task force recommendations drive system quality

The book offers specific strategies for engaging the executive leadership team:

- Gaining buy-in throughout the system by defining the blue-sky vision and the climate for change
- Designing detailed features of transformation—specific steps for gaining sponsorship and champions throughout the system
- Budgeting for transformation—how the efforts involved in the change are accounted for in budget priorities
- Establishing broad structures and processes for ongoing dialogue to make the model live
- Prizing, valuing, and growing in all dimensions of the system—outcomes management

Specifically addressed are two critical aspects of health care system communication. The first focuses on internal communication and reporting strategies that maximize effectiveness of the organization. This includes leadership tone, presence, visibility, and consistency, recognizing the influence of each aspect on sustained and effective forums for collegial dialogue and action. The second focuses on communication between patients/ families and members of the system—nurses, physicians, other professional providers, and ancillary service providers; and between and among all participants in the system in relation to health care delivery. This includes methods for including and involving patients and families as active and valued members in designing the care experience they desire and deserve. At Mission Health, we have found the inclusion of patients and family members to be particularly transformational in nearly all aspects of care redesign.

With so much time and energy focused on transformation, health care leaders and participants would benefit from a careful read of this book, before passing it along to friends and colleagues. Regardless of one's entering perspective—whether hierarchically driven, finance focused, consumer centric, or otherwise—the insights and lessons from *Health Care System Transformation for Nursing and Health Care Leaders: Implementing a Culture of Caring* will cause you to pause, reflect, stay patient centered, and stay caring in all that you do. After all, isn't that why we entered this field in the first place?

Ron Paulus, MD, MBA
President and CEO
Mission Health Systems
Asheville, NC

REFERENCES

Committee on Quality of Health Care in America, Institute of Medicine (2000). *To err is human: Building a safer health system.* Washington, DC: The National Academies Press.

Mangione-Smith, R., DeCristofaro, A. H., Setodji, C. M., et al. (2007). The quality of ambulatory care delivered to children in the United States. *New England Journal of Medicine, 357*(15), 1515–1523.

McGlynn, E. A., Asch, S. M., Adams, J., et al. (2003). The quality of health care delivered to adults in the United States. *New England Journal of Medicine, 348*(26), 2635–2645.

Preparing for the Dance of Caring Persons: Why Transformation Is Needed and Why Caring Is the Essential Value to Guide Successful Transformation

Section I provides the foundational information used to frame the subsequent practical approaches (Sections II and III) that apply caring values and the Dance of Caring Persons model as essential guides to successful health care transformation. Section I addresses the complex issues inherent within health care systems that are prompting efforts at transformation, and provides an exposition of a model of caring as a credible, powerful, and essential guide for meaningful whole system transformation, in the context of cultural transformation. Section I provides the framework for moving health care systems from a focus on continuous subsystem changes, often defined by external regulatory and accreditation bodies, to a whole system transformation focus guided by a unifying framework. The authors of this book have heard the call for whole system transformation that is authentic, values based, practical, understandable, achievable, meaningful, and generative. Our goal is to help readers of this book become confident using the language of caring as credible, strong, and integral to successful transformation of the health care enterprise using the Dance of Caring Persons as a model. Each author has specific experience with the whole system change based on caring.

Chapter 1

Challenges to the Effectiveness of Health Care Systems

What are the challenges to the effectiveness of health care systems, and why is transformation needed? This chapter addresses the multiplicity of issues facing health care organizations that prevent them from focusing on their primary service mission of caring and patient-centered care. Some of these issues include quality, safety, lack of coordination and collaboration among nurses, physicians, and other health care providers and units of care, stressful workplace environments, inefficiencies, hospital–physician alignment and reimbursement, and monetization/output/revenue imbalances. The chapter is organized in sections that address the following issues:

1. A historical perspective about the carative or caring and curative traditions in health care that have helped to define the current state of health care systems
2. A framework for examining the challenges in today's health care system, organized according to seven initiatives proposed in 2003 by a leading health care system chief executive officer (CEO) and a chief medical officer (CMO), a proposal that calls for more accountable care rather than our current ineffective, inefficient, and costly system (Halvorson & Isham, 2003)
3. Our own perspective on Halvorson and Isham's accountable care framework, along with highlighted comments made from a national gathering of health care CEOs meeting to dialogue and reflect on changes in the health care system
4. An invitation to you to contemplate health care's current standing in achieving this more accountable health care system and your insights as to how that may enhance or obscure a way for caring to be acknowledged substantively as an essential foundation in the provision of health care services

HISTORICAL PERSPECTIVE

Health care used to be a local service and is now a global enterprise. The challenges and opportunities facing the health care system and health care providers involve whole system transformation. How did we evolve from a local community service to a global enterprise? What are the implications of that evolution for the caring foundations of health care?

The health care system was largely a cottage industry prior to the 1980s, when health care began to be structured within the business model of managerial corporations. As a cottage industry, each community defined and provided health care services for the catchment area served. Although larger health care systems and academic medical organizations with broader missions existed, for the most part health care was a local service.

The cottage model, with its local service characteristic, changed as the managerial business model became more embedded and as reimbursement for services became more complex. Diagnostic-related groups (DRGs) began to operate on a prospective payment system, putting hospitals and associated providers at greater risk for the care episode for patients, rather than for the quality, satisfaction, and cost of a specific unit of service. Hospitals received a set fee for a given diagnostic category—and if they were able to reduce the length of stay and the overall costs for an entire episode of care, the difference between the cost per DRG and the payment for it could be retained. Payment incentives structured in this manner drove organizations to search for efficiencies in care delivery through implementation of care pathways, which in turn called for standardized treatments and specialized care teams. As a result, one of the most sustained effects from this era was to reduce variations in care that arose through individual physician practice preferences. Significant variations in care were subject to peer review, which applied accountability through the expectation that practice or science-based evidence be used to support variations in practice rather than individual practitioner preference alone.

This prospective model was born from calls for cost accountability from a coalition of large manufacturing companies that were seeing more of their budgets going toward health care and interfering with their competitive positioning in the global market. Over time, increased calls for cost accountability led to more emphasis on capitated-managed care insurance plans that were expected to manage both costs and quality. Capitated-managed care means that a fixed insurance fee is paid per-member per-month based on a set number of enrolled members covered in the insurance plan. If the overall health of members in the plan is good, and costs and expenditures are controlled, the per-member per-month fee can be moderated. However, managed care plans experienced considerable consumer and provider backlash in which the insurance company was seen as a barrier to decisions that should be reserved to be between patient and provider. Though costs for health care were stabilized during this era, this model at its height became unacceptable to most.

Health care organizations searched for ways to maximize revenue streams through niche services, horizontal integration (multiple same type of service sites aggregated into one larger organization, e.g., hospitals or cancer centers), or vertical integration (in which a single entity merged with units of service across the continuum of care). Organizations are complex adaptive systems and as such are constantly evolving to new models of service care delivery that serve simultaneously as an opportunity for growth and a challenge to the traditional forces within the health care system. The corporatization of health care is said to have spawned interdependency across health care sectors, sometimes labeled as the medical industrial complex. These multiple and interdependent aspects of the health care system together account for a large percentage of our gross domestic product (GDP) when considered as costs, while at the same time driving employment opportunities that ultimately are intended to serve societal growth needs. These factors, in addition to the aging population, increased technology, aversion to rationing, and so on, all shape the health care system we face today and provide momentum for transformational change. On the one side of the equation, traditional health care costs have outstripped the ability to pay for them and ultimately this affects the overall health of our national economy. Evidence of this is seen in the number of uninsured persons in the United States (over

48 million, according to the 2010 U.S. Census)—persons who might be employed, but whose employers do not sponsor health care insurance benefits due to cost. The cost of employer-based health care insurance is rising at a rate that affects the viability and competitiveness of all industries.

Because health insurance has been associated with employment, or government-sponsored programs such as Medicare or Medicaid during the Great Recession of the first decade of the 21st century, the care access problem has become more acute for both the providers of health care and patients alike. This reality has led to calls for wholesale transformation of the health care system to realign health reimbursement payments toward lower cost and illness prevention, with a shift of access to health care insurance away from employer-based models to more community-based models open to all citizens. These dynamic forces have contributed to the passage of the 2010 Patient Protection and Affordable Care Act (ACA). The ACA has used a phased-in approach toward making this shift with an ultimate goal of providing coverage for all citizens while at the same time improving quality and controlling costs. The opportunity to improve quality through this large-scale national ACA initiative will promote transformational changes in which each health care discipline can exert significant leadership.

Leadership during this time of historical circumstances leading to passage of the ACA calls for widespread transformation of our current systems. We are at a crossroads—our current system emphasizes fee-for-service revenue streams, specialization, and volume-based care, while there are simultaneous calls for a different system, one that focuses on person-centered care, prevention, and lifestyle changes related to chronic conditions and illness. In addition, there is a consumer movement toward holistic health—a multibillion dollar industry, focused on personalized services, a large segment of which exists outside the parameters of the traditional health care system. Though there are some points of integration of complementary health care practices within "mainstream" health care, they are inconsistently available and largely uncompensated through traditional payer mechanisms such as third-party insurance. Thus, consumer desire for personalized, holistic access to care and the costs of delivery of care create inconsistent and contradictory expectations for personalized health. In the United States we spent 17% of our economy on health care in 2011 (Bloomberg News, June 13, 2012), more than any other nation, and yet our health care rankings do not reflect good value for the money invested. For example, we are 29th in the world for healthy life expectancy and 30th in infant mortality (Zakaria, 2012).

As spelled out in Valentine's (1988) historical analysis of the carative tradition in nursing and health, our mainstream health care system has increasingly become a movement away from holistic care focused on the person toward fragmented care focused on the segmented service provided by each discipline. This trajectory away from caring has led to increased emphasis on specialization and curing, and less emphasis on caring, integration, and care coordination. Business models have evolved to focus on specialized dimensions of the health care industry, eliminating less profitable centers in favor of those that have a greater return on investment. High-tech fields tend to be more costly and better paid than low-tech fields and are often associated with more specialization and treatments, not necessarily coordinated care that crosses the continuum from acute to home care. Thus, we have a health care industry that accounts for about 17% of the economy and because of its size and complex interdependencies, presents as a major factor in political discourse about how public dollars should be spent. Procedural care, based on a fee-for-service model focused on volume, has dominated our health care climate. However, the question is raised, is this the best way to approach the dilemma of high cost and poor outcomes in the future?

In his classic predictive study of health near the end of the 20th century, Selby (1974) wrote that in the future, as chronic conditions become the focus in health care, there would be less delineation between health and social problems. Just as during the industrial revolution there were public health efforts to deal with clean water, workplace safety, and food safety, in today's world there is again an emphasis on workplace safety (the hazards of sedentary work, pollutants, chemicals) and the food supply (highly processed, calorie-dense food) in relation to the epidemics of diabetes, obesity, heart disease, cancer, and memory disorders. Thus, it becomes even more imperative to assure that healthy food choices, safe water, and opportunities to exercise are all part of the healthy community equation.

A FRAMEWORK FOR HEALTH CARE POLICY CHANGE

More recently, leaders within major health care systems offered a perspective on what is needed to move toward a more holistic, health-oriented system. Our analysis of the need for health care system reform is organized around Halvorson and Isham's (2003) framework for health care policy change. A brief introduction to the background of these two leaders in the management of integrated health care systems will make clear the significance of their call for "safer, better and more accountable health care" (p. 1). In 2012, George Halvorson was completing his 10-year leadership role as the CEO and chairman with Kaiser Permanente, the largest not-for-profit integrated health care organization in the United States. Prior to that he was the CEO of HealthPartners where Dr. George Isham served as a medical director. Together, in 2003, they offered a still-relevant perspective on the challenges of the overall health care "nonsystem." In that work, they proposed seven major initiatives needed to move toward a health care system that improves the health of citizens through measurable outcomes that make a difference in the quality of life. These seven initiatives are:

1. Improve quality of care and patient safety
2. Address consumer choices, creating an improved market model for buying and selling health care
3. Improve population health
4. Prevent monopolistic and anticompetitive behavior
5. Create workable framework for dealing with the uninsured
6. Fund training, medical education, medical research, resupply of the health care workforce, re-engineering of health care delivery particularly in hospital settings
7. Adopt an automated health care record to give point-of-care information for consistent delivery of best practices based on known evidence (pp. 156–157)

A decade later, and with the new Patient Protection and ACA in place, what is the status of the health care "nonsystem" relative to these initiatives? These initiatives will be used to frame further discussion related to the need for health care transformation.

DANCE OF CARING PERSONS MODEL: ITS RELEVANCE TO 21ST-CENTURY HEALTH CARE INITIATIVES

The Dance of Caring Persons is a model to guide the whole of an organization, including the functioning of human systems, in a way that is person centered and caring focused. Core dimensions of caring represented in this model include the following:

- Acknowledgment that all persons have the capacity to care by virtue of their humanness
- Commitment to have respect for persons in all institutional structures and processes

- Recognition that each participant in the enterprise has a unique and valuable contribution to make to the whole and is present in the whole
- Appreciation for the dynamic, rhythmic nature of the Dance of Caring Persons, enabling opportunities for human creativity

These dimensions of the Dance of Caring Persons taken together and sometimes individually are the touchstones for transformational strategies, some that are known and some yet to be imagined. This model, which will be more thoroughly described in Chapter 2, represents the values-based unifying framework we propose for the transformation of health care systems in the 21st century. Now, more than ever, there is a call for creative integration of values that on the surface may be considered incompatible. A major strength of the Dance of Caring Persons model is that it offers solid ground for transcending seemingly insurmountable differences between for-profit values and altruistic values. As we present the analyses of the seven initiatives, we invite you to contemplate how the model might be evident in the changing health care system of the future. How might:

- Acknowledgment that all persons have the capacity to care become evident in the design and delivery of an accountable care organization (ACO)?
- Respect for persons in all institutional structures and processes be reflected in the partnerships that are formed within and across health care organizations and within provider/patient relationships?
- Recognition that each participant in the enterprise has a unique and valuable contribution to make to the whole change the way that we form interprofessional teams, our communication, and governance structures?
- Appreciation for the dynamic, rhythmic nature of the Dance of Caring Persons enable opportunities for human creativity, ultimately improving quality, access, and cost dynamics in a way that humanizes the care experience for all partners in the dance?

Proposed Initiative: Improve Quality of Care and Patient Safety

Overall there is a desire to have patient-centered organizations rather than patient satisfaction-focused organizations. Focusing on the patient as person improves both quality and satisfaction, while focusing on satisfaction alone leads to organizational compliance without necessarily understanding the underlying values. A truly patient-centered organization has patient and family engagement evident and welcomed as an integral part of the culture. Patients and families play an active role in improvement activities. The Institute for Healthcare Improvement is a leader in helping organizations address the question: Is our organization engaged in "patient-centered leadership...or patient-satisfaction leadership?" (American College of Health Care Executives, 2012).

Forces are converging to begin a shift from the recent emphasis on fragmented and isolated parts of the health care system to a demand for ACOs. Both the federal and state governments are adopting new payment and delivery system models aimed at improving the quality of health care services and reining in costs. Identification of patient-centered medical homes (PCMHs) and ACOs are aligned to follow the course of a person's condition beyond an immediate procedure and include coordination throughout an episode of care. For example, treatment for the person with diabetes involves not only the acute situation in which the patient might enter the ER in crisis, but the continuum of services also includes helping the person begin to bring his diabetes under control to prevent such hospitalization in the future. An example about diabetes and the dynamics involved in shifting incentives from volume-based services to value-based services is presented in the Resources section.

PCMHs tend to be primary care practices, while ACOs focus on partnerships across several medical homes and across a continuum of care services from inpatient through rehabilitation, including social services. In the new model, ACOs will be paid to coordinate care. The expectation is that a focus on prevention will allow more people to be served before acute exacerbation of illnesses, will save money, and will increase quality of life. What is transformative about this initiative is the attempt to align payment incentives to organizations that allow them to move away from an emphasis on isolated services paid on a fixed fee to caring for the whole person and populations of persons experiencing a chronic condition (Guterman et al., 2011).

In addition to a wide range of reforms enacted in the Patient Protection and ACA, some states are also seeking policies and processes to align with the goals of the ACA. The challenge will be coordinating between federal, state, and private initiatives to assure that the coordinated care system meets its care delivery and payment goals in providing patient-centered, effective, and efficient quality care.

Though the Supreme Court of the United States struck the mandated state expansion of Medicaid as proposed within the ACA (Kaiser Family Foundation, 2012), there still will be considerable expansion of the number of persons eligible for Medicaid. The way that the ACA unfolds will be very locally determined within communities, based on their culture and their resources. By 2019, "up to 25% of Americans could receive coverage through the program (Medicaid), and it could account for as much as 20% of national health care spending" (Bachrach, Bernstein, & Karl, 2012, para. 3). Medicaid expenditures account for over 70% of states' health care expenditures and constitute the first- or second-largest item in the budget of every state. Implementing coordinated, accountable delivery systems could help contain costs and achieve better outcomes for Medicaid beneficiaries (Bachrach et al., 2012).

The debate about the public/private nature of the health care system was very evident in the American presidential election process of 2012. With one candidate vowing to repeal the Patient Protection and ACA "on day one" after the inauguration, and the other having championed the act toward its full adoption in 2014, the two worldviews were sharply contrasted relative to market versus public/merit good. A market good is one that responds to the dynamics of supply and demand. A public or merit good is one that is available to all. In the United States we operate from both a market and merit perspective. We allow market forces to drive access to some care (elective, specialized, cosmetic), yet we do not deny care to anyone in an emergency and cover that through public funds (i.e., everyone merits access to health care in an emergency). Thus, eventually the cost of health care is paid by all citizens often in an ineffective, inefficient manner and at the costliest point of service, such as an emergency department.

Though the reelection of President Obama gives momentum to enact the ACA health care legislation, its adoption will be uneven and fraught with controversy as it is enacted on a state-by-state model. The ACA does signal the beginning of a systemic shift in all sectors of the health care industry to prepare to share the risk for providing services for "low-power, low-tech" chronic conditions such as obesity, diabetes, and Alzheimer's. Some prevention and payment for annual wellness exams is already initiated, along with other mandated prevention services (women's health) offered without copays. For example, Medicare now also provides payment for visits focused on obesity (previously denied as an acceptable code for reimbursement). Simultaneously, hospital organizations will be asked to be accountable for patient outcomes across the continuum of care. These changes begin to acknowledge that care for chronic conditions related to lifestyle and longevity requires personalized treatment focused on the person rather than on the diagnosis. Lifestyle changes are made at the personal level of choice and behavior, amidst the array of choices available within the environment.

Proposed Initiative: Address Consumer Choices, Creating an Improved Market Model for Buying and Selling Health Care

There is an increased awareness of the need to focus on consumer needs versus system needs and to create "patient-centered" care. At the 2012 Huron Healthcare CEO Forum, a gathering of top health care system CEOs, consumer choice was acknowledged as an important focus. Kate Walsh, CEO of Boston Medical Center and former COO of Brigham and Women's Hospital and Novartis, noted that "we need to think of service lines from the perspective of the patient's experience, not our experience" (Huron Healthcare, 2012, p. 10).

The Institute of Medicine (IOM) defines patient-centered care as "health care that establishes a partnership among practitioners, patients, and their families…to ensure that decisions respect patients' needs and preferences, and that patients have the education and support they need to make decisions and participate in their own care" (Barr, 2009, slide 2). There is substantial evidence that health systems that have a strong primary care foundation deliver higher-quality, lower-cost care overall, and greater equity in health outcomes. Research also shows that patient-centered primary care is best delivered in a medical home—a primary care practice or health center that partners with its patients in providing enhanced access to clinicians, coordinating health care services, and engaging in continuous quality improvement (Commonwealth Fund, 2012).

Proposed Initiative: Improve Population Health

Health care systems are at the beginning of the adoption curve toward ACOs in which ACOs take responsibility for a defined population, coordinate their care across settings, and are held jointly accountable for the quality and cost of care. In a national survey of hospitals' readiness to participate in accountable organizations, the necessary infrastructure was lacking for many organizations and less than one third of hospitals have implemented population-based health management (Audet, Kenward, Patel, & Mauliks, 2012). Reasons cited included having the capacity to initiate population health management through the predictive identification information systems. Almost half of health care systems noted a lack of financial strength to take on the financial risk of becoming accountable for outcomes. The accounting systems to track costs and utilization combined with tracking revenue streams are complex. Current information systems often separate cost and clinical information, making tracking difficult. Aspects of care found in population health include the following:

1. Telephonic outreach to discharged patients
2. Case management
3. House calls by MDs or ARNPs
4. Safe and seamless transitions—sharing information summary of acute care stay

These would be minimal investments to obtain the necessary performance measures related to clinical quality, satisfaction, utilization, and financial measures. The challenges within population health management are to reduce clinical care variation and cost of care while developing and maintaining partnerships across social and health care organizations and providers (Audet et al., 2012).

Community health centers and nurse-managed centers are seen as the precursors to the PCMH. The National Committee for Quality Assurance (NCQA) provides this definition:

> A healthcare setting that facilitates partnerships between individual patients and their personal physicians, and when appropriate, patients' families. Care is facilitated by registries, information technology, health information exchanges and other means to assure that patients get the indicated care when and where they need and want it in a culturally and linguistically appropriate manner. (NCQA as cited in Community Volunteers in Medicine, 2012, p. 22)

Federally qualified health centers, recognized community health centers, and nurse-managed centers are early adopters of the type of provider entities that combine social and health services and assume accountability for the continuum of services. A national organization called Community Health Partners for Sustainability (2013) aims to strengthen health care for residents within public housing through coordinating care and social services. This organization is an example of partnerships forged across sectors of the social and health care systems. For example, Independence Blue Cross (IBC) Foundation of Pennsylvania provides some of the funding for the organization and also supports pilot programs that promote patient-centered care through the patient PCMH. The focus of the pilot is to be sure that when the patient does come for a primary care visit, it is coordinated around what matters most to that person. Between visits, care managers, nurse educators, and patient navigators consult with patients related to follow-up and care coordination for tests, services, and medication. Electronic health records help to coordinate across providers and settings. This type of medical home only works if the payment systems are aligned so that the cost of coordinated care can be covered in the payment. The Chronic Care Initiative by IBC showed significant clinical outcome improvement related to diabetes, cholesterol, and blood pressure measurements (Snyder & Gerrity, 2012). Pilot participants also included nurse-managed centers with interprofessional teams and these too showed the clinical outcomes as well as increased quality of life, lower anxiety, and better vitality. These pilots "present a return to truly personal care, supported by modern technology, and information improving the quality of care and leading our region and nation to a brighter, healthier future" (p. 6). These types of initiatives are committed to a "culture of caring," in which it is recognized that "how persons are treated is as important as the medical care they receive" (Community Volunteers in Medicine, 2012, p. 22).

Health care executives recognize the challenges of population health. One CEO participant at the Huron Healthcare Forum (2012) put the situation in very direct terms, saying that "healthcare systems are currently working on the 'spoiled child' model—spend what you want and expect the best. We will have to move to an accountability model with a focus on relevant levels of care and getting out in front of big expenses by taking responsibility for population health. At the end of the day, the hospital is accountable, but we are not reimbursed to support this model" (p. 8). Another CEO at that conference expressed the view that "we as a society need to have a greater understanding of the impact investments in social infrastructure could have on public health. For instance, we need to start helping very young grade-school age children develop the capacity to manage their lives in healthy ways by investing in things like education and housing" (p. 9).

The key challenges that CEOs face are presented by the transformation from a volume-based system to a value-based system as the care delivery model is changed and there is greater emphasis on wellness and prevention services. They see that it is the right thing to do for patients and that it is an economic necessity. A key dimension of the success will be the ability to partner with physicians and other providers to meet the goals of cost containment, access, and improved quality (Huron Healthcare, 2012). Before sharing risk, ACOs have to first establish the care coordination and management infrastructure so that population health will evolve from focusing on individual services to meeting the needs of persons over the long term and prioritizing care needs. Chronic conditions do not occur in isolation but are often clustered together (e.g., diabetes, heart disease, and arthritis), which put individuals experiencing these at risk for access to coordinated care. Having access to predictive tools and using them is not yet a widely adopted practice. A combination of health, cognitive, and social needs that affect poor health outcomes remains to be identified and acted upon in order to affect population health in a meaningful way.

Proposed Initiative: Prevent Monopolistic and Anticompetitive Behavior

Health care CEOs gathered for the Huron Healthcare Forum in 2012 reflected on the challenges of the current health care system. They were in agreement that the existing model of health care would not be sustainable in the future, and acknowledged that they will be required to transition from a fee-for-service model to one in which affordable, higher quality care is delivered at lower reimbursement rates within an economy that is emerging from what has been labeled the great recession (see https://www.russellsage.org/publications/great-recession). Regardless of the specifics of the Patient Protection and ACA, the business model shift from volume- to value-based services is the biggest challenge that CEOs identified. However, designing strategies to successfully meet this challenge was recognized as both a matter of survival and an opportunity to substantially reform health care for the better and for what matters most to patients. Making this transition, or more accurately this transformation, will require a greater emphasis on partnerships focused on wellness and preventive care while driving out waste from the system. The United States National Health Expenditures (NHE) are projected to account for 19.3% of GDP by 2019 according to Centers for Medicare and Medicaid (CMS.gov, 2011, p. 7). The issue in this transitional stage is running competing models at the same time; one that is volume based and one that is value based as measured by health outcomes and community health status. Halvorson and Isham (2003) cautioned that consumer expectations for miracle care at budget prices without engagement in changes related to lifestyle and chronic conditions are not sustainable.

CEOs see that the current model is not sustainable, and they recognize that there has to be care coordination, clinical and financial alignment, and a seamless delivery model supported by a robust information technology (IT) system. Current organizational structures include hospitals, Medicare, some insurance providers such as Blue Shield of California, and free-standing physician and specialty practices. The shift away from traditional payment toward an emphasis on prevention and health promotion is difficult to accomplish simultaneously with the current model of payment. Despite that, Medicare announced 150 ACO contracts and another 400 organizations are planning to apply in 2013 (Evans, 2012).

The mechanism for the payment model is found in the Patient Protection and ACA. The Centers for Medicare and Medicaid (CMS) has funded 32 Pioneer ACOs already experienced in coordinating care across settings. The payment models are:

- Simple shared savings: share savings from payer sources without penalties if cost targets are exceeded
- Shared savings with shared risk: in this model, organizations lose revenue if costs exceed targets
- Global payment: fixed payment per patient, which involves sharing some financial risk for some patients but does not apply to all services

The technical aspects of actually determining the payments, adhering to quality measurement and reporting requirements, and the tracking of expenditure benchmarks all must be successfully addressed in order to make the shift to value-based and Medicare-shared savings programs (Evans, 2012). It is expected that over time there would be a decrease in fee-for-service and an increase in hybrid fee-for-service and shared savings approaches. Over time, private pay systems would reflect the ACO payment features. The most likely participants are hospitals that are larger, urban, teaching, and nonprofit. Of concern to organizations are current antitrust laws that could be called into play during the transitions from volume to value models. Additionally, the *New York Times* reported that physicians concerned about integrated care models may allow "too much concentration of power over every aspect of the medical pipeline, dictating which tests and procedures to perform and how much to charge and which patients to admit" (Creswell & Abelson, 2012, para. 5). This type of consolidation that limits competition and raises prices is the warning that Halvorson and Isham cautioned against in 2003.

Organizations will be expected to have the required skills and staff to do case management, while managing relationships between primary care and specialty physicians in order to achieve performance measures on these five variables:

1. Emergency department visits
2. Admissions
3. Readmissions
4. Length of stay
5. Network care coordination

Major challenges in the transformation from volume to value base is the ability to motivate physicians to participate in developing and sustaining a common organizational culture dedicated to reducing clinical variation and costs, while increasing the population served through a team model. Developing leadership capacity in both physicians and nonphysicians to make the transformation as well as setting up governance structures to reflect provider and patient partnership are also challenges. The financial investments required at a system level will require capital in order to build the capacity for care. The question will be where will this capital come from?

Proposed Initiative: Create Workable Framework for Dealing With the Uninsured

The mechanisms for dealing with the uninsured have to happen at the broadest levels of federal and state government. Though charitable care is part of the safety net of services within many communities, it still does not address the lack of access to affordable insurance for the broader population. The reimbursement rate for many states is so low that providers restrict or decline to see Medicaid patients within their practices. Raising the reimbursement rate is a strategy enacted with the anticipation that more providers will agree to see more patients. This assumes that there are providers available to offer services, a problematic assumption because of projected shortages of physicians, nurses, and other health care professionals.

Proposed Initiative: Fund Training, Medical Education, Medical Research, Resupply of the Health Care Workforce, Re-Engineering of Health Care Delivery Particularly in Hospital Settings

Health care executives contemplating the future of health care pointed out that it will be necessary to assure that licensed personnel (such as NPs and physician assistants [PAs]) are practicing to the full extent allowed by their licenses in order to have the capacity to provide preventive, population-based health care. "More and more care will be delivered by providers other than doctors; nurse practitioners and physician assistants are well equipped to deliver care and are an excellent way to leverage our increasingly scarce physician workforce" (Huron Healthcare, 2012, p. 11).

This kind of interprofessional team approach will help to match the needs of the patient with the skill of the caregiver. Though care is rendered by many different disciplines within a health care setting, it does not necessarily follow that the model of care is designed intentionally as a team-based approach. Within ACOs this intentional coordination of members of the team will be taking a team approach—getting more people working up to license level. The chief executive's role within health care environments will be to lead the efforts and to "model optimism" as new partnerships and patterns of care delivery are developed. This will require attracting talent to the workplace with diverse skills.

At a 2012 conference for the Fifth Annual Retail Clinician Education Congress panel on executive and health systems leadership colloquium in Orlando, Florida, an interprofessional panel discussed trends in primary care. They represented various health care disciplines and shared their perspectives about what will be required of interprofessional teams within ACOs and the health care system in general. Scott Shipman, MD, MPH, of the American Association of Medical Colleges and Dartmouth Institute for Health Policy and Clinical Practice, projected that primary care is the backbone of the emerging system and that primary care physicians will have an increased role to play relative to population health. However, attracting new physicians into primary care is difficult because of the relative reward and reimbursement differentials associated with payment. Given the cost of medical education and associated loans, new physicians often choose specialty care. Dr. Shipman projected that medical students trained in primary care "as a team sport" will be attracted to the benefits and ability to affect health outcomes.

Dr. Kenneth Miller, associate dean for academic administration in the Catholic University of America School of Nursing, also on the same panel, discussed the vital role family nurse practitioners (FNPs) and other advanced practice NPs play in primary care. They are currently providing services within primary care and at a level that has been shown to deliver safe, cost-effective health care. NPs work closely with the medical community; but scope of practice issues vary by state, in ways that either enhance or hinder the ability of NPs to fully apply their skills to the needs of the population served. This is an issue that CEOs identified and believe needs to be resolved as well. Challenges for the supply of the NP workforce relate to the faculty available to teach, salary issues in academic nursing, and availability of clinical sites for training. Dr. Miller sees that eventually scope of practice issues will be addressed through a national license to overcome unnecessary variations in scope of practice defined at a state level. The possibilities for interprofessional education with new medical students and NPs may be able to facilitate the growth of team-based primary care.

Additional members of the interprofessional panel at that conference included physician assistant Ann Davis, PA-C, senior director, State Advocacy and Outreach American Academy of PAs and P. J. Ortman, RPh, MBA, Medvisors, LLC. Both PAs and pharmacy representatives each have a role in the interprofessional team. For example, PAs have one national curriculum and exam. There are currently 84,000 PAs in the workforce with about 6,000 being added per year, with approximately 54% practicing in primary care (Davis, 2012). Though rules about practice supervision are determined locally, most are able to fully prescribe medications. The role of the pharmacist in the interprofessional team is crucial to medication adherence. Within 6 months of prescription about 50% of patients fail to take the medications prescribed. Medications are often an important aspect of chronic care management. Finding ways to successfully engage patients in this aspect of health care provider–patient collaboration is important to overall health outcomes.

Since nurses are the single largest group of health care providers, other major organizations also see the development of NPs as part of the effort to improve health care delivery. This includes the Robert Wood Johnson Foundation (RWJF), the IOM, and the American Association for Retired Persons (AARP), groups that worked together to identify pathways for the "Future of Nursing" (Institute of Medicine [IOM], 2011). There is a projected nursing shortage that has been obscured during the great recession, yet it is projected to increase between 2013 and 2020. In the past, nursing shortages were addressed by increasing supply of new graduates. Now, nursing faculty is in short supply and the problem will get worse because nursing faculty is older and retiring at a faster rate than previously. Senior faculty represents the greatest loss in part because compared to other disciplines, nurses receive terminal degrees at an older age and, therefore, have shorter academic careers. Fewer senior faculty limits the ability to prepare an increased supply of advanced practice graduates. To address this situation, these foundations have sponsored the formation of action coalitions aimed at increasing the number of doctorally prepared nurses for research (PhD) and practice (DNP), both of whom could fulfill roles as faculty in preparing the next generation workforce.

These same foundations (IOM, RWJF, and AARP) are also looking at ways to increase the development of interprofessional team-based care. RWJF has a national center for interprofessional education and practice with the aim of addressing quality, access, and cost issues. Together with the Health Resources and Services Administration (HRSA), the Josiah Macy Jr. Foundation, and the American Board of Internal Medicine Foundation (ABIM Foundation), the RWJF convened an expert panel from the Interprofessional Education Collaborative (IPEC) formed in 2009 with representatives from six national educational associations of schools of health professions:

1. American Association of Colleges of Nursing (AACN)
2. American Association of Colleges of Osteopathic Medicine (AACOM)
3. American Association of Colleges of Pharmacy (AACP)
4. American Dental Education Association (ADEA)
5. Association of American Medical Colleges (AAMC)
6. Association of Schools of Public Health (ASPH)

This expert panel reviewed prior efforts to define interprofessional competency in the United States and Canada. Two appointees from each association formed a group that worked to develop a set of core competencies for interprofessional professional practice, published in 2011 (IPEC, February, 2011). This gives some indication of the relatively new or renewed focus on interprofessional education and collaboration. The group identified four competency domains:

- Values/ethics for professional practice: "Work with individuals of other professions to maintain a climate of mutual respect and shared values" (p. 3)
- Roles/responsibilities for collaborative practice: "Use the knowledge of one's own role and the roles of other professions to appropriately assess and address the health care needs of the patients and populations served" (p. 4)

- Interprofessional communication: "Communicate with patients, families, communities, and other health professionals in a responsive and responsible manner that supports a team approach to maintaining health and treatment of disease" (p. 5)
- Interprofessional teamwork and team-based care: "Apply relationship-building values and principles of team dynamics to perform effectively in different team roles to plan and deliver patient/population-centered care that is safe, timely, efficient, effective, and equitable" (p. 6)

These competencies and their associated behaviors apply to each graduate of health professions schools and each should be able to be performed within the context of patient care and population health across the full spectrum of care (IPEC, 2011, p. 2). In general, the team approach being called for will become increasingly important as demand for services grows concurrently with a shortage of physicians as well as other health professionals.

Proposed Initiative: Adoption of an Automated Health Care Record to Give Point-of-Care Information for Consistent Delivery of Best Practices Based on Known Evidence

The health care CEOs gathered through the Huron Group agree that "cost savings can come from standardizing care at the bedside; evidence-driven care will reduce unnecessary care variation," indicating that currently too many wrong decisions are being made at the discharge process (Huron Healthcare, 2012, p. 15). Halvorson and Isham (2003) are advocates and early adopters of electronic health information systems that support the goals of population health improvement and reduce unnecessary clinical variation. Kaiser Permanente has made a major investment in its integrated health care system that serves over 8 million members across nine states (Porter & Kellogg, 2008). They are often compared to the Veterans Administration and the United Kingdom as having the largest integrated health information system. Given their point of view, it is not surprising that they see the automated health care record at the point of care as essential to health care transformation, particularly the vital role it could play if it performs well enough to reap the benefits of patient information and clinical management for improved health outcomes and financial data.

The necessity for this technology adoption is evident within ACOs. Electronic medical record (EMR) adoption and other related ITs are of concern to CEOs because of the cost and complexity of their implementation.

Despite the challenges, it is well recognized that operational IT substantially improves health outcomes. A study conducted within Kaiser Permanente showed that the use of a population health panel support tool (PST) integrated in its electronic health system significantly improved primary care teams' performance on preventive care, monitoring, and recommendations to patients based on therapeutic evidence. Improvement was seen at each measured 4-month interval and sustained over 20 months (Zhou et al., 2011). This type of decision support is desirable and yet difficult to achieve in less tightly integrated health care systems.

Health information systems that enable collecting, aggregating, analyzing, and applying health information for health improvement across different health and social systems present technical as well as privacy issues for patients. Yet, it is widely accepted that mechanisms need to be in place to do just that through health information exchanges.

Health information exchanges facilitate sharing of information across different types of software and across different sites of service to maximize continuity of care. This is an area ripe for technology innovation, while simultaneously focusing on protecting patient privacy and patient rights.

Current health IT systems are often locally hosted and provide local results, yet the desire is there to integrate data with a larger pool to monitor quality and health outcomes. As health care systems adopt electronic health record systems, incentives have been offered to underwrite part of the cost if "meaningful use" (CMS.gov, 2013) can be demonstrated, that is, if the system is helping to track and monitor outcome data and contribute data to a larger data pool. To be effective health IT systems must: (a) help primary care providers follow practice guidelines, (b) provide disease registries for individual care planning and population care management, and (c) provide feedback to physicians and other health care professionals about performance (Zhou et al., 2011). Each of these features hold technical challenges for keeping guidelines current, and data relevant, retrievable, comprehensive, and personalized enough to be applicable to use to counsel patients during the patient care visit. Finally, it is helpful for providers or provider teams to receive feedback about their management of the patient and patient population so that the information can be used for quality improvement. Though 40% of medical practices now report using some sort of electronic health record, the level of integration required for ACOs is not widely available.

CONTEMPLATING THE DANCE OF CARING PERSONS MODEL AS AN ESSENTIAL FOUNDATION FOR HEALTH CARE SERVICES

Based on Halvorson and Isham's proposal in 2003, it appears that there is significant and yet varied movement in each of the seven initiatives throughout the health care system. It also is clear that the ACA is structured in a way to further develop transformation in these areas. (For a summary of alignment between the ACA and the Halvorson and Isham's proposed initiatives, please see the Resources section.) Health care CEOs are recognizing the challenges and realizing this is a likely and necessary direction for the future. Similarly, professional associations are also seeing that their educational and practice initiatives both individually and interprofessionally must reflect these trends and directions. This is no small task and partnerships, integration, and collaboration are essential to success. What we must contribute to this future transformation is the Dance of Caring Persons model, as a means to keep caring centered as a substantive, meaningful foundation that will help guide these efforts and assure that health care system transformation is authentically and truly person centered. What follows is a patient's story reflective of his experience of being the person around whom care was centered by an interprofessional team.

As you read the story we invite you to contemplate, as we have, how the story reflects the foundational values of the Dance of Caring Persons. In what way does Mr. Whittington's story support or refute the idea that members of his health care team created an experience that:

- Acknowledged that all persons have the capacity to care by virtue of their humanness?
- Demonstrated respect for persons in all institutional structures and processes?
- Recognized that each participant in the enterprise has a unique and valuable contribution to make to the whole?
- Appreciated the dynamic, rhythmic nature of the Dance of Caring Persons as an enabling opportunity for human creativity?

An Open Letter to My Medical Team at UMMC
By Chris Whittington

To the team responsible for saving my life:
There's not really a way for me to begin this letter other than to say the one thing that it is meant to convey.
THANK YOU!

I ask your apologies for sending you this letter in typed format. I assure you that if you had received a hand-written letter from me, you would have probably only been able to read about two-thirds of it and may have never known what I was trying to say to you.

As I sit here with my fingers on the keyboard typing this letter—a letter that has been months in the composition stage—I realize that it has been exactly four months since the team wheeled me from the ER into the operating room. It's been four months since I had a left leg.

I made some really bad choices and those choices led to my losing that appendage but there are three choices that I've made in my life that I can most assuredly tell you were good ones. The first choice, made when I was a teenager, was the one that has given me the promise of eternal life through my Lord and Savior, *Jesus Christ*. The second, made on October 25, 2000, was to spend the rest of my life with Cristy. The third decision, one that I made the morning of October 8, 2012, was to have Cristy take me to the University of Mississippi Medical Center. I want to tell you all that those second and third decisions were mine and mine alone, but the truth is that I believe wholeheartedly that the first decision set me on the path to making them.

Most of you already know that *Dr. Boland* came out of the operating room and told my wife to contact my family and prepare for the worst. He truly didn't have much hope that I would make it out of the hospital alive. I guess Dr. Boland didn't realize that God isn't finished with me—and to tell you the truth, I didn't either.

I've had the chance to thank Dr. Boland for taking care of me and saving my life. I showed him a video I posted on YouTube. The video, shot exactly 1 month ago today, showed me on my first day at the gym with my physical trainer/therapist. Dr. Boland had tears in his eyes when he told me that he could take credit for being the team leader and being the surgeon, but—as he pointed to the video—he told me that I was the one responsible for dragging myself up and reclaiming my life.

I've had some time to digest that statement and realize there's some truth to it, but without all of you, I could have never done it.

I laid in the bed for the first couple of weeks and felt completely hopeless, but thanks to the tireless dedication of the team that you are part of, I was shown the light.

Every single one of you reading this letter, and probably many more that I was too sedated to remember, played a part in my journey from the darkness, but there are four people that I want to mention here.

The first is *Nurse Ron.*

I was having a tough time with the pain after the initial amputation but one night in particular was extra hard. I'd been having trouble getting to sleep and was receiving doses of Benadryl intravenously. I had finally fallen asleep that night and somewhere about 4 o'clock in the morning, I rolled over in the bed and hit my stump on the bed rail. The pain was excruciating. I tried to call out to Cristy, who was asleep across the expanse of room 327, but I had no voice. It was that kind of pain. I pressed the "call" button and could only get the word "hurt" to come out faintly. Ron came rushing into the room a few seconds later—it seems that I was one of only two patients he had that evening (Thank the Lord). He saw the tears falling from my eyes and tried to understand what I was trying to say. He finally surmised that I had banged my stump and told me to wait just a few. He left the room and returned with a dose of morphine and then sat by the bed and held my hand until I fell asleep again.

I will never forget that tenderness. I will always strive to live up to that example.

The next person is *Wendy*, the physical therapist.

Wendy is a ruthless woman who can look into the soul of a person and see what they're capable of. Maybe that doesn't sound ruthless, but that comes into play when she demands that you—no matter that you don't believe that you're capable—accomplish the task that she wants done. Whether that task is getting out of the bed, sitting on the toilet or walking across the hall, you're gonna do it and there's no giving up allowed. She pushed me to the edge of sanity but was there to catch me before I fell into the abyss. She (with the tireless assistance of the love of my life) showed me that I was capable of much more than I could see at that point.

I will never forget the look in her eyes—those beautiful, all-seeing, ruthless eyes—the first day I made it across the hall. Those ruthless eyes were welled up with tears, but she never let me see her cry. I will always remember that and will strive to push myself and others to limits like that, knowing that I am capable of catching both myself and others before they fall into a darker place.

The third person is *Dr. Thompson*, from Dr. Boland's vascular team.

I was having tremendous difficulty with depression and realized that I was in desperate need of talking to a counselor. I mentioned this to her one day and she put in the request to have someone come by. The chaplain, Jeff Murphy, came by, but the psychology and psychiatric departments both refused to see me. That's when Dr. Thompson did something really creative. She contacted Harry at University Rehab and asked his assistance. She asked him to contact the psych department and ask them to evaluate me, claiming he was worried that I was not "stable" enough to come to rehab. It worked.

That level of creative problem solving is not something I had ever seen from a doctor before. I will forever be grateful that Dr. Thompson was that creative. Without it, I would have never met Dr. Manning or my therapist, Daniel, and may have not been able to begin to deal with my depression and other issues until it was too late.

I will always strive to be as creative in solving problems that I'm facing, and sincerely hope that Dr. Thompson keeps that spark. I believe that it will truly set her apart from her peers as she grows into the leader I can see in her.

The fourth and final person I have to thank for pulling me from the darkness (besides my wife and mother) is *Nurse Becky*.

Becky was the first nurse I came in contact with who realized that I actually had a sense of humor and she constantly worked on appealing to that side of me. That tireless effort, even though she knew how dark things seemed to me at the time, actually helped me to get back to being myself much faster than therapy (physical or mental) did. Becky, regardless of my mood or pain level, would walk into the room with a smile on her face and would make jokes and poke fun. I guess she subscribes to the belief handed down to us in the bible: "A merry heart does good, like medicine, but a broken spirit dries the bones."—Proverbs 17:22.

Much like Becky, I've always had a sick, twisted sense of humor…so much so that I asked Dr. Boland for the last piece of bone he cut from my leg so that my friend could attempt to turn it on his lathe and make a duck call out of it. I have her to thank for making that sense of humor reappear inside me.

I will never forget my "MB"—ask Becky if you're curious about that nickname. She taught me the true importance of laughter and reawakened a spirit I truly thought was dead. I will always strive to bring that sort of light into any room I walk into.

Now just because I mentioned those four people, does not mean, under any circumstances, that the rest of you reading this letter played any lesser role in my recovery. To the contrary, you all are responsible for getting me to the point of writing this letter.

I'll begin with the last face I saw before leaving the hospital for my home.

Nurse Lacey actually took the time to wheel me downstairs and aid Cristy in loading our things into the van. It was a bit cold and rainy that night so she and I sat in the lobby while Cristy fetched the van from the garage.

Those of you who know Lacey will enjoy this story. The first time I met her was Halloween night. She was wearing a pair of *Grey's Anatomy* scrubs when she came into the room and informed me that she would be my nurse. She checked on my IV and then bounced out of the room as swiftly as she'd come in. I looked at Cristy and told her that she needed to call security because we had some trick-or-treating teenager acting like a nurse. Cristy laughed and tried to reassure me that Lacey was actually a hospital employee. I, in all seriousness, looked at my wife and tried to explain that this child who was just in our room was definitely not a nurse. First, the scrubs were obviously a Halloween costume, seeing that they were from a TV show. Second, Lacey had the legs of the scrubs rolled up like the girls in my high school used to roll their jeans.

Between Halloween and November 28th (the day I got to come home), Lacey was the nurse most often assigned to my room. Cristy and I got to develop a friendship with her that I will treasure until the day I leave this mortal coil. As we sat in the lobby talking about Lacey's upcoming days off—days she was looking forward to such as celebrating the birthday of one of her children—I realized that I was going to miss being in the hospital almost as much as I was looking forward to getting home to my dog and my own bed.

Cristy pulled up out front and we lugged all the stuff out to the van—and yes, even though I was in a wheelchair, I helped... not much, but I did. Lacey started to lean down to give me a hug and say goodbye and I told her to wait. I stood up, holding on to one of the columns for balance and gave her a big hug and thanked her for her care and friendship. Lacey was smiling and tears began to fall from her eyes as she quickly turned her head and walked over to hug Cristy.

It's that kind of compassion—a compassion that was not uncommon from each of you—that will stay with me forever.

There are lots of nurses who took care of me during my stay on 3 North. I'm absolutely positive that I'm forgetting some of you, even though I began writing names down almost as soon as I came home. Pain meds are great for controlling pain but not so much for the memory center of the brain!!! If your name isn't on this list, I apologize... it's not like I'm not thankful, but there was a great deal of time—especially those first two or three weeks—that seems jumbled together in my mind, as if it were only a couple of days.

Delorise—I know things got off to a really rocky start and that my attitude toward you (and everyone else) was less than stellar. I thank God every day for your patience and understanding and will never forget all the times you stuck your head into my room just to say hello, even though you weren't my nurse!

Jennifer—I know there are two of you, but I want you to know that my mom fully expects you to take her up on the offer of a room and a tour guide to Colorado. All you have to do is let her know when you want to come! I'll look forward to hearing all about your trip. Thanks for listening to me whine and letting me know that it's okay to be scared.

(The Other) Jennifer—Don't ever let your smile leave your face. You truly do brighten a room when you walk in. Thanks for your endless devotion to your patients.

Linda—You scared me half to death one morning. I was totally gone. Sleeping is not the proper word for what I was doing. You came into the room and I wasn't expecting it and I honestly almost had to have my bed changed! Your positive attitude helped pull me out of some really dark places as well... don't ever lose it!

Wendy—I don't know if you remember walking in on me having a pity party one day. I tried to hide it, but you sensed something wrong. You stood in my room for much longer than you could afford to and talked to me until I was doing better. I can't thank you enough for taking the time to do so.

Mioshi—There's a lot that I could say about you, your attitude, your smile, but I want to thank you first and foremost for making me a glass of tea. Cristy was at home and her brother was staying at the hospital with me. He had just started talking to his new girlfriend and spent hours away from the room. I had been wanting something to drink and was too drugged to get out of bed. You will never know how good that tea tasted! Thank you!

Bryce—You are too bubbly for your own good. One of these days, those bubbles are going to pop and you are going to kill someone with kindness! Thank you for infecting me with your bubbliness. Spell check just told me that isn't a word, but I can't think of a better way to describe you!

Parminder—You have a terrific personality! Don't ever hide that from anyone! Your warmth is something that endears you to patients and that kind of feeling means far more to us than you can possibly imagine!

The other nurse I have on my list is not on 3 North, but rather in Pre-Op.

Paula (my second wife)—I had a total of 12 surgeries at UMMC. I believe that you were there for all but the first one. Your care is second to none and I thank God every day of my life that you were there to hold my hand before surgery and let me know that everything was gonna be alright. Your tears, welled in your eyes on the day of my skin graft, speak more about your soul than you will ever know. Thank you!

There were five Patient Care Technicians that I can remember sharing my stay at UMMC. To *Rhonda, Sally, Cynthia, Linda* and *Calvin*: Thank You! Letting me sleep through some of those vital sign checks was wonderful . . . even the times when you got my vitals in spite of my sleep. You guys are a wonderful support to both the patients and the staff on the floor. I will never forget any of you!!!

My other physical therapist, Alyssa, was just as ruthless as Wendy, but she didn't have to dig me out of the deep hole like her predecessor. It is because of their tireless work (and immense patience) that I was able to transition from the hospital to home without having to go to rehab in between. Being able to show her the video of my workout at the gym put a smile on both of our faces. I hope that I was able to convey to her how truly grateful I am for keeping me on my toes and making sure that I didn't give up! Randy, my occupational therapist, really helped me along in being able to skip the rehab part of the journey, too. Thanks to Randy's innovative exercise routines, I was able to build some extra upper body strength and that has made a world of difference in my life.

Dr. Manning assigned his assistant *Daniel*, whose last name I believe is Ray, but I could be mistaken, to be my therapist. Daniel helped me to find a better place in my head and taught me how to stay there. There is no level of gratitude that will ever be enough for that. Daniel, please don't ever lose the "it-factor" you have as a therapist. God gave you those talents for a purpose and I believe you will go on to help many others, many worse than I was, to find there [is a] better place. Do me one favor though . . . buy yourself an MP3 recorder and don't worry about trying to figure out smart-phones!

Jeff Murphy was the chaplain assigned to me. His guidance and compassion helped me to see that God had not forsaken me. I got to see him during my last visit to the hospital and was truly happy to do so. He is an inspiration to me and, no doubt, countless others. Jeff, THANK YOU. Whether it was praying over my sleeping self after one of my surgeries, praying with me, listening to me cry about my life or providing a shoulder for my family and friends. Your kindness will never be forgotten and I am sure that God has a special place reserved for you in His Kingdom! God Bless and keep you in his arms!

Finally, I'd like to thank the entire team of physicians who cared for me during my stay—and beyond.

Doctors Dinning, Sparkman, Richardson, Lange, Wofford, Atchley and the many, many more who I cannot name . . . I owe you my life and my unending gratitude for leading me to a life beyond October 8, 2012!!!

I hope that each and every one of you had a joyous Christmas and New Year's; 2012 kinda sucked for me, given the fact that I had two legs and a job when it started and now I'm one less in both of those departments, but 2013 has begun and I have my life and a brand new family to thank for leading me here.   (Whittington, 2013)

REFERENCES

American College of Health Care Executives. (2012). *The healthcare executive's role in ensuring quality and patient safety. Policy brief.* Approved by the Board of Governors of the American College of Healthcare Executives on November 12, 2012. Retrieved February 2013 from http://www.ache.org/policy/exec-ensure-patsafe.cfm

Audet, A., Kenward, K., Patel, S., & Mauliks, J. (2012, August 17). Issue brief. Hospitals on the path to accountable care: Highlights from a 2011 national survey of hospital readiness to participate in an accountable care organization. *The Commonwealth Fund, 22*. Retrieved from http://www.commonwealthfund.org/~/media/Files/Publications/Issue%20Brief/2012/Aug/1625_Audet_hospitals_path_accountable_care_ib_v2.pdf

Bachrach, D., Bernstein, W., & Karl, A. (2012, November 16). High-performance health care for vulnerable populations: A policy framework for promoting accountable care in Medicaid. *The Commonwealth Fund*. Retrieved from http://www.commonwealthfund.org/~/media/Files/Publications/Fund%20Report/2012/Nov/1646_Bachrach_high_performance_hlt_care_vulnerable_populations_Medicaid_ACO_v2.pdf

Barr, M. S. (2009). *The patient-centered medical home and health 2.0.* Slide presentation from the AHRQ 2009 annual conference. Retrieved from http://www.ahrq.gov/about/annualconf09/barr.htm

Bloomberg News. (2012, June 13). Retrieved from http://www.bloomberg.com/news/2012-06-13/health-care-spending-to-reach-20-of-u-s-economy-by-2021.html

CMS.gov. (2011). *National health expenditure projections 2011–2021.* Centers for Medicare and Medicaid Services. Retrieved from http://www.cms.gov/Research-Statistics-Data-and-Systems/Statistics-Trends-and reports/NationalHealthExpendData/Downloads/Proj2011PDF.pdf

CMS.gov. (2013). *Meaningful use.* Retrieved from http://www.cms.gov/Regulations-and-Guidance/Legislation/EHRIncentivePrograms/Meaningful_Use.html

Commonwealth Fund. (2012, August 20). *Home sweet medical home.* Retrieved from http://www.commonwealthfund.org/Infographics/2012/Medical-Homes.aspx

Community Health Partners for Sustainability. (2013). Retrieved February 9, 2013, from http://www.chpfs.org/chpfs/index.php

Community Volunteers in Medicine. (2012). The evolving concept of community health centers. *The Journal of Change, 1*(2), 20–23. Independence Blue Cross Blue Shield Foundation, Philadelphia.

Creswell, J., & Abelson, R. (2012, December 1). A hospital war reflects a bind for doctors in the U. S. *New York Times.* Retrieved from http://www.nytimes.com/2012/12/01/business/a-hospital-war-reflects-a-tightening-bind-for-doctors-nationwide.html?pagewanted=all

Davis, A. (2012). *Presentation at the fifth annual Retail Clinician Education Congress panel on executive and health systems leadership colloquium; Session 1 trends in primary care.* Orlando, FL: American Academy of Physician Assistants.

Evans, M. (2012). The early returns on accountable care. Newly minted ACOs grapple with allocating resources and adjusting operations to put the theory to work. *Modern Healthcare, 42*(31), S1–S5.

Guterman, S., Schoenbaum, S., Davis, K., Schoen, C., Audet, A., Stremikis, K., & Zezza, M. (2011, April). High performance accountable care: Building on success and learning from experience. *The Commonwealth Fund*, Publication No. 1494. Retrieved from www.commonwealthfund.org

Halvorson, G. C., & Isham, G. J. (2003). *Epidemic of care: A call for safer, better and more accountable healthcare.* San Francisco, CA: Jossey-Bass.

Huron Healthcare. (2012). *Leading through transformation: Top healthcare CEOs perspective on the future of healthcare. Insights from the Huron Healthcare CEO Forum.* Retrieved from http://www.healthcareceoforum.com/download-report

Institute of Medicine (IOM). (2011). *The future of nursing: Leading change, advancing health.* Washington, DC: The National Academies Press.

Interprofessional Education Collaborative. (2011). *Core competencies for interprofessional collaborative practice: Report of an expert panel.* Washington, DC: Author.

Kaiser Family Foundation. (2012, August). *A guide to the Supreme Court's decision on the ACAs Medicaid Expansion.* Retrieved from http://www.kff.org/healthreform/upload/8347.pdf

Porter, M., & Kellogg, M. (2008). *An integrated health care experience* (Vol. 1, No. 1). Kaiser Permanente: RISAI 2008.

Selby, P. (1974). *Health in 1980–1990. A predictive study based on international inquiry.* Basel, Switzerland: S. Karger.

Snyder, R., & Gerrity, P. (2012). Back to the future: More coordinated primary care-medical homes make medicine more personal again. *The Journal of Change, 1*(1), 4–6. Independence Blue Cross Blue Shield Foundation, Philadelphia.

Valentine, K. L. (1988). History, analysis, and application of the carative tradition in health and nursing. *The Journal of the New York State Nurses' Association, 19*(4), 4–9.

Whittington, C. (2013, January 11). An open letter to my medical team at UMMC. *Vicksburg Daily News*. Retrieved from http://vicksburgdailynews.com/2013/01/11/an-open-letter-to-my-medical-team-at-ummc

Zakaria, F. (2012, March 26). Health insurance is for everyone. *Time Magazine*. Retrieved February 9, 2013, from http://www.time.com/time/magazine/article/0,9171,-2,00.html

Zhou, Y. Y., Unitan, R., Wang, J. J., Garrido, T., Chin, H. L., Turley, M. C., & Radler, L. (2011). Improving population care with an integrated electronic panel support tool. *Population Health Management, 14*(1), 3–9. doi:10.1089/pop.2010.0001

Response to Chapter 1

Zane Robinson Wolf, PhD, RN, FAAN
Dean Emerita and Professor
Nursing Programs, School of Nursing and Health Sciences, La Salle University

What is the value of a caring-based perspective in health care transformation?
The value of introducing a caring-based perspective into the transformation of health care is undeniable. In part, some of this work is currently being accomplished by Magnet nursing initiatives since some health care agencies/systems have emphasized nurse caring and added nurse caring and nurse self-caring agendas to their missions, visions, and strategies. What the impact of the Magnet phenomenon is on the perceptions of nurse caring by patients, families, and communities is difficult to estimate.

Some acute care agencies have recognized the impact of nursing care, perceived as caring, on patient satisfaction. Within the current focus on relationship-based and patient-centered care exists an opportunity. The time may be ripe to clarify practice models that operationalize a culture of caring. Caring-based perspectives can start where many health care facilities and nurse leaders are already working to disseminate patient-centered care. Maybe this is the beginning of a paradigm shift that will welcome a transformation to a caring culture. Perhaps a look at Duffy's model and others is worth the attention. She and others have piloted an intervention, but not in a hospital setting. In addition, Watson's work as operationalized by exemplary nursing service organizations already has some lessons learned. An old article by Joiner noted that when caring was on the agenda within a nursing service organization, the other departments wanted to join and they did. The values were advertised in a simplistic way as I recall.

I think it is essential to examine what is meant by a culture of caring. Cultures have beliefs, norms, and values, and the building of an interdisciplinary culture of caring may start with shared values. A strategy to put this into action could begin with teams of providers in dialogue about the meaning of caring as well as formal presentations on the elements of a culture of caring.

Many providers believe that their agenda is the welfare of the patient, but few seem to have work like Gaut's on which to base their assertions. Intentionality and authenticity are crucial.

Chronic illness, sometimes a combination of chronic illness diagnoses and disadvantaged, poor populations, has challenged our health care system to transform.

Although the Affordable Care Act will shift care to lifestyle changes and prevention of illness and disability, this will be a difficult path and reimbursement will evolve with rewarding quality services and outcomes. Public health initiatives that emphasize prevention are essential; those of us who are spoiled and who order many expensive diagnostic tests will not be very happy, but we will adapt.

It is not an impossible goal to achieve cost containment, patient-centered care, perceptions of caring services, and caring providers. Hopefully the paradigm shift has begun toward this goal, and nurse leaders, once onboard with transforming health care to a culture of caring, will move service delivery closer to this end point.

Health care agencies, very dependent on outcome measures and dashboards, will need measures of perceived caring that businesses like Press-Ganey will need to incorporate into their surveys and analyze and present the results back to subscribers.

Stories can be powerful agents for change. Maybe caring stories will predominate and one, two, or three good ones receive national attention and accomplish an initial shift to promote the desire for a culture of caring.

In your experience, what would have to be in place in order to bring the ideas presented to fruition?
Start with exemplary nurse education programs that have caring theories as part of their foundational thinking. Publish examples of their curriculums and try to discern the effect of graduates from programs that have been strong "in caring" for some time. Determine this: Have their caring ways affected changes in organizations? Write about the substantive knowledge gained from this and make it a part of fundamental nursing textbooks, as well as other disciplines' fundamental textbooks.

Model the caring culture phenomenon on organizational change theory, create a consultation business that creates culture of caring "packages," and disseminate the model. This means that the model must be based on the caring literature, stellar organizations known for caring, and cultural theory presented in a manner to convince health care agencies to purchase your product.

Since strong primary care practices may be the best foundation of a more affordable and lifestyle-changing health care service, start here. Nurse practitioners are becoming increasingly more appreciated by patients and families as effective primary care providers and could be effective leaders in this transformation.

What ideas would you like to contribute to making the content even more practical?
The language of caring needs to be included in electronic health records. These projects need to go forward and I believe that they will, given recent articles I have reviewed for the *International Journal for Human Caring*.

The Dance of Caring Persons: A Values-Based Model for Health Care Systems Transformation

*A*dopting an explicit value system as the foundation for refining and transforming health care systems is a long-held ideal approach. This ideal is nearing reality because of policy statements by The Joint Commission and other influential health care leadership groups, who are now calling for values-based models. Health care systems have historically been grounded in explicit value systems. The most prominent examples are the hospitals operated by various religious groups as a visible expression of institutional values held in highest esteem. An example of a values-based model from the 19th century is Florence Nightingale's work to reform the health care system of the British military establishment. Nightingale's work in health care systems was grounded in values of service to a higher calling and the centrality of the environment to the health of populations.

More recently, significant segments of health care institutions are operated by for-profit corporations, so that a new value priority gained prominence in the last two decades of the 20th century. It is important to note that concept of "for-profit" is itself a value and needs to be understood as such in order to forge a satisfying alliance between economic values and humanistic values. As a growing body of research findings suggests that humanistic care is a key element in patient satisfaction and in staff retention, the two values of economics and humane, formerly considered divergent value systems, are now converging on a shared interest.

ECONOMIC VALUES/ALTRUISTIC VALUES

Let's examine the concept of health care that is grounded at least partly in the value of economic profit. We'll follow that with a look at humanistic, altruistic values as we propose a values-based unifying framework for health care systems that is realistic for the 21st century, a framework that honors widely held expectations of "care." But at the outset, let's make clear what we are not attempting to do in this book. We are not attempting to argue the social and economic pros and cons of public/nonprofit health care versus for-profit health care. Those arguments are important to the ongoing societal dialogue about access to health care, and have been succinctly summarized in forums such as the

Markkula Center for Applied Ethics at Santa Clara University (http://www.scu.edu/ethics/publications/iie/v1n4/healthy.html) and continue to be addressed by scholarly think tanks such as the Hastings Center, the Kennedy Institute of Ethics at Georgetown University, and the Society of Health and Human Values.

Economic implications for caring and health care systems have been addressed by several nurse researchers and leaders and are considered essential to the future of health care (Ray, 1989; Turkel, 2001; Valentine, 1988, 1997). Caring has often been aligned with traditional female role attributions and associated with "women's work" and has not been systematically and explicitly valued within our current health care system. The historical traditions of aligning nurses' work with direct care and not being associated with academic preparation is still the norm, even as more and more doctorally prepared advanced practice nurses enter into advanced practice. Such traditions have affected nursing's widespread explicit adoption of caring as the core competency of the profession and have also affected nursing's relationship with other disciplines in health care.

As we saw in Chapter 1, health care services account for 17% of our economy. Health care and its delivery through both governmental and private markets position health care as a major focus in economic reform and political debate. Witness the 2012 U.S. presidential election as an example of the fervor with which arguments are made that health care is either more of a market-driven good or more of a governmental subsidized service. In an Institute of Medicine (IOM) report on patient safety, health care organizations have been admonished to base operational functioning on "evidence-based" management as well as evidence-based clinical services (Kohn, Corrigan, & Donaldson, 2000). Thus tools for science-based management are increasingly used to guide cost and quality decisions. For example, advocates trained in the Six Sigma process of systemic root-cause analysis and rectification, using principles of quality borrowed from the manufacturing sector, are solving operational processes within complex health care systems. Plsek (2003) suggests that the managerial model based on "machine" as metaphor is problematic within complex health care systems. Frederick Taylor's Scientific Management focused on the relationship between parts, and linear deterministic functions of structures and processes. Differences from expected structures and processes are seen as a failure of the system, problems to be solved and related risks mitigated (Plsek, 2003). This "machine" metaphor continues to dominate operations within health care systems even as other metaphors consistent with complexity science emerge. For leaders seeking transformation in health care systems grounded in caring, it must be noted that Taylor's Scientific Management emerged from a value system grounded in the value of efficiency and the model of "man as machine," rather than one grounded in human caring. Thus it is essential to recognize and appreciate distinctions between "scientific management" and "science-based management." The two relevant bodies of science we are concerned with here are management science and caring science—and from the perspective of the model of Dance of Caring Persons, the values grounding caring science must be the final arbiter of "fit" when drawing on management science.

It is widely accepted that the values of an organization are made visible in institutional budgets, where priorities are established by the allocation of scarce resources. Nursing leaders within complex health care organizations are accountable for some of the largest budgets and greatest number of staff, and thus a great deal of emphasis is focused on cost savings within nursing departments. The Advisory Board Company, a global research technology and consulting firm in Washington, DC, provides leadership development for executive nurses across the country. They have listed 13 areas that nurse executives need to attend to within health care system transformation (Advisory Board Company, 2012):

1. Enhance performance on measures tied to payment
2. Prevent unnecessary readmissions

3. Pay the appropriate dollars per worked hour
4. Flex staffing for actual demand
5. Innovate on the Inpatient Staffing Model
6. Elevate role of nurses in outpatient settings
7. Achieve zero defect for preventable complications
8. Embed risk assessment for utilization into staff workflow
9. Preempt unnecessary hospital utilization
10. Redistribute siloed patient care tasks to a cross-continuum navigator
11. Drive individual accountability—underlying components of peak performance
12. Strengthen interdisciplinary collaboration
13. Position nursing as a Best-in-Class Partner for IT—benefits of IT integration in nursing

Source: From Advisory Board Company, 2012.

These are "patient-care services" and speak to the competencies of financial account-ability, but what is not evident is the patient-care model and how scope of practice and role competence factor into the patient-care experience. Knowledge and skill of the discipline of nursing are not evident in these priorities. A core competency for the discipline of nursing is to use theoretical and scientific breadth and depth of knowledge to provide clinical care performed to a standard (O'Rourke, 2003). It is also a standard of nursing practice to apply this knowledge to the patient's benefit in an integrated fashion with other care providers who deliver care from that discipline's scope of practice. We have argued that the integrated practice should be guided by principles of caring. Caring and cost are not opposite poles on a continuum. Caring and cost can both be advanced to the benefit of patients and staff. The presence of caring has been measurably linked to cost, quality, and satisfaction outcomes (Valentine, 1997). Clinical leaders must be able to articulate and advocate the power and possibility of caring as strongly as financial and system priorities. The public trust earned as licensed professionals requires the full appli-cation of disciplinary knowledge, including caring science. Values, vision, and action can be aligned within the practice environment.

Since for-profit health care systems are ultimately accountable to shareholders and not to religious or geopolitical communities, it will be essential to the goals of this book that we propose a model that explicitly includes shareholders as stakehold-ers in the enterprise. Many for-profit, investor-owned health care systems continue to engage in what are known in the language of health care economics as cross-subsi-dies, activities that enrich the larger health care enterprise and that do not necessarily produce an immediate favorable effect on the "bottom line." Cross-subsidies involve "spending money on research, teaching and as part of a broader mission of service to the community" (Kuttner, 1996, para. 10). It must be acknowledged though that not all for-profit health care systems have articulated a mission that speaks to any form of altruistic valuing.

Health care systems that are explicitly grounded, at least in part, in altruism, usu-ally express their mission in terms such as general welfare, community orientation, social justice, and a balance between the "bottom line" and the "common good." Services pro-vided under the auspice of health care systems, whether for-profit or nonprofit, are either directly delivered or at least planned and managed by health professionals whose profes-sions ascribe to explicit altruistic and humanitarian values. Therefore, it makes sense that in some genuine way, investor-owners of for-profit health care systems respect and ratify those professional values. Otherwise, the system is at internal cross-purposes and the objectives of neither group are likely to be met.

THE DANCE OF CARING PERSONS: A MODEL FOR CULTURAL TRANSFORMATION OF HEALTH CARE SYSTEMS

The Dance of Caring Persons is a model to guide the whole of an organization, including the functioning of human systems, in a way that is person centered and caring focused (Figure 2.1). The model emerged from the experience of grounding the structure, services, and administration of a life care facility in a specific nursing theoretical framework, the Theory of Nursing as Caring. Core dimensions of caring that are represented in this model include the following:

- Acknowledgment that all persons have the capacity to care by virtue of their humanness
- Commitment to respect for persons in all institutional structures and processes
- Recognition that each participant in the enterprise has a unique and valuable contribution to make to the whole and is present in the whole
- Appreciation for the dynamic, rhythmic nature of the Dance of Caring Persons, enabling opportunities for human creativity

These dimensions of the Dance of Caring Persons taken together, and sometimes individually, are the touchstones for transformational strategies, some that are known and some yet to be imagined. This model represents the values-based unifying framework we propose for the transformation of health care systems in the 21st century. Now, more than ever, there is a call for creative integration of values that on the surface may be considered incompatible. A major strength of the model, Dance of Caring Persons, is that it offers solid ground for transcending seemingly insurmountable differences between for-profit values and altruistic values.

Effective use of the model of Dance of Caring Persons as a unifying framework for transforming the culture of health care is facilitated by an understanding of the origins of the model. The model was created originally for use with a particular theoretical framework to organize and guide the study and practice of the discipline of nursing. The nursing theoretical framework, called the Theory of Nursing as Caring, was originated by two of the authors of this book, Boykin and Schoenhofer (2001). Underlying assumptions of

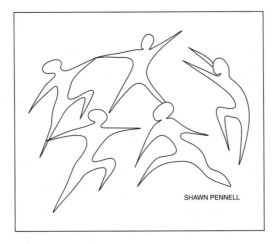

FIGURE 2.1 The Dance of Caring Persons.

Source: From Boykin & Schoenhofer, 2001, p. 37.

the nursing theoretical framework that have particular relevance to the Dance of Caring Persons model underpin this model, and include:

- Persons are caring by virtue of their humanness
- Persons are caring, moment to moment
- Persons are whole or complete in the moment
- Personhood is a process of living grounded in caring
- Personhood is enhanced through participating in nurturing relationships with caring others

The core dimensions of the Dance of Caring Persons model, together with these underlying assumptions about persons and caring, constitute the unifying values-based framework that will be used to guide the design of specific strategies for transforming the culture of health care systems so that a culture of caring permeates all aspects of those systems. Although most health care systems will address a common set of issues, the way in which issues are addressed will of course reflect the prevailing values of members of the system. The current state of health care systems—divergent and fragmented in purpose, mission, organization, and leadership—clearly has led to dissatisfaction with health care from all stakeholder groups, from consumers and direct care providers to financial investors and underwriters of health care systems. The model that will guide strategy in this book, the Dance of Caring Persons, is a direct response to the call for a unifying values-based framework that has been expressed by the IOM, The Joint Commission, and other health care leadership groups.

John Baldwin, a nurse leader and former nurse manager of the emergency department at Boca Raton Community Hospital, shared this reflection on his own journey into the Dance of Caring Persons.

In creating and supporting a model of care grounded in Nursing as Caring, it was essential for me as a nursing leader to understand, embrace, and clearly articulate, in words and lived experiences, the core assumptions of this theory. Modeling in this fashion helped to capture the hearts and hands of nursing service personnel who truly are the front line interface with patients and significant others.

In the beginning, Nursing as Caring was so totally unique in its conceptual foundation that I found myself to be resistant. I realized that I had not come to know myself as caring person. It is crucial the leader first know self as caring person and identify personal ways of living and growing in caring. Through this knowing, one can more easily "see" others (both professionally and personally) as living caring and honor their unique expressions. Commitment to knowing myself as caring person opened for me the opportunity to know staff as caring persons and to realize how important my role was to nurturing their living and growing in caring. I had to let go and trust staff and not exert my positional authority. I had to see myself as one of the performers in the Dance of Caring Persons, but not as pre-eminent. Everyone had equal value and contributed to the dance we were creating. As I continued to immerse myself more in the theory, I came to see the total practicality and "obviousness" of its tenets. It was then much clearer to me that the implementation of Nursing as Caring could indeed transform the practice of nursing.

It became my role to create an environment, or "culture," that promoted, supported, and sustained caring as the foundation for nursing service. In reality, this is the very focus of all nursing (whether it be at the service level or at the administrative level) to nurture persons living and growing in caring. In order for this transformation to occur there must be a commitment to intentionally focus on creating this caring-based culture. That is, time and effort must be afforded in a planned fashion in order for change, and then maintenance, of this nature to occur. Individuals must have opportunities to dialogue on Nursing as Caring. They need support from leadership to make explorations into this new territory—explorations that will expectedly not always be successful in and of themselves, but will certainly yield discoveries and learning that will eventually lead to success over time.

The exemplar of the nursing situation you encountered earlier was a direct result of the culture change in our department as a result of exploring Nursing as Caring. In fact, over time, many of the staff today share their nursing situations in staff meetings and, through the dialogue, we are growing in our understanding of the unique expressions of living caring in practice.

We have made a number of changes in our department as a result of implementing Nursing as Caring. The following questions guide our decisions: "What is the right thing to do, being grounded in the values of Nursing as Caring?" "What is best for the patient or staff?" The answers to these two heavy questions do not always provide easy answers, but they do offer a compass to guide us through the maze of possible answers. (Boykin, Schoenhofer, Baldwin, & McCarthy, 2005, pp. 18–19)

HISTORY AND BACKGROUND OF THE MODEL

The Dance of Caring Persons model was conceptualized by Boykin and Schoenhofer during the years 1981 to 1982, as an organizational chart for a privately owned life care facility. The developers of the model were invited to share their philosophical framework for nursing practice, which would ground the primary service of the facility in the values of caring, which was to be the provision of nursing in congregate residential care. The owners wanted their entire enterprise to be explicitly grounded in the values of caring. Initially, all employees of this start-up company were invited to participate in weekly development dialogues. Each person, representing organizational roles ranging from owner and chief administrator to groundskeeper and custodial services, and everyone in-between, was invited to share a story of how their own work contributed to the overall culture of caring that was being created. Eventually, a model for an organizational chart was presented to the entire group. It consisted of a series of color-coded overlays that represented each department in the organization; as the contributions of each department to the culture of caring were discussed, additional overlays of dancers were revealed, until the entire organization was represented by a colorful array of dancers representing the Dance of Caring Persons. At the time of that original work, residents had not yet been recruited, although planning was carried out with residents and their extended families also considered as part of the dance.

Persons in Relationship: Health Care Systems

Let us briefly consider each of the assumptions underlying the Dance of Caring Persons, as it might be lived in a health care system. It should be noted that all the chapters in Sections II and III of this book describe strategies that are grounded in these assumptions, but for now, we will lay the groundwork through examples of how the assumptions of the model underpin a culture of caring in health care systems.

Persons Are Caring by Virtue of Their Humanness

This assumption is basic to the entire model. Although we recognize that it asserts a value that is not always readily perceived as supportable, holding this assumption is essential to the integrity of the model. It may be important to answer the question that many ask and that you may be thinking as well, "What about the rapist or murderer—how can one say they are caring?" Our belief is that persons are innately caring, although one may intentionally choose not to manifest that caring. This assumption speaks to a fundamental belief about being human. A Canadian leader in nursing and hospital administration perhaps has said it best: Caring is the human mode of being (Roach, 2002). There has never been a dispute about health care as a moral enterprise. "It is a moral enterprise because it establishes relationships with moral bonds involving duties and responsibilities" (Roach, 2002, p. 2). In earlier eras, when the organization of health care systems was undertaken by military, government, and religious institutions that avowedly accepted responsibility for the moral nature of the enterprise, a value system grounded in caring was not contested. In order for today's health care systems to thrive and achieve the purposes expressed in vision and mission statements, it is necessary to situate economic values in a way that is complementary and not antagonistic to caring values. Perhaps the bottom line here is that both sets of values are human values. Understanding what it means to be human, and how to structure successful human systems, systems that respond to values humans hold dear, will require that we relinquish the restrictive idea that caring and economic values are irreconcilable opposites.

The Dance of Caring Persons model offers a way to reconcile these seemingly divergent values by inviting all those involved in the enterprise to have the freedom to offer their unique gifts and to recognize, appreciate, and honor the gifts that each person brings. This does not mean that all ideas and suggestions must automatically be adopted by the system, but it does ensure that all ideas and suggestions are considered in ways that are creative and humane. This particular value that all persons are caring and thus have a contribution to make to the enterprise is expressed in the example of creative organizational structures, such as councils that have representation from all role functions within the system. One of the struggles in actualizing the value underlying an open input system is to ensure that correspondingly open structures exist so that persons risking participation are genuinely welcomed as contributors. Several later chapters in this book will suggest specific strategies designed to genuinely encourage and honor participation.

Persons Are Caring, Moment to Moment

Again, we turn to Roach (2002) to enrich our understanding of what it means to be caring. Boykin and Schoenhofer (2001) relied on Roach's discussion of persons as caring, asserting that caring "entails the capacity to care, the calling forth of this ability in ourselves and others, responding to something or someone that matters, and finally actualizing the ability to care" (p. 2). Further, "the potential to express caring varies in the moment and develops over time. Thus caring is lived moment to moment and is constantly unfolding. The development of competency in caring develops over a lifetime" (Boykin & Schoenhofer, 2001, p. 2).

Philosophers and researchers have contributed to the development of a "language of caring" that facilitates the conceptualizing and describing of caring being lived moment to moment in situations. Mayeroff (1971), in his brief though profound book *On Caring*, identified eight expressions of caring that contribute to a basic language, providing substance and form to discussions of caring. These expressions provide a practical understanding of what it means to live caring:

- Knowing: there are different ways of knowing: personal, empirical, ethical, aesthetic; knowing that, knowing about, and knowing directly
- Alternating rhythm: the rhythm of moving between broader and more focused views
- Patience: an active participation with others in which we give freely of ourselves
- Honesty: genuineness and openness to truly seeing
- Trust: allowing others to grow in their own time and in their own way
- Humility: recognizing the need for continual learning about self and other; being ready and willing to learn more about self and other

- Hope: an expression of the moment alive with possibilities
- Courage: the willingness and ability to take risks; to go into the unknown (Mayeroff, 1971)

In coming to know self as caring, one might ask, "Who am I as caring person? How do I reflect my knowing, alternating rhythms, patience, honesty, trust, humility, hope, and courage moment to moment...at home, at play, and at work?"

Roach (2002) addresses nursing as the professionalization of human caring and offers a language of caring for nursing. The attributes of caring she describes are often referred to as the 5 Cs: compassion, competence, confidence, conscience, and commitment. She later added a sixth "C," comportment, to incorporate symbols of caring that are important in professional roles. The 6 Cs answer the question, "What is the health professional doing when caring?" The following is a description of these attributes:

- Compassion: a quality of presence that allows one to share with and make room for the other
- Competence: having the knowledge, judgment, skills, energy, experience, and motivation necessary to respond to the demands of one's profession
- Confidence: the quality which fosters trusting relationships
- Conscience: a state of moral awareness; a compass directing one's behavior based on what *ought* to be
- Commitment: includes devotion and is a "complex affective response characterized by a convergence between one's desires and one's obligations, and by a deliberate choice to act in accordance with them" (p. 62)
- Comportment: symbolic expressions of dress, language, and demeanor

Swanson (2010) proposed five caring processes that expand the language of caring for health care professionals: knowing, being with, doing for, enabling, and maintaining belief. From a meta-analysis of 130 works on caring, Swanson proposed five domains of caring to help organize discourse for nursing practice, and these domains appear to also be applicable to discourse pertaining to any and all participants in the Dance of Caring Persons. Swanson's domains are leveled and discourse at any one level presumes inclusion of all lower levels. The domains are labeled as follows:

Level I: Descriptions of capacities and characteristics of caring persons
Level II: Concerns and/or commitments (values) that lead to caring actions
Level III: Conditions that enhance or diminish the likelihood that caring will occur
Level IV: Caring actions
Level V: Consequences—intentional and unintentional outcomes of caring and noncaring (Swanson, 2010, p. 436)

Persons Are Whole or Complete in the Moment

One of Mayeroff's major themes as he discussed caring was the idea that caring means helping another grow, in his or her own time and way. In order to truly contribute to the growth of self and other, it is important to accept the person where he or she is at the moment *and* to simultaneously entertain authentic hope that growth in the capacity to express caring in meaningful ways can occur *while* offering authentic patience that allows the person to grow in caring in ways that are true to the self. One emphasis of this particular assumption, that persons are whole in the moment while simultaneously growing in wholeness or completeness as caring person, calls for us to give up the idea that in helping another to grow, we "diagnose" gaps in caring capacity and "prescribe" methods of correcting those "deficiencies." When we take that position, we are moving out of the circle represented in the Dance of Caring Persons and ascending the ladder of hierarchical privilege. As the humanistic psychologist Rogers (1961) so powerfully taught, effectively promoting the growth of self and other persons requires an environment of unconditional positive regard. In order to nurture persons as caring, it is necessary to enter into the world of the other in order to know the person as uniquely living caring ways and expressing dreams and aspirations for growing in caring (Boykin & Schoenhofer, 2001). How this assumption might be lived in practical ways in health care systems will be spelled out in later chapters on specific strategies. One area in which the assumption would need to be taken from the merely ideal (out-of-reach) to the highly practical is in performance evaluation. In many health care systems today, there is at least some recognition given to the importance of self-evaluation and shared goal setting; fully implementing the Dance of Caring Persons model would enable authentic expression of these and similar practices.

Personhood Is a Process of Living Grounded in Caring

Personhood has been addressed in many disciplines; however, we will propose an understanding taken from the theoretical underpinnings of the Dance of Caring Persons (Boykin & Schoenhofer, 2001). Personhood means living the meaning of one's own life, "demonstrating congruence between beliefs and behaviors" (p. 4), "being authentic, being who I am as caring person in the moment" (p. 4). Summarizing the nursing literature, Touhy (2005) identified attributes of personhood: wholeness, peacefulness, joyfulness, contentment, self-worth, self-esteem, purposefulness, and spirituality. Boykin and Schoenhofer (2001) explained that personhood is processual. That is, rather than being viewed as a series of sequential steps leading to becoming, personhood unfolds in everyday living. From this same theoretical perspective, Touhy (2005) succinctly explained that personhood is "fullness of being human...expressed as persons live caring uniquely day by day" (p. 45).

For health care systems to be experienced as environments to promote personhood as living the meaning of one's own life grounded in caring, authenticity must be nurtured. In general terms, this means that there must be a genuine valuing of freedom for human imagination to flourish and generate creative solutions. How this freedom can be lived in the context of institutional structures and goals requires considerable creativity. Intentionally living an authentic commitment to the values of the Dance of Caring Persons model generates space for imagining possibilities and designing feasible practices that nurture the freedom and support necessary to a viable culture of caring in health care systems. Specific strategies that nurture and honor personhood will be explored in succeeding chapters.

The following is an example of practice from the perspective of Dance of Caring Persons that illustrates the value of freedom and creativity in inviting the person cared for to lead in the "dance." The story was shared by Donna Linette, a nurse who has led the creation of nursing practice frameworks grounded in Nursing as Caring in several health care systems.

> "Jan" (patient with chronic mental illness) went to the canteen in the afternoon as she did most every day during her 18-month hospitalization. The canteen was on the furthest corner of the hospital grounds from her residential unit. Walking there on her own was a privilege that she earned and she was so proud of this independence.
>
> As soon as the afternoon shift checked to be sure everyone was present and safe, those with this grounds-level privilege were permitted to go to the canteen. Most patients (or "persons served" as we refer to patients) so looked forward to this free socialization time.

As Jan was preparing for the walk, she checked to make sure she had her pocketbook stocked with the tokens for the store, her tissues, and her wallet that contained her most prized possessions. At 4:10 p.m. the 10-minute walk ended and she was happy to find her "favorite seat" at the outside table free. She sat, talked with whoever sat down at the table, and then when the crowd thinned, went to get her cup of juice and make a purchase with her tokens.

The time to close the canteen was nearing and all persons served were reminded that the doors would close in 10 minutes, as evening curfew was approaching due to sunset. At 6:30 p.m., the doors were closing and Jan refused to go back to her residential unit. The canteen worker, a peer specialist (former patient) paged me because Jan would not leave the canteen. Bob knew that Jan and I had a relationship, as the three of us had attended a mental health benefit together off the campus the week before.

I went to the canteen and Jan was sitting on the floor and she promptly told me that she would be staying there all night. I sat down on the floor next to her and we talked about her favorite things (all in the wallet). Meanwhile, security was on standby to lock the place and I suggested to them that they could wait; Jan and I were going to have a conversation. After some time, I suggested that we put her favorite things in a safe place—the closet in her room. I extended the crook of my arm to escort her, she hooked it with her arm, and she smiled and we walked arm in arm across the campus.

Personhood Is Enhanced Through Participating in Nurturing Relationships With Caring Others

A typical organizational model depicts role-relationships arrayed in a hierarchical structure, with most relationships situated as "up/down," organized on a vertical axis, with only a limited number of relationships horizontally oriented. In organizations in which human relationships are lived hierarchically, competition and protection are dominant values of the culture. In either climbing the rungs of a bureaucratically structured organization, or in defending one's position on that ladder, it is difficult for persons in the system to "be authentic and valued as a unique person with special ideas because the risks of such valuing are often too great for the bureaucracy to bear" (Boykin & Schoenhofer, 2001, p. 36). The image of the bureaucratic ladder as an organizational structure depicts persons "who are not and cannot be open to receive other...more often than not, are viewed as objects" (p. 36). Human relationships, personal aspirations, and a sense of self-worth are difficult to foster in a vertical environment as "people are either looking up or down but rarely eye to eye," failing to "support the idea of each person as important in and to him[self or] herself" (p. 36). The Dance of Caring Persons, structured as a dynamic circle, calls for one to reflect on beliefs about relating; about being in relationship. This model facilitates participation of relationships with caring others that enhance all persons involved, with benefits accruing to the mission of the health care system.

CHALLENGING QUESTIONS

In working with the Dance of Caring Persons model in various health care settings, several questions have emerged over time, questions that will likely occur to others considering adoption of the model. The core values of the model and the underlying assumptions that ground it help give the kind of guidance to answering those questions that will retain the unifying nature of the model. For example, the question may be asked, "How are functional units of the system reflected when the model displays no hierarchical structure?"

Another example is the assumption sometimes made that the patient/client/consumer is always in the middle of the dancing circle; however, through experience and on reflection, we have come to recognize that the dance expresses the dynamic, fluid, multidimensional, and multidirectional nature of human relationships and human systems. Thus, there may be times when the patient is in the center of the circle, and other times in the circle itself, just as there may be times when a person representing any particular function of the organization may be more central to the dance. Although the patient is not necessarily always in the center of the circle, directly or indirectly, every participant in the dance has a relationship with that patient, and with every other participant in the dance.

The formal designer of a dance is generally identified as a choreographer. The Dance of Caring Persons in any particular patient care situation is choreographed by a person or persons functioning in the role(s) most central to that which matters in a given moment. Each functional role represented in the dance has specific contributions to make to the overall success of the dance, no one role is fixed in the position of choreographer. Sometimes in systems, the role of choreographer is designated by organizational role function and in order to successfully choreograph the dance, must be keenly attuned to each dancer involved directly and even indirectly.

A key question to be considered is this one: What is the purpose of the dance? When the dance in question is the Dance of Caring Persons as an expression of a health care system, whether nonprofit or for-profit, one purpose that is always operative is that of providing health services to people. Another purpose that is also present in both economic models is that the system offers a venue for the realization of dreams—the dreams of the providers, the consumers, and the underwriters of the health service. A health care system is an entity that is an expression of human imagination, undertaken for human purposes. Economic livelihood is unquestionably one of the outcome expectations shared by health care workers and system financiers alike. From the perspective of the assumptions underlying the Dance of Caring Persons model, it is assumed that all participants in the dance, whether patients, employees, or investors, are caring persons who have the capacity to imbue the enterprise with altruistic motives. One role function of recognized leading professionals within the health care system is to conceptualize and communicate shared values in ways that can be recognized and ratified by all participants in the dance. Although the move toward "commodification" of health services has not been without excesses that tend to obscure shared values, there are examples of creative approaches that find common ground in the sometimes seemingly contradictory values of service and market. We propose that grounding health care systems in a culture of caring can be maximized by the unifying framework we advocate, the Dance of Caring Persons.

REFERENCES

Advisory Board Company. (2012). Nursing Executive Center infographic. Retrieved October 6, 2012, from www.advisory.com

Boykin, A., & Schoenhofer, S. O. (2001). *Nursing as caring: A model for transforming practice.* Sudbury, MA: Jones & Bartlett and National League for Nursing.

Boykin, A., Schoenhofer, S. O., Baldwin, J., & McCarthy, D. (2005). Living caring in practice: The transformative power of the theory of nursing as caring. *International Journal for Human Caring, 9*(3), 15–19.

Kohn, L. T., Corrigan, J. M., & Donaldson, M. S. (Eds.). (2000). *To err is human: Building a safer health system.* Washington, DC: The National Academies Press.

Kuttner, R. (1996). Colombia/HCA and the resurgence of the for-profit hospital business. *New England Journal of Medicine, 335,* 362–368.

Mayeroff, M. (1971). *On caring.* New York, NY: Harper & Row.

O'Rourke, M. W. (2003). Rebuilding a professional practice model: The return of role-based practice accountability. *Nursing Administration Quarterly, 27*(2), 95–101.

Plsek, P. (2003, January). *Complexity and the adoption of innovation in health care.* Paper presented at the Conference on Accelerating Quality Improvement in Health Care Strategies to Speed the Diffusion of Evidence-Based Innovations, Washington, DC. Retrieved from https://www.niatx.net/PDF/PIPublications/Plsek_2003_NIHCM.pdf

Ray, M. A. (1989). The theory of bureaucratic caring for nursing practice in the organizational culture. *Nursing Administration Quarterly, 13*(2), 31–42.

Roach, M. S. (2002*). Caring, the human mode of being: A blueprint for the health professions* (2nd ed.). Ottawa, ON: CHA Press.

Rogers, C. (1961). *On becoming a person: A psychotherapist's view of psychotherapy.* New York, NY: Houghton Mifflin Company.

Swanson, K. M. (2010). Kristen Swanson's theory of caring. In M. E. Parker & M. C. Smith (Eds.), *Nursing theories and nursing practice* (3rd ed., pp. 428–438). Philadelphia, PA: F. A. Davis.

Touhy, T. T. (2005). Dementia, personhood and nursing: Learning from a nursing situation. *Nursing Science Quarterly, 17*(1), 43–49.

Turkel, M. C. (2001). Struggling to find a balance: The paradox between caring and economics. *Nursing Administration Quarterly, 26*(1), 67–82.

Valentine, K. (1988). History, analysis and application of the carative tradition in health and nursing. *Journal of the New York State Nursing Association, 19*(4), 2–8.

Valentine, K. L. (1997). Exploration of the relationship between cost and caring. *Holistic Nursing Practice, 11*(4), 71–81.

Response to Chapter 2

Members from the Ethics Advisory Committee of University of Mississippi Medical Center responded to Chapter 2 in a group dialogue format. The dialogue was facilitated by Savina Schoenhofer, a coauthor of this book. Participants in the dialogue include:

Rev. Ruth W. Black, EdD, Director of Pastoral Services
W. Richard (Rick) Boyte, MD, MA, Professor of Pediatrics and Director of Pediatric Palliative Care Services
Ralph Didlake, MD, FACS, Professor of Surgery and Director of the Center for Bioethics and Medical Humanities
Susan Shands Jones, BA, JD, Associate General Counsel
Mary Mixon, RN, MSN, Assistant Administrator, University Hospitals

Savina: I want to say that I really appreciate your being willing to share your thoughts on the idea of transforming health care through a focus on creating a culture of caring. Caring—I jotted a little note down on my paper here as we were sitting in an earlier meeting, somebody actually said these words: withhold care. I may have heard that differently than others in the meeting, and I did know what was meant by the term, but things like that sort of go right to my heart... and I translated that phrase because I know we don't withhold care, we withhold certain services, certain treatment. My colleagues and I decided to write this book about specific strategies for health care transformation through the creation of a culture of caring. There is mostly theoretical material in Chapter 2 that you are responding to, because it is the foundation for the whole book, and for the work that we've been doing for about 30 years—with various health care systems, nursing service organizations, but broader than that too. And so... since our approach to consultation and the work we've been doing is dialogic, the idea came forward that we should have dialogues in the book. That is why you are being invited to respond to the chapter you were sent.

So, the Dance of Caring Persons—you've had an opportunity to read the chapter. I guess you can ask me later if you want to know where it came from, but maybe we should get right to it and just start talking about these three ideas. The value of a caring-based perspective as a framework for health care, as an explicit framework, caring as an explicit concept in which to ground health care systems. And then, what would have to happen for a health care system to successfully ground everything they do in an explicit concept of caring and in particular this concept, the Dance of Caring Persons? What strategies would you have in mind that could help make the adoption of such an approach success-ful…or do you think it is even a workable idea? What do people reading this book need to think about to really make this idea work…some things we haven't even thought of perhaps, so from a real practical, "down in the trenches" point of view.

Mary: You asked about the value of the caring-based perspective in transformation of health care…I see that as high value because I see that patients and staff satisfaction is at stake, and that is a key focus—I'm sure it has always been a focus, but right now it is definitely a focus and if we had this caring-based perspective, we should possibly have the patient and staff satisfaction, I believe.

Savina: I'm just thinking of the relationship-based care approach that is being imple-mented here, and I'm not selling our ideas or our book but just asking, if that had the kind of substance behind it that is involved in this Dance of Caring Persons—what would that mean? You know, most health care systems nowadays, because of Hospital Consumer Assessment of Health Providers and Systems (HCAHPS) and all, are trying to do some-thing humanistically oriented, so how could that be brought to fruition, how could your dreams for relationship-based care be brought to fruition being underpinned by some-thing like the Dance of Caring Persons? Would it help to make that explicit?

Rick: The relationship-based care concept, I have just an overview of, I haven't been to all the classes, but the relationship-based care is the relationship with you and the patient, and you and the other staff, that's the focus, and the caring model really focuses on mak-ing sure that everybody's input is really important as well, and so they coincide and would help each other I believe. The two concepts could work together.

Ralph: I think that part of what we have to do is to determine a definition of care…every physician will say they "care" for their patients, they also would say that they care about what their hemoglobin A1c (HbA1c) is, but not necessarily care why their HbA1c is not correct, or that good control might make them better employees or better members of the community, so exactly what is encompassed in this concept of care?

Savina: What if you modified that, and asked, "What is encompassed in the concept of caring?"

Ralph: Caring as a relational act, is that what you mean? I think from a physician's stand-point, especially from the standpoint of a modern physician technologically trained, car-ing has to be very explicit. If I'm going to be attracted to a system that delivers health care in a caring relational manner, all of that is going to have to be very explicitly defined, because I am not at all trained in that…I've come to this with a background of phys-ics and chemistry and have been technologically educated, and that is really a wedge between me and the patient…so what is encompassed in my training, ability, and will-ingness to engage in this caring is really determined by what your concept of caring is, this theoretical underpinning. Now, personally, I see it as a very high value, because we're not just about controlling the HgA1C, we're about making people's lives better, and that has obvious relational elements, so if we don't "care" or don't have a perspective of caring about those relational elements, I can't do the very best for my patient. But we've got to get over this technological hurdle where I'm being valued as a provider, even reim-bursed as a provider, on the HbA1c level, and nobody cares if I'm caring.

Mary: On the back side they won't pay you if the patient is not satisfied either, so you do get it both ways.

Ralph: Yes, but is that a metric by which our current system reimburses me individually?

Mary: No, but hospitals are moving in that direction clearly...so the system has to value caring not just as a theoretical concept but it has to have a monetary value too, unfortunately.

Savina: I don't want to take up too much time with me talking, but because you brought it up, I'll share with you that a colleague of mine has developed a theory that he calls technological competence as an expression of caring, and that's exactly what you were taking about. The reason he developed this model is to help people who were scientifically and technologically trained. Because all care activities are so highly technological, we think there's a disconnect, but there doesn't have to be; if you think of the purpose for your expert technological action being your expression of caring in this moment...

Ralph: Now in this vision of a system, are we talking about a system of multiple caregivers, or are we talking about an overarching system? I think to speak intelligently about a system, I need to know what level of system we are talking about. When I was in private practice I had a "system" of caring that was constructed as follows: I would see a patient and talk about a surgical procedure, and I would do all the things that a physician is supposed to do, risk, benefits, this is how this is going to happen, and then I had the most wonderful nurse who would go in and say "this is what he said" and we would do that because I knew my technical limitations and she spoke west Alabama and she could go in there and explain very clearly what I had just said...now that is a system of caring.

Savina: And the contribution of each was valued in its own right.

Susan: ...and not hierarchical, but the circle.

Ralph: Now, how can you translate that triad of individuals to a hospital-sized system of caring?

Mary: To make the change you'd need transformation in the leadership training programs right from the top because they're trained so rigidly, transformation in physician training as well, and you have to get the hierarchy on the same page.

Susan: Not to be as hierarchical is a real challenge, in a big system like we have.

Ralph: It's just foreign to the kind of systems that we've always worked in, that we've always been a part of.

Susan: I don't do much patient care since I'm a staff member, but when I think about the ethics consult... [pause]

Savina: ...but you do have a connection to direct patient care...

Susan: I do...and it's the Ethics Committee and the consult, and when I think about it, that whole idea about the circle, and the patient sometimes being in the middle, but sometimes it's the doctor, or the social worker, or whoever called the consult, and a fact that I learned really quickly that communication is such an issue...and usually, if you'll permit me, it's the physician who so often isn't talking, and it's the social worker or the poor resident that is discussing. I don't know where...[pause]

Savina: ...where the call for caring is coming from?

Susan: Right…but when it works well, it is the circle, and everybody, they go "Well, I didn't know that" and the social worker goes "Well, I talked with the family" and then especially the doctor says, "Well, I didn't know that, this is the first time we've all been together"—that's happened a couple of times. Suddenly the Ethics Committee is working and it's not really the process, it's just getting them all together and then the caring just kind of happens. I had not thought about it in this way, but there are moments when that happens and everybody feels good about the discussion and that you've helped them. But then on the other hand, from the perspective of the legal standard of care, the first thing I thought about is, "Have you done what you're supposed to do? Are you going to get in trouble?"

Savina: Susan, how are you connected to the service mission of this institution in your role as attorney?

Susan: Well, you want the best case scenario, which is everyone gets wonderful care and everyone is caring, and you know you're getting the best outcomes because the trains are running on time…

Savina: …and you're the one that's looking out for…

Susan: …to make sure the contract is signed, all the little details that are important for the care…and it's sort of like when you work on a research contract or something, it always helps me to be able to talk to the person who is the investigator, and I think that's important for the accountant people and the grants people and all the people who don't ever see a patient, but in an academic health center, it is research and education, and health care, you need all those pieces, and I think that's an idea—do you try to do some training for the other side of the house, because you should be having good customer service, which we are getting into that now, with even the secretaries and all up and down, trying to treat everyone as a consumer and try to get more staff people to come here as patients, and get good care, and so I think we're getting that, but I don't think we've gotten that far. And I think the idea of having everybody be a better listener would be wonderful.

Mary: You advise us on care issues, and with the Ethics Committee, you come in and out of the circle depending upon…

Susan: …but it's not my type of work, but I feel like it is my type of work.

Savina: I would say you're always in the circle, sometimes you're closer to the center at a given moment, but even when you're up there looking at your law books, I would say you're still in the circle.

Mary: That's right.

Ralph: I think you're always in the circle, regardless of what you're doing at this institution, once you're on campus and in a role, the ultimate end user of your accountancy or legal work or delivering the mail or the lady who runs the cash register in the lunch room, the ultimate end user is a patient. Jo Anne has heard me say this so many times, that a patient is made vulnerable by disease or injury, and that's a moral obligation and it's probably much more difficult to see that care when you are in the cafeteria.

Savina: How useful would it be for that person running the cash register in the cafeteria to have that sense of connectedness to the institutional mission?

Mary: It's very important!

Ralph: I think it's absolutely vital, and I'll give you an example. A year or two ago there was a patient who died unexpectedly in the CT scanner, and the family was called down and informed about what happened. They started grieving very openly, loudly, demonstrably—a culturally appropriate grieving for this family. The young CT technician became frightened in the situation, did not understand the grieving behavior that this family was engaging in and felt threatened, called security. It ended up with family members, the sons of the deceased family member, arrested, handcuffed, and a gun was drawn at one point. Now, that's a complete disconnect in caring, so that the individual who normally would not have to interface with that family and that death, had she been fully engaged in a culture of caring, would have recognized what was going on or at least would have had a support system to help her recognize. So for me, I think engaging everyone including that police officer—that police officer is as much a caregiver as Rick and I are.

Mary: I have another story. I was head nurse on psych years ago, and my housekeepers saved our lives more than once. They would come out from a patient's room and say "I just heard them say that they were going to come up and hit you, or do something to you, or try to escape." They were part of the care team. They would interact with the patients and they would be able to come and be part of the team, they felt comfortable enough to tell us what was going on with that patient that day. That is incredible they were just part of our team, saved our lives.

Rick: I think this is a great conversation; it's very interesting to me. I felt like I'm part of the type of transformation you're talking about, I feel like I am actually living it…because I was very technologically based as a critical care physician. I felt like I was providing good care and was very adept at doing these kinds of things…and was thinking essentially how that care has changed for me though. The definition of that for patients was that good care was doing what they asked of me explicitly, take care of my child, do what you can to get him through this illness, that type of thing, but really, about the diseases itself. And so I think what you're trying to help us all do here, through your book, is recognize that care has a much deeper meaning and it is often about what they don't ask us, which is, nobody really asks explicitly "care for me as a person," they come into health care asking "please help me with my illness, with this disease" so I think that's what I'm starting to see. Actually this fits very nicely into what I do now with health care, because we really often talk about lowering the hierarchy, leveling the field, valuing each member's input, and having transdisciplinary care. For in bereavement, I have definitely started to see that every team member, whether they're a respiratory therapist, chaplain, social worker, specialist, physician, nurse, nurse practitioner, all need to be extremely good at bereavement…the care at the end of life, because you never know who's going to be in the room to help with grief support.

Savina: It could be a custodian…

Rick: Right, I do think it's fascinating, for the folks who aren't directly taking care of patients, like custodians, how do you get that across, from the time that you're hired to the time you retire, how do you help that employee feel like they're part of that care?

Susan: One thing we do with the politicians now and different groups is that Dr. McMullan loves to take them up to the neonatal intensive care unit [NICU] or surgery, just to be in a hospital, just to say that's why we need this bond issue or whatever. And I wonder if we should sign them up for "Friends." I do think that just physically, I go to that Friends meeting, just to see patients, and realize that's what is part of what is going on.

Mary: I have thought that as well, time and exposure...people need exposure to the concept, the caring model over time. With the health care disparities, you can't just take the recipe, you can't just write it down and give it to them, you really have to live it through readings, through engagement, speakers, and dialogues among the group over time. They need time to understand it at their own pace.

Savina: ...understand the most fundamental idea on which this model is based, the idea that to be human is to be caring...period...you don't have to prove it. If you're human, you're caring. And so where do we go from that perspective?

Ralph: Is the idea that we all have this base of expertise already, I mean, we tend to feel we always have to...[pause]

Savina: We all know something about caring. I said I wasn't going to tell you how this model came about unless you asked, but as Ralph was talking I realized it may be helpful. It came about because Anne Boykin and I were asked to consult at a congregate living center that was just being developed...it had been built, it was now being staffed, there were no patients or residents, and the owners of this place had the foresight to realize that they wanted it grounded in caring...and they had the luck I guess to call the university and asked who were the experts in caring...we were called because it was known that we had done some work in that area. We went in there and worked with them. The whole staff who was employed at the time would sit around a conference table just like this one—some of them didn't even speak much English—and we would talk. It was the gardener, the electrician, the laundry person, the owner, the chief executive officer [CEO], the chief financial officer [CFO], and the chief nursing officer [CNO]...anybody who had already been brought on staff was a part of that dialogue. How this model came about is that it was our design for an organizational chart for this company. And then we started using it in all our work and it has just sort of developed from that. As Rick was describing, in terms of story, that's mostly how we advocate bringing people in and helping them see that, yes, they are part of the circle. If I had invited an accountant here with us today, we would have gotten an even richer dialogue.

Mary: I've seen, in the 33 years I've been here, that when the CFO knows more about the care that is being provided, they respond differently. In the past they would stay in the office, and now they'll go with us and go look at the area and talk to the staff and get input. It makes a difference—it really does.

Ruth: I'm thinking of how many times I've been asked to do things of an unlikely tune. I was thinking about a family, for instance, whose mother had been a faculty member here and wanted to be an eye donor. The children didn't want it to happen, but they said "We love mother and we will do it if you will be there when the Lions eye bank guy comes to enucleate." We talked later about what that was all about, and I hoped I was prayerful and "there" with her on behalf of these children who didn't want to follow her wishes but did. The room was full, with the Lion eye bank people, the student, the chaplain, and one or two of the staff, who would come in and say [whispering] "Why is the chaplain in there?" I realized that part of what was going on was a kind of caring that she would have wanted...in fact, she was a wonderful professor with gorgeous eyes, I "get" how they didn't want it to happen. I promised we would be as prayerful as possible, and it was one of those holy times when I was part of an unlikely event, but it was about caring, and what would be, even after her death, the caring thing to do. The nurses on the floor were so respectful of that, and the physician had said if that's what she wants, that's what he wants, and we'll do it. But often I've been called into unlikely teams where basically the request is just "care," be there, and many times I just bear witness to what is happening and to people's stories as they tell them to me.

It's the unlikely team, often the one that you wouldn't picture in a business textbook, that is the caring team that begins to form something much larger than you could have envisioned. Had you begun to plan it...it just begins to happen. Often the forming of an unlikely team is something that happens in this place. The openness to that, the invitation for an unlikely committee...I don't know any other way to say it, the unlikely team. Not bound by specialty area or even expertise, but caring and focusing on the patient or the family. So it sounds as if that's the kind of concept—you want everybody to feel part of the team, invited and held together, but with the inborn ability to care...a kind of natural gift that we arrive with, and if it gets trained and developed...

Rick: That makes me think of how the act of caring can be very impromptu or extemporaneous, because in counterbalance to Ralph's story earlier about the CT scanner and how they didn't recognize bereavement, lacked ability to accept what they were seeing. I remember a couple of years ago we literally were in a palliative care consultation, when we began to hear a loud commotion outside our office, literally banging on the walls, people with loud voices, and we went out and quickly recognized that there had just been a death in the pediatric intensive care unit [PICU] and the family was very physically emoting. The staff had called security and were trying to get security into the room. I stopped them, and I said, "Please don't go in the room, I think we have this under control," and it was true, they were very physically demonstrating how they were grieving...but there was really no true physical danger to any of the staff, so yeah, I think that's true that you can happen upon something, and if you already have a base of caring, you can probably be helpful.

Savina: What are some of the biggest drawbacks to an idea like this having a chance for success? What are the hurdles, the challenges that have to be met?

Mary: I think with some of the people, with their perspective on quality, cost, and satisfaction, and everything, they need to see...you mentioned that the presence of caring is measurably linked to cost, quality, and satisfaction...I think that has to be drawn out and shown that you have the data. That's one thing that would help the analytical side to see the figures.

Rick: I have to admit I have a hard time seeing how you do that.

Savina: One example was in an article that Anne Boykin and I published. It was a home health situation, a community-based situation. It was a combination of qualitative narrative research, and gave the perspective from the patient, her husband, the home health nurse, the CNO at the home health agency, the owner of the home health agency, and the people from the ambulance service, and the local hospital emergency department, getting the cost factors, the comparative data. The crux of that story was that this was a small community in which the people felt free to call on the nurse and she would come over, they didn't have to go to the ER...and that showed some cost saving, but it was only part of the story. The article brought out the value of caring to the patient, to the nurse, to the CNO, to the owner of the agency, what was the personal human value, and then we also had the monetary values in there.

Rick: I struggle to get the institution to recognize the value of it, to find ways to demonstrate that value. For the institution I don't think they see the value of qualitative research.

They want hard numbers, they want to show cost reduction, length of stay reduction, all this type of thing. Sometimes that's difficult to do, so I think I would very much invite and want a qualitative study that talked to my patients...I hope that would come out in favor of me, but if the institution would value that as much as they would me coming up with a database that shows cost reduction, then that would be good.

Savina: That's one thing that we're trying to do in this book, although none of us have CFO expertise, but we are trying not to ignore the fact that money matters, that money counts, and especially because this book is broadly oriented and we're looking at corporate entities as well as not-for-profits or community-based health care systems, we felt like we can't just ignore the idea that money counts.

Mary: You really can't because if you're trying to appeal to everybody, if you want everybody in the circle, you're going to have to bring them in at their thought processes. I think that could be a barrier but I think that could be something that could be worked through, it just takes some time and thinking through, with the CFO types, bring them into the picture, as far as how to present that.

Ruth: There even may be a new way of doing those figures...that has not even been thought of yet. We used to laugh that many times the CFO types see chaplains as lawsuit preventers...we knew that was true...there were many times that we would be able to have people talk about their grievances in a way that would take them away from their hot anger, the "where's my lawyer" stage, into beginning to look into what happened, what the future might look like for the family member...that's not a measurable kind of thing, but we "knew." One day they were going to sue, and the next day they started thinking about that other family again and there was something that happened, a transformation of their perspective that we hadn't had any idea would be there, and we would realize later that things are being worked out in a very different way that will be less difficult for the medical center than it would have been, and less difficult for the family too. So that's not part of Chapter 8 in the business manual of how to save money, but I do think there are going to be some new measurable pieces that we don't even know about yet...but I do think it's very valuable to measure, in some way, the difference, to represent that this will make a difference. As a priest of ours used to say, "After all, money is a sacrament"...his point was that it's one way we pay tribute to what we value.

Savina: I guess that one thing in working with this book and in general, we try to avoid casting one against the other, but to always be working to figure out how can all values be honored in appropriate ways.

Mary: I appreciated reading that, I felt like that was a very good point. From my years of experience, from being in administration and in nursing, I could see the importance of making sure that it wasn't one way but not the other, that they weren't fighting each other, but that they were both important.

Ruth: Something almost like spokes in a wheel...a wheel won't roll if there's not that kind of equality of all the pieces that are holding it together, that's the picture I sort of got as I was thinking about how you get everybody there ... that was the metaphor that was present. It's not easy, is it, but it could further your vision of caring in health systems.

Savina: I think all of us share that vision, from knowing you from the Ethics Advisory Committee, that you are people who could hear what we are trying to say and who could relate to it in ways that would open our eyes farther and help others who read the book see things more clearly. We aren't seeking agreement necessarily, we don't mind "yes, but's" because some people who read this book are going to be saying "yes, but," and we want to help them to be willing to consider these ideas as well.

Rick: I do think that as Ralph reflected in the beginning of this, that we already do care. I do think it's highly important and admirable that you want to focus on narrative… I think that if you care about a person's story, you care about the person.

Savina: Just imagine if all of you shared your stories. I'm thinking of a hospital in Atlantis, Florida, where they had a wall in a hallway where people could put their stories of how they lived their caring through their work.

Rick: Knowing a person's narrative helps you understand. There are many people I have misjudged, until I found more about them through them telling me about themselves.

Susan: That gets back to that whole listening thing. I always feel like I need more training, not in "what is the role…" but in listening and being taught how to get the story from the other person until you get to the conclusion, and having the time to do that… and that would be more of your training about what is caring, how we all need to take more time, and listen more.

Savina: Time is always one of the objections that we have had throughout all of our work, and we've even written an article that asked "Is there really time to care?" Because that's always the first objection, "Well, that's fine but we don't have time for all that…"

Mary: …"soft stuff"…

Savina: …"touchy-feely stuff." This theory I mentioned to you before, technological competency as an expression of caring, is one idea that lets us know that it doesn't have to be touchy feely to communicate caring.

Mary: As long as it's communicated, that's the key. Because when it's not, that's when I have to send the team from the Office of Patient Affairs to undo all that lack of communication, and then they're spending all the time going between the doctor, the staff, and the patient and the family trying to undo that lack of communication and correct the problems that have come from it.

Savina: The jumping to conclusions that Susan was talking about, jumping to hasty conclusions.

Ruth: …sometimes when it's just a matter of making meaning for ourselves. When we can take this person, this experience, and put it into something that we think we already know about, then we can take a deep breath and go forward. That's not always the case but it helps us makes sense for ourselves of who this person is. It's sort of like when I start to put in a word in my iPhone, and it finishes it for me, sometimes that's a great help and sometimes it's just the wrong word, and that's sort of what happens. Like Mary said, you have to go and unsnarl the mess and so often when we make a decision within ourselves about a person or situation or whatever, we do a nice selling job of ourselves… each time we repeat the story, every time we think about it again, we almost have to sort of reinforce, and get to the "I'm right" sort of feeling about it, rather than asking what else is there… what else is there—in this story, person, or situation.

Ralph: You asked about barriers to establishing this model. Have you gone so far as to think how you would institute it, or how small a critical mass you would have to have for a kind of care to…not to exist, because that could be two people, but sustainable over time…because whether we like it or not, institutions have some kind of hierarchy and if I'm working every day and I really care, I care about the people I serve, I care personally about doing a good job, that's kind of a caring system, but over time if the person to whom I report is unable to express their caring in a nurturing way, I may still care but I'm going to express it differently. Or I may even internalize it completely. I'm going to challenge your thesis that everyone is able to care. I guess the sociopath, we do have some of that…but a sustainable system is what we want.

Rick: I think what you're talking about is the perception that we care. How do you go from "that's a great hospital where Dr. Didlake cares about me" to "that's a great hospital where the system cares about me."

Mary: That's it.

Ralph: Exactly.

Savina: That's what HCAHPS is shooting for, right?

Mary: Yes. We have heard over the years "we love our doctors but we're not coming back to hospital X"—we've heard that, so that's what you're saying, the system didn't care, or didn't express that in a way that met their needs.

Savina: I think it can be frustrating, demoralizing even, if we think of the system as some inanimate object, but a system as a series of evolving and dissolving relationships—after all, this system *is* a human system here.

Mary: I work from the back end. Once they're upset, then we're jumping in to show that we really did care and we're having the manager and the staff from that area contacting the person, the family, coming back and expressing a regret for not showing the care in the way that they needed at that time, which is really tough. It would be great if we did it up front! That's the grievance and complaint policy and guidelines that we're having to go back and follow up on.

Susan: On my level now we've got three huge computer systems about all the contracts and you don't get any credit for the 85 you do well, but the two that are wrong, you have meetings taking up your whole calendar, I'd much rather be talking about caring for patients. And part of it is that with the Electronic Medical Record everyone wanted to have their own system, and sometimes I think we spend the time on the bean counting and the technology and that's less time on the listening and the system things—rather than just trying to fix one little thing that messes up, really trying to find out what's wrong in the bigger picture.

Ruth: We tend not to say anything about the 85, we don't say "you've just done such a wonderful job this week with this patient and that situation. We will go quietly along and then all of a sudden somebody will do something that isn't right and that's what gets the attention. It's very much like you ran the stop sign, rather than 25 times you went down this street and stopped every time, it's a kind of legalistic, punitive system because institutions have to have stop signs, but it makes it much more difficult I think that we don't daily, in a sustained way, reward the good things, the caring that gets done, the sharing of stories.

Mary: I think there are so many different systems we have had, the one with the sticker, when you get caught doing something well, like I would come up to Dr. Boyte and caught him doing something really good today with caring and he gets an "atta boy sticker," that came and went…

Susan:…and remember the line, do they still have the telephone line where you could call the customer care connection, and now they have employee recognition…but that's not like I stop you and I say "you know, I really appreciate what I see you doing with that patient and that family today, you did something way out there."

Savina: Is that the way you would like the system that you're a part of to be?

Mary:…to recognize them on the spot.

Susan: I think the Centerview Publications people are trying to do that more in these little articles about people doing things, and not always hierarchical, not always the big name professor that has come from some fancy place but the everyday, and I think the more we can do that, the more caring we can be.

Ralph: Wouldn't the fullest expression of the system, if everyone in the system would be affirmed by good outcomes…theoretically that would be everybody's report…but it's getting everyone educated in the "micro-affirming" along the way to be effective, so that the lady at the cash register would look at the outcomes and say "I'm part of that," or the accountant…

Mary:…and for the housekeeper to say "they didn't get any more infections because of my good work." But they don't ever get that. In part of your model you talk about making sure that everybody's unique gifts are recognized, appreciated, and honored, and I was thinking about what systems we have—we have the virtual suggestion box, the customer care line, and things like that, which would get feedback. And in reading what you said about care, I think that when people put in suggestions, they probably want to talk more, they have probably just scratched the surface of what they really want to say, they want to have a concern or a discussion, or something brought out, so we're hearing them but we're hearing a little paragraph, where really maybe we need to knock on their door and say "Hey, you put something in, let's elaborate on that and tell me more." So I think that's a good way to bring this forward.

Savina: What structures can you see being created across disciplines as well as within work groups?

Mary: Whoever those suggestions go to—they go to the appropriate leader—they are screened, and they go to the appropriate leader, by one person controlling it, they'll say, "Oh, this should go to Pastoral Care," and they shoot it over to Pastoral Care, Ruth will see it and she only is "required " to read that little paragraph and give a snapshot response …

Ruth:…and no face to face, no interaction. Sometimes it really is all about what they have actually sent in, and sometimes there's something much deeper going on with the person who sent it in—that needs to be heard. But there's no time, money, or plan for that hearing to occur.

Mary: So if we did, would it be appropriate to say "Okay, Ruth, get on the phone, make an appointment" or whatever that person would need; how about instead of putting in the suggestion, just go knock on our door?

Savina: Money is something that could be budgeted down the road, time has to be carved out, so I'm wondering what structures might we envision that wouldn't take all that time…or where's the time going to be carved out from, to make these follow-ups?

Susan: We do the lunch, things like "come and read," and research sessions, but when you try to bring people together across lines, sometimes it works and sometimes it doesn't. Hearing the three people on the panel doesn't always do it for me…I'm right-brained, more than taking your compliance training on the computer, but I think that's individual learning style too. Dr. Didlake is doing great with his computer, but maybe could you say that you could have caring be a thing, like twice a month, but I don't know how you'd get it in the system.

Ralph: I'm thinking about how you're going to carve out time at the bedside. I don't know if this was an open invitation to crawl on a soapbox or not…

Savina: Yes it is!

Ralph: Over the years we've taken a trained observer, the RN, and taken that person further and further away from the bedside, and we've interjected less trained persons and technology…so rather than using the RN-trained observer as a data clerk, we can create structures that would put them back at the bedside with duties to listen and to report meaningful data, not just the text of the Epic thing. Although we have in our hospital our multidisciplinary team meetings, that's a time carve out…it would be more helpful if rather than meeting about all the patients on the unit once a day, and again, taking everybody away from the bedside, with many of the team members not being there, say okay, today, we're going to have team meetings in Mrs. Jones' room and Mrs. Smith's room, and take the team to the bedside…now that's an efficient carve out of time where you're explaining institutional care to the patient, an efficient use of time, in bringing those trained observers back to the patient.

Rick: It does work too. I used to love to do that in ICU, especially if families were present, because then they could be incorporated into the rounds, they hopefully have a fuller understanding of how we were about to care for their child, and it also offers them an opportunity to ask questions, not just to me but to the other disciplines that are there. I think that it's a terrific concept. I do agree that technology is making that less the case because we used to "round" and write our notes and document it, but now they're documenting while they're rounding, and it creates a wall between them and the patient.

Susan: That's what I had a nurse come and tell me. I know that electronic medical record is the thing, but you're not looking at the patient, you're…

Rick:…but technology is part of our lives, and we'll be forever working out how to do that so that we're still more efficient but we don't create barriers.

Ralph: I think there is a huge opportunity for nursing for that to be a rich area for research…how do we take our technologies and make them work at the bedside, rather than have something at the bedside where you walk in and you have a keyboard at the bed or whatever, to learn how to exploit our technologies in ways that bring us back to the patient and are not between us and the patient.

Mary: Today, we had a guest speaker and one of his suggestions in asking the patient questions about their sexual identity was to hand them the iPad and let them enter their information so it's not just said out loud, maybe they're not comfortable saying it, but they can themselves write it, depending upon the level of health literacy, of course. That would go into information that could lead to creating a dialogue, but the patient would have the control.

Ruth: That is an example where the technology is allowing for more, rather than less, intimacy, where they can comfortably self-designate gender or whatever they need to, but most of the time the back is to the patient.

Mary: Your concept of rounding at the bedside is wonderful, I'm still seeing the pillars in the adult critical care tower where the family is dismissed while they make rounds in the critical care…and you know, that is not okay.

Rick: It sends a message, whether it's intended or not, that there's something that is being hidden from them.

Ruth: That's a systemic piece; it has been and continues to be a systemic practice that is making it more difficult for healing…

Mary: …that authoritarian approach to medicine doesn't come across as caring.

Rick: Your iPhone analogy reminded me of something that happened recently…it really is best to look at what you're sending before you press "send." I've got a message from a first-year resident, and she asked "Are you here yet?" and I wasn't…I was actually getting in my car, trying to get the defroster to work, to get my daughters to school, and I see this message, and I type "No, I'm not there, will be in 30 minutes," and I put it down, completed my task with the car, got my daughters on the way to school, and I happened to glance down, and saw that I had not texted "No, I'm not there yet," I had texted "I'm not a tiger yet!" [Laughter]…and both statements were true. I had no idea what she thought.

Ruth: This wonderful sense of humor is a requirement for these people gathering in teams, doubt if we'd make it otherwise!

Savina: I see our time is up, and Ruth, that's a wonderful reminder for us to end on.

Chapter 3

Cultural Factors That Influence Transformation

Institutional transformation alters the culture of the institution by changing underlying assumptions and institutional behaviors, processes and products; it is deep and pervasive affecting the whole institution; it is intentional; and occurs over time. (Eckel, Hill, & Green, 1998)

*T*his chapter examines the cultural aspects of health care systems and their relationship to the experience of those within these systems. It also addresses how a *groundedness* in caring can transform an organization and especially how caring affects the *experience* of care.

In broad terms, the primary challenge for health care organizations is to identify how to strategically enact changes in ways that benefit the patient, the staff, and the overall success of the organization. It is an extremely difficult proposition, particularly since innumerable aspects of culture are relevant within the discussions of health care systems.

As the future of health care affects all, a caring-based philosophy applied to organizations that produces measurable, dynamic change benefits the system as a whole, organizations and people. The Dance of Caring Persons model recognizes this potential, the direct effects of an organization's culture on the experience and performance of all who are a part of that system, and each cultural component active within the organization, from whatever source. This model thus provides a framework for changing the fundamental culture and institutional perspectives within health care organizations, which addresses and improves care for every individual contributor within the system.

The philosophy underlying the Dance of Caring Persons is reviewed, along with a demonstration of how, in practical terms, an organization can adopt this model to create a dynamic core change. Stories further illustrate the effect of this model within real-world situations in health care.

CULTURE: ITS MEANING

A brief look at organizational culture will provide a framework for understanding the culture of health care.

No universal definition of culture, or even of health care culture, exists. A broad swath of current and historical literature affirms the complexity of cultures, as well as their positive and negative influences on organizations. Some examine culture as an attribute, something an organization "has"; others examine culture as what an organization "is."

Nevertheless, a review of the attributes of culture in anthropology, psychology, and sociology suggests certain commonalities. Across the disciplines, a culture is defined to be socially constructed and thus affected by the environment and history; composed of many symbolic and cognitive layers; and potently invested with shared, accessible meaning that helps those within the organization interpret events, symbols, and rituals so as to arrive at an understanding that can be shared, or at least be broadly considered reasonable or just (Tharp, 2009).

However, in no human organization is culture or understanding uniform. Any definable group with a shared history can have a unique culture, and within it many subcultures likely abound. A culture is for this reason distinguished as dominant when its values are widely shared among its subcultures. Every dominant culture has numerous subcultures, some of which may support the dominant culture's assumptions and beliefs and others that may oppose them.

Not, incidentally, embedded within all cultures are social controls that influence decision making and behavior of its members. In organizational culture, these controls are particularly visible in regulating permissible pathways toward judgment and behavior among the organization's employees.

Of note here is that it is through the confluence of cultural assumptions and beliefs with social controls that the creation of shared meanings within work life is possible (Davies, 2002). That is, the assumptions, beliefs, and regulations of organization cultures become a way of interpretation and understanding that permit the creation of the meaning of work.

In sum, culture, which is indeed comprised of widely shared values or attributes that may appear static, is instead an active process that will contribute interpretations influencing the daily creation of meaning in work.

Further, culture viewed through the lens of its attributes provides a means of measuring and managing critical aspects of an organization—such as its structure, strategies, or processes—in order to create change (Scott, Mannion, Marshall, & Davies, 2003). In discussing this dynamic, ongoing potential, we will refer to culture according to its common attributes: assumptions, beliefs, and values; styles of leadership; definitions of success; symbols; language and stories; and rituals.

The ambiguous nature of workplace organizations can make delineating the cultural constructs of an organizational culture difficult. Organizations with short histories or rapid turnover of members may understandably have little or no culture, whereas those with a long history of shared experiences may have a strong one. In any case, however, a useful approach to organizational cultures consists of assessing and defining those basic assumptions that a group has learned as it solved problems of external adaptation and internal integration. Over time, these are the assumptions that prove their worth; become the basis of teaching new members to perceive, think, and feel in relation to problems (Schein, 1990); and underlie such further developments as certification, accreditation, recognition, and the emergence of the organization as one to be emulated.

LEADERSHIP AND ORGANIZATIONAL CULTURE

Leaders of organizations wield significant influence by embedding their views within their organization's culture. Schein (1990) identifies five primary ways that leaders of organizations embed their views into organizations:

- What leaders pay attention to, measure, and control
- How leaders react to critical incidents and organizational crises

- Deliberate role modeling and coaching
- Operational criteria for the allocation of rewards and status
- Operational criteria for recruitment, selection, promotion, retirement, and excommunications

An additional five secondary ways in which leaders embed views into organizations include their impact on

- the organization's design and structure
- organizational systems and procedures
- the design of physical space, facades, and buildings
- stories, legends, myths, and symbols
- formal statements of organizational philosophy

In considering the impact of leadership, it is important to distinguish between organizational culture and organizational climate. Culture emphasizes that which the members of the organization share (assumptions, beliefs, and values; styles of leadership; definitions of success; symbols; language and stories; rituals). In contrast, organizational *climate* reflects employees' perception of the organizational culture. These perceptions of organizational climate are as diverse as its members (Siourouni, Kastanioti, Tziallas, & Niakas, 2012).

Scholars of organizational culture describe culture as something that is learned. As such, effective ways to transmit cultural values, assumptions, and beliefs over time exist. These approaches can be used to strengthen the meaning and growth of the organization.

HEALTH CARE CULTURE

Just as the concept of culture in general is complex, so too is the concept of health care culture. This culture differs from others because of its management and organizational structures.

Health care cultures are situated within the broad context of the health care system. These cultures cross many institutional settings, such as hospitals, community-based care, clinics, and other health delivery systems; however, within them all, patient safety and quality care are priority concerns. One recent study conducted at the Veterans Administration (VA) focused on the relationship between hospital organizational culture and safety; it determined that the higher the level of group culture, the higher the level of safety (Hartmann et al., 2009).

A contributing factor to this finding was a strong group culture and a way of being that emphasized mutual respect and civility. As a result, individuals felt safe to openly discuss problems. This stood in contrast to a hierarchical structure that resulted in poorer outcomes, as members of the organization were reluctant to bring forth issues for fear of blame (Hartmann et al., 2009).

A unique relationship exists among health care culture, the environment, and organizational performance (Mallak, Lyth, Olson, Ulshafer, & Sardone, 2003). Health care organizations with strong cultures have been found to achieve higher performance and improved clinical outcomes. Strong cultures result from "consistent, visible role modeling and leadership, consistent feedback on performance—positive and negative, constant communication about what is important in the organization, and sharing stories of how the organization's culture played a critical role in patients, staff or visitor experience" (Mallak et al., 2003, p. 35). Basing all decisions and actions in the values prioritized by the organization and effectively communicating these beliefs to all in the organization have been found to be essential to success.

Within health care cultures are numerous subcultures, each with its own unique characteristics. Further, within these cultures, large numbers of diverse health professions function within various organizations—for example, medicine and nursing. These professions encounter competing needs of patients, families, providers, administration, and external entities; diversity of patients and staff; and multifaceted hierarchies with many interacting parts (patients, families, staff, infrastructures, technology, and others).

Through this complexity and fragmentation, the health care system has resulted in increased errors and rising costs. Current trends in structure and culture do not universally support the involvement of patients in their care or collaboration across disciplines. The omission of this involvement is crucial, because, without it, what matters to patients and their families cannot be—and is not being—addressed.

An array of metrics, quantitative and qualitative, demonstrates the importance of collaboration to successful health care outcomes, as do anecdotal reports. How many stories have we heard or have we ourselves experienced in which a patient's stay in a hospital has been far less than one would have hoped for?

NURSING SUBCULTURE

As we know through our own experience, the existing nursing culture, by taking on the culture of the health care organization of which it is a part, is grounded in a biomedical approach with medical diagnosis and treatment as the guides to care. The dominant focus is often on diseases, parts, tasks, and compliance with policies, procedures, and the workplace culture. Because the nursing subculture is generally the largest disciplinary subculture in a health care system and the one we know best, we are going to specifically address certain aspects of the nursing subculture that are problematic.

Outcomes of care are expressed in a language related to industrial processes rather than human processes. This includes cause–effect relationships, with the requirement for detachment so that parts of the process can be studied. The result can be an unintended objectification of person. Unfortunately, the culture of nursing is playing a major role in supporting this dehumanizing view. When nursing accepts the language and processes borrowed from manufacturing and often adopted by health care administrators, nursing is subordinated into a way of practice that belies the professional values of the discipline. This has been referred to as "new managerialism," the replacement of professionals by managerial control (Porter, 2011).

An example of this "new managerialism" is adherence to protocols. Rather than accepting protocols as guidelines, nurses often view them far more rigidly than physicians do, seeing them as explicit instructions. Porter (2011) suggests that "guideline compliance by nurses can become an end in itself" (p. 113).

Evidence-based practice is intended to be a guide, not a recipe. Evidence-based practice requires the use of professional judgment with each person's particular circumstances (Stetler, 2003). Without this judgment and personalized decision making, the experience of "this" patient is lost. Some argue that evidence-based practice is grounded in empirics and focuses on fact finding and actions to that "which statistical manipulation of the facts indicates is on average most efficacious" (Porter, 2011, p. 106). This then becomes labeled as *best practices*. More important, nurses and other health care professionals are at risk for using this as an exclusive guide to what is important in their practice in an effort to be "scientific." Nurses, for example, often identify their contributions to a patient's well-being through participation in medical regimes such as treatments and medication, rather than through collaboration with physicians in a shared goal of providing better health care (Jonsdottir, Litchfield, & Pharris, 2004).

Our research has taught that nurses struggle daily with the conflict of nursing and other professional services focused on responding to the demands of the health care organization rather than those seeking care (Boykin, Bulfin, Baldwin, & Southern, 2004; Boykin, Schoenhofer, Smith, St. Jean, & Aleman, 2003). An explanation frequently heard is *there is no time to care.* The preoccupation with tasks and system-imposed measurements removes nurses from the bedside, often resulting in no connection to the patient. Yet, nurses more than any other health professional group have the opportunity to come to know the beauty of those for whom they care because of the invitation from patients to enter into personal space and the continuity of relationship that can be developed. Nurses want to provide individualized, humanistic care; however, it becomes the ideal and not the real. It is our belief that nursing can not only create a culture grounded in caring values, but also lead the whole of the health care organization in this essential transition.

CULTURE AS A FACTOR IN QUALITY

The Institute of Medicine's (IOM) National Research Council (2012) addresses the complexities of health care today and their impact on culture. The vision expressed in the IOM report focuses on "achieving a learning health care system—one in which science and informatics, patient–clinician partnerships, incentives, and culture are aligned to promote and enable continuous and real-time improvement in both the effectiveness and efficiency of care" (p. S-11). It calls for a culture of teamwork, collaboration, and adaptability in support of continuous learning.

Health care organization providers and administrators are well aware of the fact that organizational cultures must change. They understand the effect organizational culture has on the success of the organization. The dilemma is envisioning how these changes might occur amidst ever-changing institutional demands.

As the cost of care increases and the burden of cost shifts to the provider, organizations are pressured to focus on financial survival as their mission often to the neglect of those seeking care—which is in fact their core value and reason for their existence. As a result, those organizations that have attempted to respond in some way to the call for reform issued in the various IOM reports have still not succeeded in making substantive changes in their systems.

The reasons for this are many. The ever-growing challenges to operating margins drive health care organizations to employ various strategies to solve the problems, but the strategies emanate from a traditional view of health care. The drive to *stay in the black* results in a piecemeal approach to system change—changes that are short-lived and offer only poor or isolated performance improvements. The effects of a system's response to outside political and environmental demands trickle through an organization. Unfortunately, the system's pressures directly influence the experience of all persons within the organization and ultimately patient care.

Nurses and other health care providers are now required to do more with less. This is not an isolated phenomenon. The person needing care has the experience of not being cared for and of being objectified and unheard. Achieving patient-centered care is essential, defined in *Crossing the Quality Chasm: A New Health System for the 21st Century* (Corrigan et al., 2001) as care "that encompasses qualities of compassion, empathy, and responsiveness to the needs, values, and expressed preferences of the individual patient" (p. 48). To accomplish this, a fundamental change in health care culture is necessary.

ASSUMPTIONS, BELIEFS, AND VALUES OF THE TRADITIONAL HEALTH CARE SYSTEM

Health care cultures reflect the assumptions, beliefs, values, and priorities of the staff. The culture "influences the effectiveness of the hospital's performance including its ability to achieve the goals of high quality, safe care, financial sustainability, community service and ethical behavior" (Schyve, 2009, p. 19). Most people employed in health care organizations are there because they care and want to make a difference. Yet, the experience of those within the system is frequently just the opposite. Based on our experience and research on the topic over many years, it appears to us that the following assumptions have become ingrained in the current health care system:

- Persons assume hierarchies
- Persons are concerned about the part, not the whole
- Persons have value based solely on knowledge and expertise
- Persons are externally motivated
- Persons lack a sense of connectedness
- Persons compete for scarce resources
- Persons see caring as a luxury
- Persons do not experience a sense of commitment

CULTURE SHAPES PATIENT AND STAFF EXPERIENCES

Patients

The assumptions listed above affect the experience of being a member of the health care organization. They influence one's way of being in relationships and direct what one sees and how one acts. They also affect the families and patients we know and to whom we have committed our lives. What has been created and perpetuated is a system out of touch, an impersonal organization where caring about self is more important than caring for others.

Assumptions and beliefs influence actions and direct lives. Patient care is directly impacted. What is absent in the above assumptions is a valuing of what it means to be human at a time in a person's life when the patient trusts that those involved in health care will live caring, what Hunt (2004) calls a "sense of life," a sensitivity, a philosophy. In a strong assertion that will find resonance with our readers, Hunt declares that a "sense of life is the great professional deficit in modern large-scale healthcare" (p. 189). This deficit of caring jeopardizes the sense of life that Hunt described as "the wisdom, sensitivity and responsibility that is necessary for the authentic care of others" (p. 189). The experience of patients and staff is that technology, policies, procedures, and protocols drive modern-day *care*. The heart of modern industrial-style health care is its inflexibility and lack of fluidity and responsiveness. The common experience of patients is that they are not heard, that staff persons are busy doing other things that the organization requires them to do as part of their job. This experience of patients reflects assumptions, values, and beliefs held, purposefully or more subtly, by those within the health care organization that consequently define the culture.

Staff

Within existing health care organizations are multiple layers of a rigid hierarchical structure that make patient-centered care challenging and difficult. The concept of hierarchy carries with it the idea that there is a top and a bottom.

Because of this vertical view, individuals tend to be consumed by what they need to do on *their rung* of the ladder in order that they be rewarded by the organization or promoted within it—climbing to the next rung. The existing competitive nature of health care organizations inhibits collaboration.

Structures imply what is valued in the organization. The current view of those in health care systems is a valuing of people by what they do—namely their jobs—in the organization. Persons are defined by their work, and in so doing, there is a devaluing of the human experience. The intention is not about knowing person as person. There is little *human* connection. The intention is to ensure job performance and financial viability. The goal becomes protecting and bettering one's *part*.

Because no one wants to fall down the ladder, knowledge is protected, and suspicion and mistrust develop. The distance between those at the top and at various lower levels of the chart make it difficult to understand the importance of one's work to the whole of the organization. Persons are evaluated by position held. The success of the organization is determined by growth and profitability. The higher one is in the organization, the more difficult it is to remain connected to the organization's core purpose for existing—to serve those seeking care.

From this perspective, it is difficult for individuals to risk being authentic and choosing values, aspirations, and desires that would give meaning to their being in the organization. Some organizations have attempted to decrease the layers in the organization by developing structures that flatten it. These beginning efforts to create a *new* view of system structures continue to hold *old* ways of relating. Even though systems speak of teams and collaboration, Weinberg, Cooney-Miner, Perloff, Babington, and Avgar (2011) note that "despite the rhetoric and assumptions of egalitarianism around health care teams and collaboration in practice, decision making in interdisciplinary healthcare teams is often hierarchical rather than collaborative, as is the level of participation" (p. 716). These authors state that those at the top have the greatest influence. Those at the bottom of the hierarchy experience teamwork as orders from the top. Some persons within the system are perceived to be powerful by virtue of position, others powerless.

Power structure and path of reporting are made explicit in the system's organizational chart. Groups such as the board of trustees and titles such as president, chief executive officer (CEO), senior vice president, associate vice president, vice president, director, and the like communicate power and authority. One study of health care culture concluded that the organization of the hospital and its management, more than any other factors, retained the power to confirm and organize the overall context of the nurses' and patients' experience (Holland, 1993).

CHALLENGING ASSUMPTIONS WITHIN TRADITIONAL HEALTH CARE CULTURE: DANCE OF CARING PERSONS

The need for transformation to a person-centered caring culture is both long overdue and difficult. Some people, as in all organizations, have their own vested interests and do not want the status quo to change. Persons' experience in health care is becoming more impersonal—many in all aspects of the organization feel not cared for personally.

There is an increasing societal urgency for a different, more personal, and sustainable model that is grounded in caring values with a commitment to knowing what matters most to patients and their families, as well as to all those whose everyday work contributes to accomplishing the mission of the organization. More and more it becomes evident that for transformation to occur, the whole of the organization must change. It will require the commitment and involvement of all persons within the entire system, across all disciplines, as advocated in *Crossing the Quality Chasm: A New Health System for the 21st Century* (Corrigan et al., 2001). This document specifically calls for "change at all levels, including the clinician and patient relationship; the structure, management, and operation of healthcare organizations; the purchasing and financing of health care; the regulatory and liability environment; and others" (p. 33).

The Dance of Caring Persons as described in Chapter 2 is the view proposed for transforming the culture of health care organizations. It is a radical idea and calls for a complete reconceptualization of understanding health care systems. By its very nature as a radical idea, it calls for a core change. It is different. The Dance of Caring Persons returns us to our deepest roots—that we are all related, that we all are caring. It is an idea that, we have come to believe through our experience, does transform one's way of knowing and being.

Adopting this perspective changes an organization from a task-oriented, mechanistic, fragmented focus to one that is humane and integrated. The assumption that all persons are caring implies that all persons within the health care culture are caring persons. One of the responsibilities of all persons in the system is to come to know each other as caring and to nurture and support each other to live caring. The concern is focused on persons and understanding what is important to them. This commitment centers on knowing and valuing each other: person nursed, families, the community served, nurses, health care workers, administrators, doctors, housekeepers, all persons.

Each person in the organization is celebrated for the gifts they bring to the person cared for and all roles within the organization are recognized as equally important—at any time, the person occupying a given role, from CEO to housekeeper, could be the key contributor to that which matters to a person seeking care. Each person has a voice and is encouraged to speak up on behalf of the patient.

All persons in the organization are envisioned to be members of the circle. For example, represented in the circle would be the members of the governing board, the president and CEO, chief financial officer (CFO), vice presidents, directors, benefactors, families, patients, community, and all persons employed within the system. There is no "power over," no competition. Relationships between roles and lines of responsibility and accountability are symbolized by solid or dotted lines.

COMING TO KNOW SELF AND OTHERS

The commitment to know other as colleague breaks down the many traditional *silos* in health care. There are the traditional silos of disciplines and units/departments, particularly in hospitals. Each is focused on its own performance with differing standards of performance and measurement.

Historically, medicine has emphasized autonomy and independence resulting in a long-standing cultural divide between medicine and administration. The clinical culture of medicine as formed in medical school is based on biological sciences, cause–effect relationships, responsibility for individual patients, and professional autonomy in determining actions. In contrast, the managerial culture of health care is based on social and behavioral sciences, less emphasis on clear cause–effect relationships, longer time in planning, and focus on groups and populations.

Managers tend to view physicians and other health professionals as being the means to achieve the goal of patient care; physicians tend to view organizations as being the means to achieve goals for their patients and to advance their careers. This conflict has made physicians resistant to managers' efforts to impose rules or standardize practices (Ferlie & Shortell, 2001). Because of the business nature of the relationship between physicians and administrators, physicians (unless employed by the hospital) are viewed as *customers* of hospitals.

This view further impacts the existent professional hierarchy within health care systems. Interactions among groups tend to be guarded, making collaboration difficult. Wesorick and Doebbeling (2011) make the point that no single discipline determines quality of care, but rather it requires a "strong partnership with each other and those we serve" (p. S53).

Moving from silos to a perspective of oneness requires an understanding of different disciplines and their scope of practice. An interprofessional team model results in the clarification of a discipline's scope of practice, understanding each other's scope, and identifying the overlaps. This new knowing helps to "eliminate duplication and repetition and assures integrated, individualized care" (p. S54).

Moving from a conglomeration of independent practices to a team approach to true patient-centered care will require a new way of being in health care. Patient-centered care requires that providers come to know their patients' stories, what matters to them, and to invite them to be full partners in their care. It calls for collaboration among disciplines with those cared for.

The transformed culture is built on shared values, and respect for and inclusion of all persons. Creation of a caring-based culture is a commitment to humanizing health care, and as such it requires the daily living of this commitment.

A CULTURE OF CARING

The assumptions and beliefs that form the basis for transformation to a culture of caring are as follows:

- All persons are caring
- Caring is lived uniquely moment to moment
- Personhood, or the living of caring, is enhanced through participation in nurturing relationships with others
- Persons are at all times whole

These are the beliefs that persons within a transformed system of health care would hold about person. All aspects of the organization—mission, vision, policies, procedures, and so on—would convey a valuing of being human. Relationships would be transformed through valuing and knowing other as caring person. These assumptions are not congruent with those of most health care organizations today. Table 3.1 illustrates the differences.

The assumptions, values, and beliefs of members of an organization are what make a strong culture. When caring is the core value, the relationship of those within the organization is grounded in the importance of person as person and person as caring. There is an ongoing intention to know those with whom we work and for whom we care as caring persons. This way of being is a way of valuing other and supporting that which matters. The experience of being in the organization is that of being cared for.

For most persons in the organization this way of being will require a transformation of the mental model one holds of health care organizations (Senge, 1990). Mental models are defined as "deeply ingrained assumptions, generalizations, or even pictures or images that influence how we understand the world and how we take action" (p. 8). Transformation begins by refocusing the lens for one's existence.

Entrenched ideologies and cognitive frameworks that form today's traditions will have to be let go. Rather than view health care as a service delivery model with a focused goal of economic profitability, the transformed view would make the person cared for at center and visible. For nurses, as well as other health care providers, this change will be challenging.

TABLE 3.1 Comparison of Assumptions of Current Health Care Systems and Assumptions of Dance of Caring Persons

ASSUMPTIONS OF THE CURRENT HEALTH CARE SYSTEM	ASSUMPTIONS OF THE DANCE OF CARING PERSONS
Persons assume hierarchies	No person is better than another; each is respected and valued as person as person
Persons are concerned about the part, not the whole	All persons are committed to knowing other as caring; all are committed to the one cared for
Persons have value based solely on knowledge	There are different ways of knowing and expertise; each person is valued for his or her unique contribution
Persons are externally motivated	Persons are committed because they care
Persons lack a sense of connectedness	All persons are called to live and grow in caring
Persons compete for scarce resources	Decisions reflect "what ought to be"
Persons see caring as a luxury	Caring is our gift; our way of living
Persons experience a lack of commitment	Persons are nurtured in caring relationships

Because the authors are nurses, we can speak with greater certainty about the experience of nurses. These experiences may or may not be shared by others in the system. We have observed that nurses, especially in hospital settings, have become comfortable with structuring practice from a problem-based, medical, or nursing diagnosis approach. We are knowledgeable and skilled at identifying and fixing problems. As comfortable and good as we are at this, it leaves the experience of truly nursing empty. We have been told many times that it is this *emptiness*—knowing that one has not nursed but rather performed tasks—that has led many nurses to leave nursing. There is a growing sense that a similar situation exists in medicine and other health care professions.

We have also witnessed that when nurses practice from the perspective of Nursing as Caring, they return to the *soul* of nursing. Rather than seeing nursing as focused on a part, or a diagnosis, the focus is on person and coming to know the one cared for as person, as human, as caring. The purpose of nursing is clear. There is a commitment to making explicit nursing's unique gift to those seeking care, which is to offer our caring service. It is caring that is offered every time a nurse enters a nursing situation. The nurse is intentionally present to know and to nurture the wholeness of person and to know other as person living caring uniquely in the moment. No longer is nursing defined by *doing* things.

LEADERSHIP, CARING, AND DEFINITIONS OF SUCCESS

Leaders

Leadership exists throughout the complex structure of health care. The two most referenced styles of leadership are transactional and transformational. Judge and Piccolo (2004) have characterized transactional leadership as stemming from a traditional view of leading, a way characterized by power and authority relationships. This style is characterized by contingent reward, management by exception–active and management by exception–passive. The difference between management by exception–active and management by exception–passive is the timing of the leader's response. Active implies action before a problem develops and passive is action after the problem has occurred (2004).

Aspects of transformational leadership include "charisma or idealized influence, inspirational motivation, intellectual stimulation, and individualized considerations"

(Judge & Piccolo, 2004, p. 755). Charisma or idealized influence is the ability of the leader to inspire others to connect through behaviors. Inspirational motivation is the ability to articulate a vision that is appealing to others. The leader communicates hope and provides meaning for work. Intellectual stimulation is the degree to which the leader takes risks, challenges assumptions, and invites ideas from others. Individualized consideration is the ability of the leader to attend to what matters to others. As such, the leader listens, mentors, and coaches.

The leader sets the tone for what is experienced and determines or ratifies definitions of success in the health care organization. If the leader values a transactional approach to health care that is grounded in a business vantage point, attention will be on compliance and control in order to ensure that *bottom line* or profitability is met. The experience of those in the system is one of objectification, distance, and anonymity.

The determinants of success are targets achieved. These targets might include patient and staff satisfaction scores, morbidity and mortality rates, meeting performance measures set by The Joint Commission on Accreditation of Healthcare Organizations (JCAHO), full-time equivalents (FTEs) per occupied bed, profitability, and so on. There is no doubt that these outcome measures are important as they provide valuable information about the viability of the organization. The concern is that these processes and measurements are disconnected from persons. The true gauge of determining the significance of outcome measures must be those served.

If the leader values transformational leadership and lives the value of caring, the central concern will be persons. All persons will be understood as having inherent worth. The leader in the dance is not at the top but in the circle. The focus is on coming to know person as caring and what matters most to each person. There is a commitment to creativity, to knowing and supporting persons within the organization, to instilling hope for the future, and honoring the collective gifts of each person.

The experience of those within the system will be quite different because the culture will be different. The way of being, manifested by this leader, would demonstrate the living of caring values essential for transformation. Success would be measured by the experiences of those within the system. These experiences would reflect the valuing of person as person and of person as caring. It is the relationship that is the driver—not the bottom line. Because the quantifiable outcomes are directly influenced by values lived, they are met.

Governing Boards

Since transformation requires a new lens for all in the organization, let us look at the role of the governing board, the *highest* rung of the organizational chart, as an example of how caring values might guide or reframe the approach to their work and influence the culture of the health care system. Governing boards are ultimately responsible for safety, quality, and the financial health of institutions. Their purpose is to guide and provide oversight to the organization. Board members are chosen based on the special expertise or opportunities that they bring and for their dedication and commitment to the vision and mission of the organization. (It is interesting to note that rarely is there a nurse leader on these boards.) This void is a concern. Hamilton and Campbell's (2011) work shows that "nurses' knowledge is routinely altered as it is worked up into institutionally useful information" (p. 2). These authors further contend that "boardroom knowledge" of health care is constructed with "different priorities than is the knowledge of direct care on which nurses' safe, efficient, and effective care relies" (p. 2). Who is better to bring the voice of the patient to the table than a nurse?

The general composition of the board includes prominent community members, a few lay persons, physicians who serve in leadership roles, and persons from the hospital who are there by nature of their role in the organization. Typical board meetings address a range of items: review of minutes, various committee reports that are generally statistical in nature, medical executive reports, discussion of budget; and detailed discussion of the measurements of success that influence the organization's ability to secure incentive or reward dollars from state or federal sources. These discussions are important.

But what is missing? What is absent is the reason for why they are there. All persons and groups within a health care system are there to respond in their special ways to those seeking care. The patient/family experience should be the situational context for all that happens at board meetings as well as everywhere else in the organization. However, it is the actions of board members that communicate their priority to the CEO. If the board members are primarily focused on the financial reports, it is this which will then become the priority for the CEO. In order to remain connected to the caring mission of the institution, board members need to intentionally bring the patient/family to the boardroom. What strategies might support this connection?

BOARD STRATEGIES FOR CONNECTING FISCAL STEWARDSHIP AND CARING

Quality of care directly corresponds to the patient's experience. Patients' experiences directly relate to their satisfaction and their decision to return for future care. Therefore, governing boards that focus on quality and satisfaction are being good fiscal stewards as well. Cost, quality, and satisfaction are inextricably linked. Patients' and nurses' perceptions of caring correlate with cost, quality, and satisfaction (Valentine, 1989). A governing board that focuses on caring is providing sound stewardship to the organization.

When new members are appointed to the board, an orientation program is generally provided. These orientation sessions typically point the board's attention in a particular direction or focus, generally to fiscal and legal viability, and sometimes even focus on those aspects of institutional viability in light of the expressed mission of the organization. What is missing in most instances is an orientation to caring, the service mission of the health care system.

We believe it is essential to provide substantive knowledge and affective experience of caring and caring science as a key component of the orientation program for the board. Although it is accepted that all persons know caring in some way in their own hearts and their own experience and live caring in their own way, providing broad leadership and direction to an enterprise that has caring as its fundamental service mission requires more than a casual, everyday acquaintance with caring.

As part of learning about caring—not merely health-related activities, but caring, the board should be oriented to the way in which various professional roles in the delivery of this core service express caring. This would include orienting the board to the caring mission of nursing as a discipline and the core service of nursing as a profession. The same orientation would also be conveyed for other disciplines. With caring and caring roles incorporated as an important aspect of board orientation, those persons whose role in the dance is to provide broad viability and direction to the health care system would be prepared to make decisions based on all aspects of the system that figure in that role, most notably the human, caring aspects of the enterprise.

One of the quality measures discussed at board meetings is the Hospital Consumer Assessment of Health Providers and Systems (HCAHPS). The purpose of this survey is to measure health care quality based on the consumers' experience. This report is essentially about a person's health care encounter and notably often focuses questions through the lens of the experience with nursing. Questions asked of patients are as follows:

- During this hospital stay, how often did nurses treat you with courtesy and respect?
- During this hospital stay, how often did nurses listen carefully to you?
- During this hospital stay, how often did the nurses explain things in a way you could understand?
- During this hospital stay, after you pressed the call button, how often did you get help as soon as you wanted it?
- During this hospital stay, how often did doctors listen carefully to you?
- During this hospital stay, how often did doctors explain things in a way you could understand?

Questions are to be quantifiably answered on a scale from never to always. The response of *always* brings reimbursement to the organization. Some organizations have resorted to *scripting* what health care providers say to influence a patient's response to that of *always*. The HCAHPS results are important, but would provide more meaning if they were in the context of a patient's story of care received. Through the patient's expressed experience, members would come to know not only the lived experience of the patients, but also the experience of those providing direct care.

The following is a story of a nurse practitioner reflecting on her experience of a health care situation from a caring framework. Let us listen as Susan shares her story and then we will suggest some ways a governing board could work with the story to understand in a very real way the whole of the health care situation, including ways the board could be involved.

It was 3 o'clock in the afternoon. I entered an exam room. I was exhausted. The patient was distraught. We both quickly assessed and understood the nursing situation at hand, but we kept it locked in the corners, failing to appreciate or acknowledge it within the pattern of the nurse/nursed relationship that unfolded. Nursing as caring had broken down, as neither of us was fully present within the moment.

My mind was reeling, bogged down with the stress of the day, work, and family. Clinic had started with a vengeance at 8 a.m. and had not stopped. Clients, prescription refills, lab reviews, follow-up, a grant report deadline, and managing the implementation of a drug research study in seven clinics the next day weighed heavily on my mind. I had just come back to work full-time, 6 months after having my second child. I had a 2½-year-old and 6-month-old at home. Sleep was a commodity of which I didn't have much. I hadn't yet eaten and I wasn't sure if I had gone to the bathroom. My mind raced with thoughts of: "How many more clients were waiting for me in the waiting room? Was I going to be able to pick up my kids by 5:30? Was I going to have time to look at document edits from a colleague? Did I have everything together for the meeting in the morning? What did we have at home for dinner?" I was cranky and preoccupied to say the least.

The client, let's call her "Lily," was there on the exam table, fully clothed, rocking back and forth with her hands on her abdomen. She looked pale and scared. She went on about how she had been (vaginally) bleeding heavily for over a week and was weak and tired. She was telling me "I've never had this before. I know I'm not pregnant. I keep wondering if and when it's going to get better. What's causing it?" Lily's significant other was there and silent, but the look on his face revealed that he was truly concerned and at loss as to what to do. Then Lily said, "but I think it's getting better...I'm still in pain, but *less*. I'm still bleeding, but *less*." Lily then grabbed on to her next biggest concern, money. "I don't have any money. I can't afford to go to the ER. I can't pay you today. How much is it going to cost? Will you bill me? Do you know where I can go and not pay? I don't have health insurance or a job. Is there anything you can do?"

As a nurse practitioner, I knew how to visually assess a person in acute distress. I knew when someone was in pain through observation and physical examination. But I chose not to see it. I wasn't present. I was thinking of all of my other responsibilities and not the responsibility to care for the person in front of me. I narrowed in on the word *less*. I remember thinking, "She feels like she is getting better. She said the bleeding and pain is subsiding. She really doesn't seem to be pale. Her conjunctiva looks nice and red. Capillary refill seems good. She can't be in too much pain if she can sit here and have a conversation with me." I focused on the words, "I can't afford it." I told her that this was a fee-for-service clinic, so if I were to touch her I would have to charge her.

I explained that if I were to find anything I was going to have to send her to the ER. "This is only an outpatient clinic," I said, "and I'll send you to the ER or GYN for a D&C or ablation if intervention is needed. I can only treat you medically with hormone therapy, iron supplements, dietary suggestions, labs, referrals, and follow-up. If it is really bad, it won't be enough. It's going to cost you a lot of money and the ER will treat you regardless of your ability to pay. You really should go to the ER."

Lily asked, "What do you think I should do?" I replied, "Go to the ER." "I can't," she said looking terrified. "I can do an exam and go from there, but if I touch you I have to charge you." Lily looked like a deer in headlights, "No . . . no exam, is there anything else you can do?" "Well," I said, "if you really think you're getting better, you can wait it out, but you have to promise me that if you get any worse you will go to the ER. If it is still a problem tomorrow or the next day, you need to come back to the clinic for a full assessment at minimum." Lily promised she would come back if it persisted and assured both herself and me by saying, "Yes . . . I really think I'm getting better. I just can't pay. If I'm not better I'll come back."

I left the exam room. I didn't examine her, I didn't charge her, I simply made a quick note in the chart and forgot about her. I did Pap smears, gave out birth control, edited a document, went to the bathroom, had some crackers and a drink, picked up my kids and became a mom. I left, but I was never there in the first place and I am not sure that Lily was either.

A week later I was reminded of Lily and every detail of the visit returned into my head. Lily came back to the clinic 2 days after I had seen her. I had not been there. The nurse practitioner she saw was present and actively assessed, listened, and cared for Lily. She was still bleeding and her hemoglobin had dropped below 7. She went to the hospital, had a D&C, and 2 units of blood.

She had been in crisis and I hadn't cared. I had chosen to listen to her comments about feeling better and her inability to pay, rather than listening to her true concern. She was bleeding so heavily and was in so much pain that she was scared to deal with it. She was convinced that it had to be something very bad, maybe cancer, and she didn't have a job, money, or insurance. Her fear and attempts at denial made her convince herself that she was getting better and that her lack of a job and money were more important than her health problem. I was not authentically present to listen to and care for the true health crisis at hand.

Susan's story could be the focus for part of a board meeting, or even a board retreat, as a strategy to enhance the culture of caring in the health care system for which the board had broad governing responsibilities. Board members can come to know Susan as a person, and they can come to know "Lily" as a person, and to understand that every employee of the system and every patient who enters a system is a person, with their own lives and their own concerns. Board members can identify with the very human attributes displayed in Susan's story and in this way realize a connection with Susan and Lily, and every other person who is involved in the institution . . . including each other and themselves.

This profound sense of connection alone can have long-ranging transformative resonance, particularly if there are opportunities to be reminded that all involved are persons in our lives like those in our lives for and with whom we care. When board members are considering what matters to them in the moment, this experience of connectedness has the potential to reawaken personal commitment to maximizing the culture of caring in the health care system for which they have governance responsibilities.

When a sense of connectedness happens, board members can genuinely realize that HCAHPS is only a sign of what really matters, and not what the real value of care and caring is. Another strategy that could be employed at a board meeting would be to invite a board member to share his or her own story of caring. In what way is caring lived in his or her role as a board member? Some examples of living caring might include the following:

- Engaging with direct care providers and patients to understand their experience
- Risking asking questions that link the quantifiable measurements of quality to the patient

These examples are intended to illustrate strategies for changing the way one views his or her role. Strategies to transform other aspects of the health care system follow in subsequent chapters.

Given the organizational focus on the nursing experiences as a measure of quality and satisfaction, nurse leaders play a fundamental and essential role in transforming the culture of nursing as well as that of the whole health care organization from a detached world to one rooted in caring. The success of this change is directly linked to the values held and to (for the nurse leader) one's understanding of nursing as a discipline. Relational care calls for health care professionals to be free to practice without the constraints of focusing only on achieving outcomes predetermined by the health care system (Jonsdottir et al., 2004).

Leaders are called to infuse the health care organizational culture with an understanding of what it means to be human and what it means to be caring. A commitment to actualizing a vision where the environment has been created to support all care providers to effectively live caring is foundational to the transformation. Leaders must understand that a key component of their role is to hear what matters to those cared for through the voices of those providing direct care; to understand how to nurture and support those providing direct care; to understand what is needed to truly live out the organizational mission of *care*; and to secure the necessary resources. Leaders must create and support practice environments that reflect the valuing of person as person regardless of role.

The living of caring brings one intimately into the lives of others where through intentional presence focused on knowing person as caring, the experience of care is transformed. Expressed commitment to the assumptions of the nursing theory, Nursing as Caring, directs a way of being that honors personhood. We believe that though the theory was developed within and for nurses, it also has relevance for all of those who provide direct care. It returns to the core value held dear...that of person. The direct care provider's role is to come to understand persons and their experience; to understand what matters to them; and to provide care that reflects this knowing. The nurse leader's obligation is to create ways of nurturing and supporting direct care providers to accomplish this. Strategies for accomplishing these desired ends will be addressed in Chapter 7.

THE ROLE OF SYMBOLS, RITUALS, LANGUAGE, AND STORIES IN HEALTH CARE CULTURES

Symbols

Assumptions, values, and beliefs of persons within health care cultures are communicated through symbols, rituals, and language. Symbols are simply things that represent something else. For example, symbols in nursing are many and varied. Though we speak of nursing symbols, symbols are present within each discipline. They include the representation of one's educational level (PhD, DNP, MSN, PharmD, MD) and the meaning of that academic credential to practice. Ethical obligations for nurses are reflected in the American Nurses Association (ANA) Code of Ethics, and for physicians these are in the American Medical Association (AMA) Code of Medical Ethics. Commitment to integrity in research, such as through the informed consent process; handoff reporting in practice, as an important way to communicate essential aspects of care of persons; the dress of hospital workers in hospital and other settings; and language all serve as symbols of valuing person.

Health care cultures are replete with symbols that tell us about the meaning of something in regard to the organization. These symbols may be verbal or nonverbal, written or spoken. They communicate the values of the organization and sustain traditions. They are observable artifacts that influence how one sees and experiences the organization (Schein, 1990). Symbols are "things that stand for the ideas that compose the organization" (Rafaeli & Worline, 1999, p. 95). These physical representations of an organization take on important meanings. Symbols play four functions in an organization as follows:

- Symbol as a reflection of organizational culture
- Symbol as a trigger of internalized values and norms
- Symbol as a frame for conversations about experience
- Symbol as an integrator of organizational systems of meaning

Symbol as a reflection of organizational culture refers to the physical manifestations that provide a tangible, sensory way of coming to know an organization. In health care settings there are many examples of this. They might be uniforms, visiting hours, room design, physical layout of space, volunteers, furniture, pictures, annual reports, and so on. Encountering these symbols generates feelings and establishes a way of knowing and relating to the organization. For example, an elaborate office may be a symbol of one's status on the organizational chart. More extensive physical space and furnishings often reflect one's higher position within the organization.

Symbol as a trigger of internalized values and norms refers to one's response to a symbol. A frequently cited example in health care is the white coat or business attire of a physician that elicits a certain response of respect. Certain symbols result in specific behaviors as appropriate to the situation.

Symbol as a frame for conversations about experience refers to the framework through which one sees. These frameworks for understanding particular symbols can be shared and discussed. In health care, budget cuts may require the layoff of some employees. The budget is the symbol that invokes a value-based discussion about who should be laid off. Or, for nursing, the symbol may be dress. A focus on dress, whether it should be scrubs, street dress, or uniforms, invites a dialogue that reflects philosophical differences and values among nurses.

Symbol is an integrator of organizational systems of meaning. Symbols integrate complex and various systems of meaning. They help build shared understandings. An example of this from our research is reflected in the following situation.

A for-profit healthcare organization that had adopted caring as a framework for the entire organization wanted to make explicit to the community its commitment to integrating caring values into the whole of the organization. At the end of Nurses Week and the beginning of Hospital Week the organization issued "An Invitation to Caring" to all internal and external constituents of the hospital to participate in forming a circle around the hospital. All disciplines were represented as well as patients, families, firefighters, police and others—as it was intended to demonstrate the connectedness of all persons living caring uniquely in their roles.

Each person in the circle held hands as a sign of a strong sense of community, of shared values, cooperation, and responsibility. A revealing picture was taken from the air depicting the unity of persons in the organization. This treasured artifact hangs proudly in the hospital and prompts many responses. (Pross, Hilton, Boykin, & Thomas, 2011)

This circle of a group of people joined by a commitment to live caring values became a powerful symbol that demonstrated that caring is the common ground among all persons. This example also highlights the importance of understanding symbols in the context of the organization. If one did not know the intent of the circle surrounding the hospital, there could be various and misleading interpretations. Powerful symbols tend to have immediately recognizable universal meaning, and part of the power of symbols comes from the dialogues they generate. What meanings do you and your colleagues immediately recognize as you envision the circle surrounding the hospital in this story? What symbols might your unit, department, or system create to express the culture of your environment?

Understanding symbols of particular health care organizations requires one to come to know and understand that organization (Pratt & Rafaeli, 2001). It is this understanding that leads to meaningful interpretation of the symbols. The hospital circle example illustrates how the organization has defined what it does—its essence—as caring. This shared meaning was expressed through symbolic action.

Disciplinary philosophical frameworks, "grand theories" that frame practice in a discipline, are also symbolic representations of a reality where meaning is constructed both by those who develop and use the theory in practice and research (Pilkington, 2005). For example, nursing theories offer a specific statement of focus for nursing, communicating the intent for practice. It makes explicit why one is there as nurse. The symbolic representation of a nurse practicing from the lens of Nursing as Caring would be visible—a sign—in the way the nurse lives caring uniquely, in each particular nursing situation. Although the intention of all nurses practicing from this framework is to know person as caring, the caring responses reflect the individual nurse's unique living of caring in the moment.

What might be the new symbols of nursing and other health care disciplines one could consider if the health care system were transformed and focused on persons seeking care? Perhaps every room would hang a philosophy on its wall reflecting the valuing and honoring of person; perhaps persons would feel embraced in their health journey by the exquisite aesthetic expressions of direct care providers that surround them; perhaps persons would be the orchestrators of their care and, as such, be actively engaged in the dialogue and decisions; perhaps each practice space would have pictures and names of staff; perhaps policies and procedures would be flexible to allow for the uniqueness of the situation; and perhaps nurses and other direct care providers would be viewed as a symbol of caring and healing.

At times, symbols speak more eloquently than words, a smile, holding a patient's hand, an embrace—all bespeak the profound gift of hearing and caring. These simple yet universal symbols employed daily as a part of our care communicate a universal language so vital in the direct care or nursing situation. Symbols allow others to speak and be understood, even if the given languages between the person providing care and the patient are different.

We may have had the experience, perhaps in the ER, where an older person is brought in who does not speak English and radiates fear and uncertainty, and is calmed with a nod of the head, which says that I am here for you...I will not leave you alone. Perhaps in no other than this setting, where the issues of life and death are dealt with daily, is the manifestation of the signs/symbols of caring most necessary. They have the potency to reach within us at our deepest level of feeling to tell us that someone is there for us.

A patient told the story of his reconstructive surgery for his knee.

> While he was waiting for the nurse to complete the paperwork prior to surgery, an aide came in the room to see how he was doing. As the aide was leaving she said "Everything is going to be all right—I prayed for you this morning." He did not see this person again, but he said he would never forget her caring. He did not know her religious affiliation— nor did she know his—but her sign of belief and concern filled him with such a feeling of the goodness of others that it transformed his stay in the hospital.

Such a simple sign of her caring, certainly not one prescribed as part of the hospital's protocol, affected him greatly.

Rituals

Rituals are another powerful way to communicate culture and affirm values in a health care organization. They are similar to language in that they create a shared meaning about events. For groups building cohesiveness, the rituals may be rather elaborate. Once this shared meaning is created and the group becomes closer, the elaborate ritual is less important. The rituals are ways to express collective beliefs and values (Douglas, 1978). Rituals occur in every aspect of life and are enacted on a regular basis. Rituals are formal patterns of cultural behavior that are an integral part of every human community. They are the ways through which groups celebrate what is important to them (Helman, 1990).

According to Smith and Stewart (2011), rituals serve nine interdependent functions. They provide meaning, manage anxiety, exemplify social order, communicate values, improve group solidarity, include and exclude others, reflect commitment, manage work structures, and prescribe and reinforce significant events. Rituals significantly influence the instilling of beliefs and are embedded within symbolism (Smith & Stewart, 2011). The putting on of the nursing uniform represents a meaningful ritual. The nurse takes off clothes belonging to the outside world and puts on clothes of the nursing subculture to which he or she belongs. This same ritual around uniforms is experienced within many disciplines. It is a part of creating reality and meaning (Holland, 1993). Another example of creating meaning is the Blessing of the Hands during Nurses Week or Hospital Week. This ceremony involves the pouring of warm water that has been scented with an essential oil over hands. This ritual is a symbol of a renewed spirit. It unites health care professionals who are committed to caring.

The effectiveness of a ritual is dependent upon those who participate in it. The receiving of a nurse's pin, a badge, or a diploma does not of itself make that person a better nurse, policeman, or student. It is in the participation of the meaning of the ritual that one is moved to become a more committed person. Some daily rituals in organizations run the risk of becoming less meaningful because of their frequency—such as reciting the pledge of allegiance or uttering brief, rhetorically intended greetings like "How are you?"

Rituals alleviate anxiety over uncertainties because of their associated meaning. For example, if a beloved nurse leader retires from an organization, there is a ritual to affirm the value of the person to the organization. This ritual though is coupled with an understanding that this is also a time of transition and as a result may be an anxious time for members of the organization. Ritual practices protect the nurse from anxieties arising as a result of encountering human suffering (Wolf, 1988) and serve as a defense against making decisions that are a part of care (Strange, 2001).

Rituals also serve to strengthen groups and reinforce social structures such as hierarchies in health care organizations. People in hierarchies know what is expected of them and this power relationship is perpetuated as ritual. Within this social structure communication is also a ritual. There is a language that is understood only by certain groups within health care systems.

Rituals and routines are strongly embedded in nursing and other disciplines' history and have been important in transmitting culture. They express symbolic meanings important to groups of people within a culture or subculture. Rituals such as bathing, postmortem care, and administration of medication have been identified as symbolic healing actions, whereas the change of shift report is more an occupational ritual. The change-of-shift report was a way of exchanging patient information creating a sense of unity and understanding of what it means to be a nurse (Wolf, 1988). This meaning attached to the change-of-shift report could be an unintended barrier to fully engaging in new ways to exchange patient information. Thus, understanding the meaning of rituals can allow for new behaviors and rituals to emerge.

Rituals are an important aspect of structuring time and tasks. Time is central to the daily activities. Holland (1993) describes this focus on time as "something done, day in and day out, same routine, same methods, something you've always done, daily reports, same thing every day" (p. 1467). These routines done at certain times control practice and ensure a structure for completing tasks. Routines of care focus on what needs to *get done* in order to meet various mandates. They are not guided by the world of the person cared for. Today the practice of health care seems to be grounded more in routines than rituals—routines that conflict with the idea of person-centered care.

Attention needs to be paid to new rituals that hold at their center, the person cared for. An example of this is interprofessional rounding with patients as the center of the dialogue. This ritual of a team of professionals intentionally being present together with the person cared for, in order to know the person as caring, to hear what matters, and to co-create meaningful responses—would return care to its core.

Language and Stories

Organizations are heavily dependent on language and stories. Organizations create their own language that allows people to understand the world in which they live and work. Those in control of the organization effect the direction of the organization through their deliberate use of language and stories. Language does more than facilitate communication of thoughts and ideas. It shapes the way one feels, builds trust, and influences the experience of belonging.

One way to view the role of language and stories in an organization is from a socially constructed viewpoint. Social construction maintains that "organizations are dynamic, living human constructions whose fate is a reflection and extension of the relationships of the people within a system (the community) and the language that they intentionally create within the context of the system" (Ricketts & Seiling, 2003, p. 33). The conscious use of language serves a vital function in "setting the stage for organizational change processes to be effective and long lasting" (Ricketts & Seiling, 2003, p. 33).

The growth and direction of an organization is dependent on the language used within it. The modeling of leaders, especially by the language used, directly affects the life of the organization.

Stories may best convey the power of language. Stories communicate the norms and values of the organization. They exemplify shared ideals and purposes and are most powerful when described from a lived experience. It is our experience that the sharing of stories that reflect caring is an effective way for nurses and others to come to know colleagues as caring persons and to transmit essential values.

> When professionals and nonprofessionals alike share stories through which each person's caring practices are made visible, each person comes to a clear appreciation of how every role within the organization and every person within these roles contributes to an overall caring environment. (Boykin & Schoenhofer, 2001, p. 5)

Participating in the stories of others is an essential way to connect to core values. This is a story told by a CFO in a for-profit hospital when invited to share how he lived caring in his role.

> After several days in the ICU, it was determined that the patient should be transferred out of intensive care into a general medical bed. It was at this point the husband called me to meet with him and his boys at her bedside. While in his wife's ICU room, staff members were explaining that they were going to transfer her to another room, but that the breathing apparatus couldn't be transferred with her. Staff planned to assist her breathing by bagging her during the five minute transfer. They assured her that the new room and the transfer would be okay. His wife made it clear by her gestures that she was frightened to have the apparatus removed, and her husband looked over to me as if he expected me to try to stop the transfer. As we were discussing options, staff stepped outside the room and began to talk about her deteriorating condition and the likelihood she wouldn't last long whether transferred or not that evening. The family members, as well as the patient, could hear exactly what I was hearing from the staff's conversation. I stepped out of her room to address this with the staff. The decision was then made to defer the transfer, and the family felt relieved that she wouldn't be disturbed. I left for home. About an hour after leaving the hospital, I received a call that she had passed away. The next day, the husband stopped by my office and related the events that had happened later that evening. Within 15 minutes after I left her room, she had asked for something to write on. She wrote "Time" on the note pad and held it for her husband to see. He told her it was about 5:45. She nodded and said "No, it's time." She died within 30 minutes. He thanked me repeatedly for being with them in her final moments and said it meant a lot to them that I was there to help. (Pross et al., 2011)

A simple story about the most important minutes of a family's life reveals the understanding of caring persons that greatly affected the final time a mother had with her family. It is notable in this recounting that a CFO could be available and would go to the ICU himself as he listened to the family's situation and the staff's deliberation of what should be done to best care for this family. He supported the hope of the family and professional judgment of the staff.

Within health care settings multiple languages are communicated either verbally or nonverbally. All professions such as medicine and nursing have language that arises through their scope of practice and educational preparation. Medicine's language comes from a view of biomedical science. The concern is with diagnosis and curing. Nursing's language arises from a bio-psycho-sociocultural framework, and although it reflects something of the language of medicine, it is at its best, a language of holistic practices. The language based on biomedical science, by its research traditions, renders a person objectified by diseases, numbers, and conditions.

Nursing has long struggled to articulate its unique contribution to health care through a universally accepted practice language. This is captured by Orem (1997):

> The lack of language has been a handicap in nurses' communication about nursing to the public as well as persons with whom they work in the health field. There can be no nursing language until the features of humankind specific to nursing are conceptualized and named and their structure uncovered. (p. 29)

Language ought to convey the discipline's view of their phenomenon of concern—person. One of the values of nursing theory is that nurses using a particular theory share a collective identity and shared language. For example, nurses practicing from the theoretical perspective of Nursing as Caring would use language that communicated caring and person as caring such as that described in Chapter 2.

Because nursing professionals are so central to transformation of the culture of health care, let us speak directly to nurses for a moment. We must return to a language of nursing in order to convey nursing's unique role in health care and to accurately and effectively portray outcomes of nursing care. Nursing's language is the language of caring—"it is human, it is personal, and it is at the core of the organizational purpose" (Boykin & Schoenhofer, 2001, p. 6). The language of nursing is best conveyed through the stories of practice. Through stories, meaning is created in knowing self and other as caring. When nurse leaders invite nurses to share their stories of practice, nursing and the language of nursing is articulated. The following story of a nurse, Adam Meyers, conveys the values and language of caring.

I came into work that Friday morning with some reservations inside. It was the beginning of a long 5-day run of 12-hour shifts, which always seemed to lengthen as each day passed. I walked into my pod in the ICU where I had been working for over a year to receive report on the patients for whom I had been assigned care that day, and most likely all 5 days. Bobby, I'll call him, was lying there in bed in the small room filled with monitors and equipment. A series of lines and tubes protruded from his face and were connected to a few machines whose screens illuminated the dim room. His chest moved in and out as the ventilator pushed oxygenated air into his lungs. His eyes were rolled back into his head; he was unaware that I was there. I learned that he had suffered an injury to his head from complications of extreme hyperthermia for over 12 hours due to a condition known as Neuroleptic Malignant Syndrome. Bobby had taken antipsychotic medications for a Bipolar Disorder for years and suddenly slipped into this severe condition. He had been transferred overnight from an outlying facility but the damage had already been done. I stared, saddened by the appearance of this young 27-year-old lying helplessly before me. I thought, how unfortunate to suffer for years from a condition in which the treatment had now caused a more severe complication. The day proceeded as days most often do with my becoming acquainted with every aspect of the situation. Soon it was visiting time and I waited for families and friends to enter to see their loved ones.

As I approached Bobby's room I could see all of his family, including his mother, sisters, brothers-in-law and even a few friends, standing in the room next to his bed. His mother, I'll call her Martha, ran her hand across her son's face as a tear ran down hers. Bobby was loved, that was very clear. This large, young man lying in bed looked nothing like the small-framed sisters and mother that were standing in front of me. As we visited, his family explained that Bobby was adopted; however, no less a member of their family. There was little to do in hopes to save the life his loved ones had once known. A few medications were given; a cooling blanket system to control his body temperature, a ventilator and pulmonary toiletry was maintained, along with some basic care needs. The weekend slipped into a new week and my 5-day stint in the unit was nearing an end. Bobby's family attended every visitation provided, waiting anxiously for any sign of improvement. My next 5-day shift came and I found myself assigned to Room 10 again, Bobby's room. I found him there again, looking somewhat more deteriorated than before.

Saturday came and it was a somewhat slower day in the unit. I looked at Mary Beth, the nurse assistant, and told her that today Bobby was going to get the whole treatment. Scruff now rested on Bobby's jaw line, his hair mangled and his lips were chapped with dried skin peeling off layer by layer. For 2 hours we washed and cared for Bobby. He now had a clean-shaven face and hair that was clean and combed over to the side, the way it naturally fell. His face was no longer oily and his lips were once again free of the dried skin and saliva that had accumulated there. His teeth and mouth had been brushed with toothpaste and fingernails had been trimmed. His skin smelled like the berry-scented body wash Mary Beth kept on hand for certain occasions with her patients. Along with a new hospital gown, new bed linens draped across Bobby's lower body. Martha and her family passed through the doorway. Rather than proceeding to the head of the bed like usual, she stopped before reaching the foot of the bed. She stared at her son lying in the bed as tears began to trickle down her face. She hadn't seen Bobby in this manner for over 2 weeks. She walked across the room to where I was standing and embraced me tightly. "He looks good," she expressed and then moved to his side. I spoke with them briefly and then left so not to monopolize their visiting time.

The next day Martha came to me and expressed that the family had made some decisions. Bobby's kidneys had failed as many other areas had done due to immense complications. "We've decided not to do dialysis," she explained. I nodded my head as she continued to express her feelings. "Tell me we're doing the right thing," she begged as she continued to look at her son. I took Martha by the hand as I expressed to her and the family that I accepted and understood their decision. I expressed in a soft, gentle voice that this would more than likely be Bobby's life connected to machines and tubes even if he survived. The pain in her eyes demonstrated how hard this decision had been to come to. Later on that day after a long discussion with Bobby's primary physician, I helped move him out of the ICU to the respiratory floor so that his family could be with him at all times. I checked on him before I left on Sunday evening and again on Monday. But on Tuesday morning word came that Bobby had passed. I didn't have the opportunity to see Bobby or his family that day before he passed. But nearly a year later, at a local college football game, a young woman stopped me outside the stadium. Her face was very familiar and before she could explain who she was I assured her that I knew she was Bobby's sister. We talked for a while and I asked about her mother. You could tell things had been hard by the tremble in her voice, but she expressed that they were doing well but that they certainly missed her younger brother. I often think of Bobby and his family and the couple of weeks we spent together. And when I do reflect on that time, I hope and pray I made an impact on their life, the way that Bobby and his family did on mine.

This story, shared by Adam, needs no interpretation to communicate the power of caring, within the family and between Adam and Bobby, and his family. The story can be used by board members and other groups in a health care system as a way to come to know, in a very personal way, why effective nurse caring has been found to be correlated with favorable patient satisfaction scores (Valentine, 1989). The sensitivity conveyed in Adam's careful languaging of this nursing situation is certainly a reflection of the sensitivity and caring that was experienced so meaningfully by Bobby's family.

This chapter presented an insight into health care organizations through the concept of culture as described by Siourouni et al. (2012). The key concepts of culture are values, beliefs, and assumptions; leadership style; definitions of success; language; symbols; and rituals. The chapter describes these concepts as currently embedded within the health care system and offers a description of how a groundedness and the intentional living of caring values fundamentally transforms systems of care.

QUESTIONS FOR CONSIDERATION

- Describe a caring experience. What about the experience made it caring? How did you come to know yourself as caring through the experience? You are invited to draw on the language of caring shared in Chapter 2 to help you with your description.
- What difficulties are encountered when one tries to know those nursed as well as colleagues in the current health care system?

- What structure for health care would best respond to what matters most to those served as well as members of the system?
- What beliefs and values do you bring to your role? How are they lived?
- What symbols reveal caring?
- What is your most prized symbol of caring in the health care organization? Why?
- What is the most meaningful ritual in the health care system? Why?
- What are the responsibilities of the health care organization to the community it serves?
- How do I (nurse, doctor, and so on) describe my practice away from the practice setting? How is nursing languaged? How is the practice of other disciplines languaged? (Physicians, physical therapists, medical technologists, admitting clerks, and each group included in the Dance of Caring Persons in your health care system can explore these questions both within and across the disciplinary group.)
- What does it mean to be a nurse? (or physician, physical therapist, medical technologist, and so on)

REFERENCES

Boykin, A., Bulfin, S., Baldwin, J., & Southern, R. (2004). Transforming care in the emergency department. *Topics in Emergency Medicine, 26*(4), 331–336.

Boykin, A., & Schoenhofer, S. O. (2001). The role of nursing leadership in creating caring environments in health care delivery systems. *Nursing Administration Quarterly, 25*(3), 1–7.

Boykin, A., Schoenhofer, S. O., Smith, N., St. Jean, J., & Aleman, D. (2003). Transforming practice using a caring-based model. *Nursing Administration Quarterly, 27*(3), 223–230.

Corrigan, J. M., Donaldson, M. S., Kohn, L. T., et al. (2001). *Crossing the quality chasm: A new health system for the 21st century.* Washington, DC: National Academy of Science.

Davies, H. (2002). Understanding organizational culture in reforming the National Health Service. *Journal of the Royal Society of Medicine, 95*(3), 140–142.

Douglas, M. (1978). *Implicit meanings: Essays in anthropology.* London, England: Routledge & Kegan Paul.

Eckel, P., Hill, B., & Green, M. (1998). *En route to transformation.* On change: An Occasional Paper Series of the ACE Project on Leadership and Institutional Transformation. Retrieved from http:// www.eric.ed.gov/ERICWebPortal/search/detailmini.jsp?_nfpb=true&_&ERICExtSearch_ SearchValue_0=ED435293&ERICExtSearch_SearchType_0=no&accno=ED435293

Ferlie, E. B., & Shortell, S. M. (2001). Improving the quality of care in the United Kingdom and the United States: A framework for change. *The Milbank Quarterly, 79*(2), 281–314.

Hamilton, P., & Campbell, M. (2011). Knowledge for re-forming nursing's future: Standpoint makes a difference. *Advances in Nursing Science, 34*(4), 280–296.

Hartmann, C. W., Rosen, A. K., Meterko, M., Shokeen, P., Zhao, S., Singer, S., & Gaba, D. M. (2009). An overview of patient safety climate in the VA. *Medical Care Research and Review, 66*(3), 320–338.

Helman, G. G. (1990). *Culture, health, and illness.* Oxford, England: Butterworth-Heinemann.

Holland, C. (1993). An ethnographic study of nursing culture as an exploration for determining the existence of a system of ritual. *Journal of Advanced Nursing, 18,* 1461–1470.

Hunt, G. (2004). A sense of life: The future of industrial-style health care. *Nursing Ethics, 11*(2), 189–202.

Institute of Medicine. (2012). *Best care at lower cost. The path to continuously learning health care in America.* Washington, DC: The National Academies Press.

Jonsdottir, H., Litchfield, M., & Pharris, M. D. (2004). The relational core of nursing practice as partnership. *Journal of Advanced Nursing, 4*(3), 241–248.

Judge, T., & Piccolo, R. (2004). Transformational and transactional leadership: A meta-analytic test of their relative validity. *Journal of Applied Psychology, 89*(5), 755–768.

Mallak, L., Lyth, D., Olson, S., Ulshafer, S., & Sardone, F. (2003). Culture, the built environment and healthcare organizational performance. *Managing Service Quality, 13*(1), 27–38.

Orem, D. E. (1997). Views of human beings specific to nursing. *Nursing Science Quarterly, 10*(1), 26–31.

Pilkington, F. (2005). Myth and symbol in nursing theories. *Nursing Science Quarterly, 18*(3), 198–203.

Porter, S. (2011). Bringing values back into evidence-based nursing: The role of patients in resisting empiricism. *Advances in Nursing Science, 34*(2), 106–118.

Pratt, M., & Rafaeli, A. (2001). Symbols as a language of organizational relationships. *Research in Organizational Behavior, 23*, 93–103.

Pross, E., Hilton, N., Boykin, A., & Thomas, C. (2011). The dance of caring persons. *Nursing Management, 42*(10), 25–30.

Rafaeli, A., & Worline, M. (2000). Symbols in organizational culture. In N. M. Askanazy, C. M. P. Winderom, & M. F. Petersen (Eds.), *Handbook of organizational culture and climate* (pp. 71–84). Thousand Oaks, CA: Sage.

Ricketts, M., & Seiling, J. G. (2003). Language, metaphors and stories: Catalysts for meaning making in organizations. *Organizational Development Journal, 21*(4), 33–43.

Schein, E. H. (1990). Organizational culture. *American Psychologist, 45*(2), 109–119.

Schyve, P. M. (2009). *Leadership in healthcare organizations, a Governance Institute White Paper* (pp. 1–35). Retrieved from http://www.jointcommission.org/assets/1/18/WP_leadership_standards.pdf

Scott, T., Mannion, R., Marshall, M., & Davies, H. (2003). Does organizational culture influence health care performance? A review of the evidence. *Journal of Health Service Research & Policy, 8*(2), 105–117.

Senge, P. M. (1990). *The fifth discipline.* New York, NY: Doubleday.

Siourouni, E., Kastanioti, C., Tziallas, D., & Niakas, D. (2012). Health care provider's organizational culture profile: A literature review. *Health Science Journal, 6*(2), 212–233.

Smith, A., & Stewart, B. (2011). Organizational rituals: Features, functions and mechanisms. *International Journal of Management Reviews, 13*(2), 113–133.

Stetler, C. B. (2003). Role of the organization in translating research into evidence-based practice. *Outcomes Management, 7*(3), 97–103.

Strange, F. (2001). The persistence of ritual in nursing practice. *Clinical Effectiveness in Nursing, 5*, 177–183.

Tharp, B. M. (2009). *Defining "culture" and "organizational culture: From anthropology to the office.* Retrieved from http://www.haworth.com/en-us/knowledge/workplace-library/documents/defining-culture-and-organizationa-culture_5.pdf

Valentine, K. (1989). Caring is more than kindness: Modeling its complexities. *Journal of Nursing Administration, 19*(11), 28–34.

Weinberg, D., Cooney-Miner, D., Perloff, J., Babington, L., & Avgar, A. (2011). Building collaborative capacity. *Medical Care, 49*(8), 716–723.

Wesorick, B., & Doebbeling, B. (2011). Lessons from the field: The essential elements for point-of-care transformation. *Medical Care, 49*(12, Suppl. 1), S49–S58.

Wolf, Z. R. (1988). *Nurse's work, the sacred and the profane.* Philadelphia, PA: University of Pennsylvania Press.

Response to Chapter 3

Wendy Bailes, MSN, RN, CNE
Assistant Professor
University of Louisiana at Monroe

Can one implement the Dance of Caring Persons model in today's health care mine-field? I think the better question is "Can you afford not to?" When I began my career 20 years ago, I had the privilege of working with doctors, nurse managers, nurses, staff that exemplified caring. There was always an air of mutual respect, caring about each other and collaboration. In 2002, everything changed. The hospital changed leadership and at the same time it began to struggle with breaking even. Layoffs occurred, budgets became tight, managers changed their attitudes as pressure came from above to decrease spending, and nurses began to nurse computers with the arrival of the Electronic Health Record. I transitioned to a faculty position where I find my biggest challenge is helping students see past the tasks in order to come to know the person cared for. There is a need to infuse both—the systems of health care and education—with the philosophy of the Dance of Caring Persons.

Having experienced both transformational and autocratic leadership, I believe the transformation of cultures of care must begin with the support and enthusiasm of its leaders. Leaders do not have to set aside the bottom line in order to care for others. However, leaders will need to be open and receptive to others and involved intimately with individuals from all areas of the hospital. For example, last year one facility I am involved with underwent a change in leadership. This new leader implemented a program in which each member of her administrative team was randomly assigned to a staff member for the day. That administrator followed the staff member for the entire shift. This opportunity to directly know a staff member occurs each month and all administrative personnel are required to participate. In this situation, it is nurses; however, I believe it should be more than staff nurses. Individuals from housekeeping, maintenance, laboratory, respiratory therapy, physical therapy, and nursing assistants should be included. Nurse managers should also stop and take one day to be the staff nurse or to follow the nurse's aide and housekeeper to experience what they experience. Time is a commodity that demonstrates caring through action.

There is value in each person. If you have ever watched *Undercover Boss*, you see individuals who care in spite of working conditions, without expectations of reward. These individuals have ideas and thoughts that have the potential to benefit and improve the organization. However, they need access. As stated by the authors, all members should be represented and considered as equal within the group. Representatives from maintenance, housekeeping, laboratory, respiratory therapy, physical therapy, and nursing aides should be included when discussing hospital business. When discussing changes, their voice should be heard and considered as equal in importance to administration. The staff knows how to make the day-to-day operations successful. They can help elucidate why Hospital Consumer Assessment of Health Providers and Systems (HCAHPS) scores are not at benchmark, why core measures are not being successfully implemented, or why hospital readmissions are rising.

Research has demonstrated that when the staff members feel that their voice is heard and respected they will buy into change more readily. This means that leadership must be receptive and willing to listen. I wonder many times as to how successful an organization could be if all voices were heard and respected. Leaders of the organization must be willing to lay aside their authority in the moment. Successful hospitals have demonstrated the effectiveness of this type of leadership.

Massachusetts General Hospital is one example of leadership that stays connected with the employees. Turnover is not an issue with the hospital as they strive for excellence in all areas. This excellence has resulted in their being named the best hospital in America for 2012.

In academia there is a term known as the *ivory tower*. This implies disconnect. In many ways, health care has become an ivory tower. Each group is disconnected from the other: Administration from middle management, middle management from staff, and staff from patients. Mandates are handed down from group to group without thought to implementation or implications. Information is being collected from patients, through surveys and discharge data. Information is collected from staff/middle management through surveys. However, this information is useless if it continues to be dispensed as mandates from above to "do better." Success in changing the perspective of health care to a caring-based perspective requires the following:

1. Identifying key stakeholder(s) in each department of the organization
2. Recruiting key stakeholder(s) to actively participate in organization and department meetings
3. Laying aside role authority in the moment to hear others, especially key stakeholder(s)
4. Removing the disconnect between groups by increasing interactions, such as spending the day with selected personnel (walking a mile in their shoes)

Caring is a multiplier. When one feels cared for, one tends to care for others. When one feels valued, one tends to value others. For health care, the cycle is demonstrated through improved patient satisfaction, improved patient outcomes, decreased employee turnover, and ultimately improved bottom line.

Response to Chapter 3

Suzanne C. Beyea, RN, PhD, FAAN
Director, Center for Nursing Excellence, Mission Hospital

*A*caring-based approach provides a critical infrastructure for achieving a high-quality and safe health care system. Knowing who the patient is and providing a healing environment in which care is consistent with an individual's needs, preferences, and values serves as an imperative to nurses and all the members of the interdisciplinary team. Transformation of the health care system will not occur without a commitment to co-creating this culture of caring with patients and families.

Patients and their families deserve care that is focused on each individual's need. Each of us wants this for ourselves or our family members; however, this goal is not consistently achieved in today's health care systems. Appointments are often scheduled at the provider's convenience, waits may be excessive, and informed and shared decision making does not occur in a consistent manner. Care in hospitals may be provided by numerous different nurses and physicians, often creating a perception that no one cares for the patient as person. From a caring-based framework, each person would receive high-quality, safe care in the right place, at the right time, every time. Careful consideration would be given to how to best meet the patient's needs and wishes for continuity of care. These provide some of the essential components for a transformed health care system in which caring permeates the primary structures, processes, and outcomes.

Health care systems focused on caring can, but will not, exist without leaders who share, promote, and support such a vision. Commitment to that vision requires a holistic approach to patients, families, and members of the health care team. A sense of connectedness to one another and those served by the health care system must be created and fostered. Teamwork and collaboration must serve as critical values of the organization and be fully supported to provide the lived experience for patients and staff members. Such a nonhierarchical approach to leadership helps create, establish, enhance, and expand such a caring culture and helps eliminate barriers to high-quality and safe care.

A caring culture requires genuine and authentic leaders who emulate the full embodiment of caring. Leaders must create environments in which staff members are supported to grow and develop their individual and team competency for caring. Rewards and recognition for excellence in caring must be integral of the process. The DAISY® award provides an example of an award that recognizes nurses who demonstrate compassionate care. Recognition of staff members through programs such as this supports the "hard-wiring" and visibility of shared values focused on caring. Programs such as this should be expanded and include all members of the team. Patients and family members should serve as individuals who can nominate staff members and be integral to the selection team. In this way, caring environments are co-created by teams well advised by the individuals they serve.

Listening to the voice of the patient and the family serves as another critical link to creating a caring culture. Patient and family-centered care as described by the Institute for Patient and Family-Centered Care (http://www.ipfcc.org) provides an essential approach toward co-creating genuine caring environments. It is through the voice of the patient and their family that health care clinicians truly learn how to provide individual respect, dignity, and care that is consistent with each patient's values and preferences. Councils consisting of patients, family members, and members of the health care team provide a critical strategy in advancing this work. By including patients and families in their care and valuing their input, care and caring become focused on the individuals who are the very purpose of the health care system.

The desired future state for caring health care environments will require commitment by nursing faculty and schools of nursing to create curricula that focus on caring and how to live caring with patients as well as how to care for self and colleagues. Shared accountabilities must be created for establishing caring environments and competencies. In addition, existing staff members and leaders need an opportunity to develop their skills and competency in relationship-based care and leadership. Unrelenting support and high-level resilience must exist when individuals or the system confront challenges in creating the desired culture.

The contributions of each member of the team must be valued and each individual offered respect in his or her daily work. This includes accepting differences and supporting one another with difficult, stressful, or challenging work assignments. This may be as simple as making certain a colleague takes a break or lunch, or providing quiet rooms for staff members to relax during a busy shift. Leaders must examine and realign the organizational culture and practices to ensure that staff members work in safe and healthy work environments. Caring must be visible in all aspects of nursing work including scheduling, work hours, staffing, and work environments. These goals cannot be achieved without the valuable input of staff members and a strong commitment of leaders to address their needs and concerns.

Establishing these goals and committing organizational resources in both academic and clinical settings should offer clear evidence of the significance of this agenda. Words alone cannot transform environments. Leaders at all levels of the organization must be aligned and visibly committed to this most important core value. It is imperative that leaders advance transformative changes that ensure a patient-centered, relationship-based care environment. Success will depend on a meaningful partnership with patients, families, and members of the health care team. These same individuals will serve as the impetus for the required transformation.

Practical Relevance of the Model
at All Levels of the System

Section II addresses strategies to prepare people and processes in all organizational functions to participate meaningfully in transforming the health care system to actively reflect the values and principles of the unifying caring-based model, the Dance of Caring Persons. In this section, specific emphasis is placed on promoting readiness, initiating the design phase, and staging the phases of implementation.

Chapter 4 addresses the ways in which leaders at all levels of the organization propel the desire for change into commitment for action. The importance of leaders embracing a common value-based vision is important to drive system changes. Specific planning for how to create awareness, build knowledge, honor and manage expectations, prepare early adopters, enable and motivate all participants, build proficiency, and define benefits are presented in Chapter 4.

Chapter 5 focuses on preparing staff throughout the organization for implementation of the transformational model. Suggested steps are provided for leading the alternating rhythm between personal, local, and cross-organizational change. Readers are provided with resources for answering questions that arise throughout the process, and forums and methods for mobilizing action and successful collaboration are suggested. Questions to consider in the chapters in Section II are as follows:

- What might we do on our unit to create a caring environment so that all persons involved can experience the caring we intend? (vision)
- How might we care for self and each other as part of this process? Are we ready to embark on this journey? (readiness)
- In what way am I ready to change? In what way are we ready to change? How might this change help us meet our vision? (clarity about expectations)
- How are we going to use the resources available to us to become proficient in substantive knowledge about caring? (enabled action through preparation)
- How will this knowledge become visible within our day-to-day work? (authentic action)
- How will we know that we are making progress toward our vision? (prizing, valuing, and growing)

- How might we have a meaningful dialogue that supports our committed actions? (forums for dialogue)
- How might we optimize and then stabilize our new processes? (prizing, valuing, and growing)
- Are the experiences of our patients and families enlivened and enriched through our commitment to caring? (prizing, valuing, and growing)

Chapter 4

Readiness for Health Care System Transformation

*T*he purpose of this chapter is to assist leaders in health care systems to anticipate and embrace the joy of the Dance of Caring Persons. The fundamental question is how might we ready ourselves and others for re-forming our organization into one in which caring guides our behavior, our knowledge, and our actions with each other and those we serve? The energy evident at the end of "getting ready" is widespread commitment to engagement in an intentional change process. The change process we propose has five phases. The first two phases are about "getting ready" to embark on the journey of moving the culture toward caring as a dominant value. The last three phases are about "getting set" and "going." These phases of change are derived from many change management processes. Hiatt's (2006) ADKAR model recognizes that change happens through engaging with people by building *Awareness*, creating *Desire*, developing *Knowledge*, fostering *Ability*, and *Reinforcing* changes in organizations.

Implementation Management Associates (2010) has a model called accelerating implementation methodology (AIM), which shares some of these same features while also focusing on the organizational factors that reinforce the sustainability of a desired system-wide change initiative. In another approach, Creative Health Care Management organizes the phases of transformational change into "I2E2," which represents dimensions of change focused on inspiration, infrastructure, education, and evidence, as it works throughout the organization to implement changes related to relationship-based care (retrieved October 2012, http://chcm.com). Rogers (2003), known for his theory of diffusion and adoption of innovation, defined four elements in the process: innovation, communication channels, implementation, and confirmation. What is common to each of these frameworks is the lesson that system-wide change processes require systematic planning, communication, and sustained attention to both people and processes to bring about lasting and meaningful adoption of a proposed change.

We have organized the phases of this change process as follows:

1. Create awareness
2. Build knowledge and articulate expectations
3. Prepare the first adopters, increase the desire for change

4. Enable and motivate all users
5. Build proficiency and reinforce skill

These phases for transformation are neither linear nor tightly bounded; what they represent is the dominant work activity required to move the commitment to change forward toward the benefits that are expected. If there are no anticipated benefits from engaging together in this work, then remaining with the status quo will likely create the greatest magnetic energy for persons within the organization. It is widely accepted that organizations do not change; rather, it is the people within them that do (Hiatt, 2006). Unless a person decides to change and has the structure and resources to do so, neither the person nor the organization will change. It is all about the person. Regardless of the role or function that a person holds within an organization, in the end, it is a personal choice to change or not.

If that is true, then how does a committed leader help individuals to consider changing as a member of an organization? It is widely accepted that collective change processes require motivational energy to propel effort. When that energy is in the form of fear, the perception is that the current conditions are difficult and there is little to lose by trying something new as a survival tactic. The alternative view is to offer a compelling vision of the future with the possibility for improved conditions and "the sky is the limit" thinking about possibilities. People commit to a visionary future because it matters to them and they can see themselves in it.

Organizational leaders cannot command commitment. In the human service field, the agents of action are individuals in relationship with others. Thoughts and feelings cannot be mandated, behavior is always a choice, and actions occur in the moment and reflect who persons are, what they know, their affect, and their intended actions—in other words, what matters to them. Health care actions, in the end, are wholly dependent on the individual performing that action—no policy or procedure can substitute for human judgment. Simple rules and principles guide expected parameters within which professionals are expected to practice.

In this chapter, we focus on the first two phases of change: raising awareness and building knowledge to articulate expectations. For the purposes of this chapter, we are assuming that the reader is from the patient care services area and is likely a nurse leader. What are the reasons for that assumption? What may have attracted the interest of the reader is an interest in grounding his or her health care system in an explicit model of caring. The discipline of nursing as a health care discipline focuses on the study of caring through sustained and substantive theoretical and applied knowledge. The transformational model upon which this book is based, Dance of Caring Persons, is grounded in the assumptions that all persons by virtue of being human are caring (Boykin & Schoenhofer, 2001) and all health care professionals have a mandate to care. No other professional discipline defines caring as a substantive domain of inquiry.

With those assumptions, as health care organizations move toward evidence-based management as well as evidence-based practice, it would be likely to find nursing leading the efforts to integrate caring science within the interprofessional team. Of course, all members of the team know caring, practice caring, are caring, yet the substantive breadth and depth of caring knowledge may not be formalized within the field of study for other disciplines. The concepts of humanistic care, of patient-centered care, of empathic customer service, are concepts that are studied and resonate strongly with caring science, even as these concepts emerge from various fields of study.

As a clinical leader committed to making caring visible and substantively significant within your organization, how might you:

Engage the executive leadership team?
Gain initial buy-in throughout the system—inviting all to the dance?

Design detailed features of transformation—general pattern for the dance?
Budget for transformation?
Establish broad structures and processes for ongoing dialogue to make the model live?
Prize, value, and grow caring in all dimensions of the system—outcomes?
Manage the processes and structures needed to sustain the commitment?

This chapter addresses these questions and the importance of leaders embracing a common value-based vision to drive system changes. Through relevant stories, specific aspects related to human and technical resources are highlighted, as they relate to the transformational processes within units and the system as a whole. The challenges and opportunities encountered within these examples are also addressed.

RAISING AWARENESS

Raising awareness is an ongoing process throughout any transformational change. At the beginning of a change process grounded in caring, it is important to be clear about *what it is* that one wants others to become aware of. If the task is to raise awareness, what is it that the organization is currently blind or inattentive to? How do we know that? What harm is being done by keeping blind to the issue? What good could be served by illuminating the need for a greater focus on substantive caring? How does one raise awareness? The short answer to raising awareness is that the champion for the change must connect with decision makers at various levels of the organization around a common shared value. This section on Raising Awareness first addresses raising personal awareness of self as caring person, and then focuses on raising awareness of the organization as a caring environment (Box 4.1).

BOX 4.1 Questions to Ponder: Personal Awareness

Food for Thought, from *Nursing as Caring: A Model for Transforming Practice* (Boykin & Schoenhofer, 2001):

> Caring expressed in nursing is personal, not abstract (p. 45).
> The caring that is nursing cannot be expressed as an impersonal generalized stance of good will, but must be expressed knowledgeably (p. 45).
> Coming to know self as caring person in ever deepening and broadening dimensions (p. 15).

With these ideas in mind, consider:

> What is the meaning of "personal" versus "abstract" for you?
> What dilemmas or questions does it raise to express personal caring knowledgeably?
> What actions does it suggest?
> How might you talk about this with colleagues who are open to your interest in caring?

ASSUMPTIONS RELATED TO PERSONAL AWARENESS

If you have chosen to read this book, there is something that has drawn you to think about caring. You are likely a champion for change within your organization for building a practice environment more explicitly committed to substantive and significant caring. What energy do you hold related to caring? How might you explore your own assumptions, beliefs, and values related to caring? If caring is a human mode of being, what is your mode of being with and in caring? Taking time for reflection about your own beliefs related to caring is part of the process of coming to know self as caring person. Knowing yourself as a caring person assists in the processes of helping others to know themselves as caring persons, thus clarifying a shared value as a foundation for commitment to action together. Choosing to ignore processes for personal knowing may undermine your energy moving forward, as others question and challenge the wisdom of focusing on caring. Clarity can strengthen your own voice in articulating what matters related to embarking on the journey of transformation (Box 4.2).

BOX 4.2 Actions/Exercises to Enhance Knowing Self as Caring Person

What are the activities or processes that might help you to come to know yourself as caring person? To live and grow in caring becomes a self-embedded, ongoing internal process. You cannot make someone else believe as you do, feel as you do, think as you do. It is for each of us to discover and grow for ourselves. What we can do with and for each other is create the possibility for reflection individually and subsequently agree to share the journey with one another.

ACTIVITIES TO FOSTER COMING TO KNOW SELF AS CARING PERSON

1. Story of a nursing/health care situation: From the theoretical perspective grounding of this book, a story of a nursing situation is the story of a shared lived experience in which the caring between the nurse and the nursed enhances personhood. "Health care situation" is a term that can be used to adapt that understanding to any role in a health care system. For example, providers from other direct care disciplines, such as medicine, physical therapy, medical technology, and so on, and from supporting disciplines and services such as accounting, management, medical records, engineering, security, and custodial services, and so forth, have their own stories of living caring in their roles in a way that ultimately resonates to the well-being of the patients. So now, create a reflective space for yourself. Allow the attentions and distractions of the moment to recede as you create inner and outer stillness. Now, recall the most beautiful moment of your health care experience, a time when you felt you were living your role in a way that reflected the highest values of yourself as a person and of your professional or occupational role in health care. Bring that situation fully to life in your memory, experiencing the sights, sounds, smells, the people who were present, the surrounding space... and dwell with that scene, recapturing the fullness of the moment that stands out for you as one of your finest moments in the practice of your health care role. Focus the scene around the caring that was mutually lived between you and another—whether a patient or a coworker. Allow that sense of the "caring between" to be fully re-experienced. And after a few moments, record the story of that situation, focusing on the shared lived

experience of caring that enhanced all persons involved, directly and indirectly. Let the story be told from your heart, rather than through filters such as external expectations or an analytic "framework"—just let your heart tell the story of your caring. Record your story in writing, or with voice, or video recording.

2. Study your story, asking yourself questions such as: In what ways was caring reflected within your interactions with patients/families/colleagues in this story? Turn to Chapter 2, pages 25–50, and use Mayeroff's ingredients of caring and Roach's attributes of caring to help you put into words a description of the caring that was shared in the story. In what ways was caring different from how you imagined it might be? What insights do you gain from reflecting about that caring situation?

3. Create an aesthetic representation of the caring between you and another as expressed in the story. A way to get started with this is to read your story, and write one sentence that comes from the story, rather than being "crafted" in your head, a sentence that starts with the words...*The essence of caring in my professional/occupational role is*....And then render that essence in any artistic form you can think of—painting, drawing, sculpting, creative dance, melody, song lyrics, fiber art, quilting, poster making—any art form you would like to use to express the deep meaning of caring that was created in the situation described in your story. We are all artists, some better developed in their art than others, but we all are artists. Rendering the essence of your caring in some artistic expression can foster appreciation for yourself as a caring person and can deepen your appreciation for the meaning of caring in your life and the lives of those you encounter in your health care system and beyond.

4. Engage in dialogue, sharing your story of caring and inviting others to reflect with you on the meaning of caring in your story; invite those in the dialogue to recollect a story of their own caring, using a process similar to the one described in point 1 above. Committed time for dialogue and reflection with trusted colleagues can help to articulate and reflect on coming to know self and each other as caring persons.

5. Read scholarly literature and aesthetic reflections of caring. We have listed a fairly extensive range of theoretical, research-based, and aesthetic reflections on caring in the Resources section at the end of this book to help you get started.

6. Practice relaxation response and breathing at specified times of the day to help you remain attuned to yourself as a caring person and to nurture an environment of caring in your workplace.

7. Dwell in nature, listening to the sounds; appreciating the power and beauty in the natural world.

8. Create a place for reflection at work and/or at home—a corner, a garden, a water fountain, a candle that signals to you to slow down, breathe, and reflect, to appreciate yourself as a caring person and your surroundings as a caring environment.

Creating the Space and Time for Coming to Know Self as Caring Person Within the Work Setting

At the beginning of this journey the organizational environment may not yet have created the space or the time for you to take time out for reflection for yourself. Your reminder to care for self, to foster growth in knowing yourself as a caring person may happen in your own place at your own time. As caring comes to be understood, and the desire for caring practices grows, there may be a commitment to creating a reserved space for reflecting and engaging in a dialogue. Examples of this include a lounge, decorated by the staff in calming colors with comfortable seating and access to music, and a massage chair. Within the Christine E. Lynn College of Nursing at Florida Atlantic University, there is a room dedicated to quiet meditation, a labyrinth for meditative walking set in an outdoor garden. There is a center for intentional healing, and a room for yoga. Within the College's Memory and Wellness Center, there is a quiet, comfortable lounge with ocean scenes and a massage chair for staff to take time for themselves away from the calls for nursing that they attend to throughout the day.

Caring rounds—a moment at the beginning of the shift to share a story of caring in action related to a patient and its meaning to you. Identify an existing quiet space within the facility that can serve as a reminder of the self as a caring person. Some facilities have decorated their staff rest room to signal that one could "rest" for a moment within the daily routine.

Caring aesthetics day—a time and place where staff can gather and use art to express caring as they know it. Submit your story or poetry to an aesthetic journal such as *Nightingale Songs* (refer to Resources section) to share reflections with colleagues. Retreats with colleagues to appreciate nature and its relation to knowing self as caring person.

Sponsor specific workshops for personal growth and health for staff to demonstrate a commitment to coming to know self as caring person. The Memory and Wellness Center of the Christine E. Lynn College of Nursing at Florida Atlantic University hosted an 8-week mindfulness-based stress reduction program for staff to learn skills for mindful eating, mindful walking, breathing, movement, communication that included time at the ocean to create aesthetic expressions meaningful to the self.

ORGANIZATIONAL FOCUS FOR CARING: RAISING AWARENESS

It is now well accepted that connecting personal meaning to collective action accelerates the possibilities for sustained adoption of change in practice. The change has to matter to the person, it has to have meaning (if it is complex and dependent on judgment), or it has to be seamlessly engineered into the workflow through human factors engineering (e.g., automated barcoding). When considering human interaction and communication—judgment, choice, and action are at the discretion of the practitioner. The person has to commit to change. Consensus about an idea or approach is not the same as commitment. In conversations, people can agree to the concept of an idea to change the practice environment. Commitment differs because it requires planning, resources, a budget, timeline, and methods for appraisal of success. Forced compliance to an initiative may appear to be adoption, but most likely it elicits short-lived behavior exhibited to achieve a milestone or requirement. When focus moves away from the milestone or requirement, behavior is not sustained because it was never internalized nor truly adopted. It is the illusion of adoption, which is often the result of the "illusion of inclusion" in the decision process to move forward with a change. Illusion of inclusion is involving persons in what *appears* to be an open dialogue about which direction the participants want to move, yet in truth the direction has already been determined. It is important to be truthful about the process of inclusion. Inclusion might mean a collaborative process of decision making about what direction to pursue. Inclusion might also mean a feedback session about the pros and cons of an already determined path of action. Pseudo-inclusion undermines trust. Articulating the scope of engagement and decision making is important to building a partnership.

Commitment also requires a system to sustain change through reinforcing what matters most to the persons upon which the adoption will rely. For example, if what matters most to nurses at the bedside is to have meaningful communication with patients and families, the scheduling standards for continuity of care need to reflect that. If instead, patient assignment is determined by geographic location rather than continuity of provider, then reinforcement for an enduring commitment to that caring practice is jeopardized. Continuous and visible communication about what is different in this new way of interacting with patients is essential for it to flourish as the new state of practice. Caring between the nurse (or other care provider) and the one cared for is guided largely by the actions of that provider (or nurse) in that moment, with each patient. The caring action has to be "owned" as authentic and valued.

It is important to *hear the story* of persons to raise their awareness about an issue. How might this be done? There are abundant examples of ways to raise the awareness about the meaning of an issue to an individual person. Story is a powerful means of connecting personal commitment to larger change processes. The inner journey requires deep focus, it cannot be superficial; story allows for reflection. Campbell, Moyers, and Flowers (1988) teach us that "one way or another we have to find what fosters our blooming of humanity in contemporary life. It is within each of us to recognize the values which take us beyond survival—either economic or physical."

One example of a story used within practice innovation is found within IDEO (Kelley, Littman, & Peters, 2001), a design and innovation consulting company in Silicon Valley. That company's mission is to help organizations innovate product or process improvements. Their methods have been adopted by the Transforming Care at the Bedside (TCAB) initiative sponsored by the Robert Wood Johnson Foundation (Rutherford et al., 2008). One of us (K. V.) had the opportunity to be trained as a certified facilitator in the IDEO processes. Their process goes from the abstract and thematic to the concrete and observable.

One of the first steps is to tell a story about what matters most about the topic at hand. If the topic at hand is the organization as a culture of caring, what is a story that exemplifies the best of that caring? And what is a story that exemplifies the absence of a culture of caring within the institution? The idea is to be specific, who, what, when, where, why? What did it smell like, look like, feel like, taste like, sound like? Stories are shared with the innovation team and used as the substantive starting point for brainstorming possibilities for what might be different and then creating those possibilities in prototypes that are field tested as an innovation that moves the practice forward toward articulated values and purpose.

There is a recognition that change is constant and that the adaptive strategy for thriving in the constancy of change is to move from a focus on structure to a focus on process, and to focus on the whole versus parts (Wheatley, 2006). This focus on the whole and processes versus rules is consistent with caring theories. With information as the organizing force, the work of management is to create opportunities to diffuse information across boundaries. This will expedite interactions and networks that put people in proximity to new information to promote understanding of different perspectives, to learn through connection. The idea is to move from control to principles through which decision making is guided in complex ever-changing systems. Within this world, the "narrative" or story becomes a means for creating and exchanging information. One of the values that the Dance of Caring Persons brings to an organization is that of authenticity. So the story of the organization—its purpose, core values, mission, structure, functional processes, and so on—when grounded in the model we advocate, would authentically portray the reality of the organization, rather than a fraudulent "framing."

The power of story is generated through understanding who you are in the story, who others are, sharing beliefs by asking what meaning is in the story, and what principles merge to guide our next choices (Wheatley, 2006). The theory of Nursing as Caring can stimulate a discussion of these principles. Persons are caring:

By virtue of their humanness
Moment to moment

Being whole/complete in the moment
By living grounded in caring
By participating in nurturing relationships with caring others, enhancing
personhood. (Boykin & Schoenhofer, 2001)

How do these assumptions guide your choices and stimulate your narrative?

SEVEN STORIES OF CARING IN TRANSFORMATIONAL CHANGE

The Dance of Caring Persons—Learning to Let Go of Rungs and Hold Hands

One of the exciting discoveries for leaders involved in creating this dance is that because they are part of the circle and are not on a higher rung of the ladder, they were free to *be with* colleagues, to learn from and with each other, and to support and nurture others in what matters to them.

> One example of "what mattered" to staff on a particular unit was that work schedules were created in an objectified way—without any personal knowing of an individual staff's situation. To address this, the unit manager initiated a process for work schedules to be done collectively in order to support the unique and individual calls of staff persons. This resulted in a strong unit culture where loyalty and giving of self was lived. Only in a true emergency was there ever a planned absence from staff. Staff felt listened to and cared about.

A summary of action steps in this story is as follows:

1. Letting go of the rung takes courage and trust
2. Commitment to knowing colleagues and responding to what matters instills hope and engagement
3. Various persons lead in the dance at differing times. Here the staff led the innovation to scheduling

Sustaining a Commitment to Caring Through Ongoing Dialogue

The opportunity for continual dialogue on caring is important to ongoing knowledge development and understanding of the substantive nature of caring, to creating a caring-based culture, and to sustaining the commitment to a practice model grounded in Nursing as Caring.

> This commitment to creating a caring-based model was lived in an emergency department of a community-based hospital. A team representing all categories of staff (nurses, physicians, unit secretaries, emergency department technicians, patient/guest relation staff, and department leadership/administration) was formed to lead the unfolding of a caring-based model. The team met every two weeks and shared stories of how they and the staff were engaging in a dialogue on what it meant to live caring in practice; how they were growing in their understanding of caring; and strategies for advancing the model. The discussion and suggestions of the team were then brought to monthly staff meetings for further dialogue and input. It was a devotion to the importance of living caring in everyday practice and creating a culture grounded in caring values that kept the dialogue as the most important item on staff agendas.

A summary of action steps in this story is as follows:

1. Commitment leads to obligations to sustain a caring model
2. All persons must be engaged in the dialogue
3. Time for dialogue is essential to the success of the model

Story of Community Culture and Caring: Caring Initiative Led From Nursing, Informed Through Others, Findings Applied Within Nursing

In the 1980s, the hospital industry was on the verge of converting from a "cottage industry"—meaning self-contained entities serving the needs of local communities—to a corporate, consolidated entity. This is the story lived by one of us, Dr. Kathleen Valentine (Box 4.3):

I lived in a community that was converting three small hospitals into one larger corporate entity. It was a time of great turmoil for the community, for the employees, for the providers, for patients, and for managers. Not a single member of the community would be untouched by these large-scale changes. The compelling reason for the change had to

---

BOX 4.3 With Each Individual Interview I Asked

1. Can you recall an incident within the last six months that you think captures what your views are on caring?
   So the critical elements of caring are…?
   Are there other aspects of caring that this incident does not illustrate but that you feel are important?
2. If you were to observe a nurse and a patient in their interactions throughout a shift, how would you know that caring had occurred? What would be the critical indicators?
3. If outside observers spent a day here, what would they observe that would indicate to them that this is a caring institution? What critical indicators would have to be observed or intuited?
4. In what ways, if any, do you think that caring is linked with specific health care outcomes?
5. What resources are currently allocated to caring functions (here)? What criteria are used in making these decisions? Do you anticipate that resource allocation decisions may change in the future?
6. Do you have any issues, concerns, or ideas you would like to see addressed related to this project on caring?

Each person then told a story about an experience he or she had participated in or observed. Through reflection, the meaning of caring became personalized. These stories were analyzed, and, along with other data from document analyses and concept mapping data, were used to develop an instrument to measure caring and its relationship to outcomes. That study showed that when caring (as perceived by nurses and patients in particular encounters) occurred, postoperative complications and length of stay went down, and satisfaction went up (Valentine, 1989).

do with quality, satisfaction, and cost. Competing for duplicate services was depriving the community of necessary services and technologies. Staff, services, medical providers all were in turmoil as service lines merged, differentiated hospital care was started (babies at one hospital, neurology at another when prior to that all three hospitals had a full array of services). For the first time in the communities' history a drive for nursing unionization was brought to a vote. Though it was not ratified, the atmosphere was full of distrust between the management and the staff. Patient care was compromised. A management team was brought in to address the need for a "customer service focus" and a slogan of "we're in the business of caring" was adopted. There was a great deal of resistance voiced by the medical and nursing staff, related to a prescription for customer service through scripted interactions rather than a commitment to authentic caring.

The nursing leader of the organization allowed me to work across the organization to interview senior management, managers, nurse managers, nurses, and patients about what caring meant to them.

At the time, published literature about the substantive theoretical knowledge related to caring in nursing in health care was not prevalent. Having opinion leaders reflect and then act upon discoveries from that study helped the organization to move from slogan to substance related to making caring more significantly visible within the organization. For example, caring exemplars were part of the development of a compensation system for nursing clinical leaders. In this story the impetus for change came from nursing. It was informed by opinion leaders outside of nursing and the application of caring remained within the functional area of nursing. The overall awareness of the organization was raised (a sculpture dedicated to caring was installed in the lobby); but substantive changes based on caring science within the daily functions in other disciplines were not immediately evident.

A summary of action steps taken is as follows:

1. Promoting personal readiness through commitment and gathering knowledge from the field, identifying supportive mentors
2. Identifying and securing an internal champion situated within the organization who can facilitate access to key persons, resources, and forums for decision making
3. Focusing activity (interviews and interactive data collection) to raise awareness, and stimulate dialogue about the substantive meaning of caring
4. Following through with a project (research study) made the concepts concrete and applicable
5. Integrating results into ongoing organizational operations through using the findings in the development of a compensation system that explicitly emphasized caring practices as the expected standard of care

Organizational Change Project: Caring as a Dimension in Choosing Among Alternatives

In another large-scale hospital organization, the results of a caring questionnaire administered to nurses and patients after nurse/patient encounters were used to determine if different models of patient care delivery were more or less effective relative to satisfaction, outcomes, and cost. In this case, measurement of caring became part of a cross-disciplinary study led by nursing and joined by financial system and industrial engineering to choose which model of care delivery achieved the broadest and most sustained outcomes. In this model, caring, as perceived by nurses and patients, was included as an essential dimension of determining success for an organization-wide initiative originally situated as a cost-saving framework but then broadened to include caring. What nurses and patients perceived relative to caring was made explicit and visible.

A summary of action steps is as follows:

1. Personal commitment of high-level executive for patient care services to broaden the appraisal criteria to include caring
2. Agreement to integrate measurement of caring as an explicit component for appraising success of the different models of care
3. Organization-wide education sessions with staff about theory and evidence-based knowledge related to caring in practice
4. Participatory research methods to engage patients and families about their expectations related to caring
5. Incorporation of what was learned into the final design of care delivery models subsequently adopted within the organization

Caring as a Model of Care: Deferred at a System Level Yet Embedded Within a Suborganizational Level

A multisite, multipurpose health care organization was growing its professional practice environment for nursing and sought a model to define and frame an array of future nursing initiatives across the organization. The concepts of caring were presented to the nursing leadership group and aroused enough interest that field trips were taken to explore other organizations that had committed to adopting caring as a practice model. Multiple consulting companies that incorporated caring practices as part of their professional practice development were invited to assess the possibilities within the organization. Ultimately, the large-scale change process using caring as the core principle was not explicitly adopted at that time throughout the entire organization. Nursing leaders were unable to commit the necessary cross-organizational support, while simultaneously leading the challenges of other large-scale, mission-critical transformation processes. Smaller units within the organization advanced caring within the scope of their projects and sphere of influence. Some of these projects were then disseminated throughout the entire organization without overtly connecting it to caring science. This was a "not now" as a whole system change followed by smaller changes unconnected to a nursing theory or framework. The system was not ready for adopting a change process of that magnitude at that time.

A summary of action steps is as follows:

1. Acquire an initial sponsor to charter a data-gathering phase to determine what was currently being tested within other health care organizations related to caring and professional practice
2. Present the findings to a cross-sectional leadership group for consideration and authorization for next steps
3. Secure assessments from consulting firms familiar with the work of transformational change, caring, and professional practice
4. Consider the cost of the change process within the context of competing priorities
5. Defer system-wide change; seek smaller-scale integration within projects not requiring whole system adoption–incremental adoption
6. Revisit periodically for readiness for integration in the future

Unit-Based Change Process

A nurse manager within a hospital oncology unit attended an RN to BSN completion program and learned about different theories of nurse caring. She became energized by the possibilities that might be able to be infused within the practices on her unit. She invited nurse faculty familiar with scholarly works within caring to meet with staff on the unit and explore possibilities for changes in practice based on these theories. From these sessions emerged a commitment to listen for and to elicit each patient's and family's story and to discern what mattered most relative to their hospital stay. Nurses on the unit were encouraged to pursue their own self-care needs and some were adopted within the unit rituals such as a daily inspiration shared at change of shift and aroma therapy in the staff lounge. Ultimately, a patient advisory council was established that helped to keep staff and administration informed and focused about what mattered most to patients and their families throughout their care experience. This story starts with an individual, expands to a peer group, and ultimately to the community.

A summary of action steps is as follows:

1. Personal commitment of unit-level leader to focus on caring knowledge and to bring it to his or her role as manager
2. Enlistment of peers in exploring the literature and research related to caring
3. Small tests of change with staff, initiating a reflection space, aroma therapy in the staff lounge
4. Incorporating attention to caring within daily rounds (what matters most to Mr. Green today?)
5. Reinforcing the importance of caring to patients and families by engaging the patient advisory council in discussions related to caring

Whole System Change and Adoption—Interprofessional Partners

An organization with multisite, multipurpose hospitals and outpatient facilities was moving toward a large technology adoption through implementing a system-wide common electronic health record. The collective patient care leaders from across the organization agreed that a model of professional practice based on caring and the patients' experience was essential to developing the team culture necessary to have the adoption of technology be a success. The organization contracted with a consulting company that helped to build the system-wide capacity and developed site-specific local teams to change the way members of the interdisciplinary team communicated with one another about patient care. By appreciating new patterns of communication and designing new forums for case conferences and communication, cultural expectations shifted. Interprofessional team work, which helped all members understand each other's scope of practice, helped to assure that the patient and family received appropriate care by the designated professional. The patient's story and what mattered most to the patient became the focus of each team member's practice and documentation. Technology adoption enhanced team communication keeping the patient's need central and improving the continuity of care.

A summary of action steps is as follows:

1. The executive team at the highest level of patient care services determined that whole system change related to caring practice was a high priority to success in larger system changes related to technology adoption
2. Each executive committed sponsorship, personal commitment, and budget to the project
3. System-wide infrastructure was formed, and chartered with defined accountabilities

4. Each local site formed teams to carry out the process at a local level supported by coaching from the consultant team and central steering committee, and executive sponsors

5. The project engaged interprofessional leaders and built capacity throughout the organization from the boardroom to the bedside

SYNTHESIS OF CARING LEADERSHIP ACROSS STORIES

These stories are offered as a way to stimulate your own reflection about what "it" is that you wish to affect within your organization. Each of these examples affected the organization relative to scope, resources (human and material), and impact. Is the change process you envision local, cooperative, or an integrated system approach?

Caring and Leadership

Our U.S. health care system is broken; consumers expect, demand, and deserve reform. Rule-based control will not provide the necessary innovation to transform hospitals. Chaos, uncertainty, and complex adaptive system theories offer possibilities for reframing approaches to entrenched problems and the innovation of new care delivery systems. Principles versus rules help create patterns that shape caring cultures and cultures of safety. For example, Magnet hospital evaluation processes are pattern versus rule based; excellence is discerned from patterns aggregated from individual practitioners versus prescriptive criteria. Caring science is based on multidimensional complex patterns aggregated from the lived experience of the practitioner.

It is the role of the caring leader to participate with people to understand their beliefs/expectations about caring, to help make those explicit, and then work together to create a culture that can value and support caring practices. To advance the value of caring requires the team to secure resources in order for caring relationships to grow.

There is a growing voice of conviction related to the importance of caring. For example, failure to communicate is the number-one root cause for sentinel events (Joint Commission, n.d.). Suggested efforts to improve communication include the following:

Institute for Healthcare Improvement initiatives (Patel et al., 2012)
Structured communication, handoffs
Electronic health records
Care Boards for continuity of care
Care Rounds—which include patients in determining what matters most to them

Caring and Complexity

Plsek (1997, 2003) and coauthors (Globerman & Zimmerman, 2002; Zimmerman, Littman, & Plsek, 1998) offer insights into simple, complicated, and complex system changes. The first, simple changes, relate to activities that are recipe driven, such as baking a cake. The second, complicated changes, require coordination across teams all working on specific parts of a whole; such as sending a rocket to the moon. The third, complex system changes, is complex, such as raising a child. No child is ever the same; there is an interactive process between parent and child unfolding a unique relationship. In *Nursing, Caring, and Complexity Science* (Davidson, Ray, & Turkel, 2012) the authors make the case that humans are complex adaptive systems, living within complex adaptive organizations. Complexity is the norm. Complex, naturally adaptive systems create conditions for self-regulation through simple rules. This creates room for innovation.

The essence of professional caring is complex, multidimensional, and focused on who the nurse is (professional ethics, trust, personal character), what the nurse knows (cognitive, affective), what the nurse does (comfort, teaching, healing), and how the nurse acts in interactions with patients and families. The quality of that interaction has measured outcomes for quality, safety, satisfaction, and cost (Ray, 1981, 1984, 1989; Roach, 1992; Sherwood, 1991; Valentine, 1988, 1989, 1991, 1995; Wesorick, 1991). Standards of Caring (Wolf, Miller, & Freshwater, 2003) and Nurse Practice Acts for nine states serve as the foundation to promote professional role imperatives for each nurse's care accountability (O'Rourke, 2003, 2006; O'Rourke & White, 2011).

As a response to Kingston and Turkel's (2012) chapter on complexity science and administrative practice, D'Alfonso provides a framework for looking at caring leadership from the complexity science perspective. He presents a particularly useful chart to help reflect upon the self within caring leadership (D'Alfonso in Kingston & Turkel, 2012, p. 189, Figure 1). One way of expressing a unitary view of caring is to consider it as a synthesis of knowing, being, and doing. Alfonso gives examples of what one might consider in self-reflection: "Knowing in light of noble values" includes ideas such as integrate a vision of love, compassion, caring and wisdom, honor, authenticity of being and becoming in all relationships, communication, and leadership actions. Words related to "being" include resilient, curious, grateful, courageous, and knowledgeable, and words related to "doing" include protect the joy and spirit of others, lead by continuous living example, uphold excellence in stewardship of resources, and a climate of caring economics. Table 7.1 (Kingston & Turkel, 2012, pp. 192–193) is a great resource for providing a crosswalk of caring science concepts within sample leadership sources.

Caring Leadership in Practice: An Opportunity

There are opportunities to change the culture within organizations. One means for action is the pursuit of Magnet hospital designation. This is the highest honor that a hospital can earn and it recognizes excellence in nursing practice. Just 7% of hospitals hold this designation. Magnet-designated hospitals and those based in caring share similar patterns of excellence. The fact that more hospitals are seeking Magnet designation reflects a search for both quality and reputation. An increase in Magnet hospitals will accelerate the likelihood that there will also be evidence of increased caring in health care systems.

Magnet hospital evaluation processes use quantitative measures and "narrative stories" to provide evidence that the principles have been internalized by each practitioner and that they permeate the organizational culture. This evidence demonstrates that the organizing principles have been internalized substantively rather than merely superficially. The Magnet designation focuses on transformational leadership, structural environment, exemplary professional practice, new knowledge, innovation and improvements, and empirical quality results (American Nurses Credentialing Center, 2012).

Both Magnet designation and a caring-based framework for professional practice focus on the lived experience between the nurse and the patient. Both use similar evaluative criteria focused on the structure, process, and outcome of the care experience and each recognizes nursing as a discipline and a profession. As a discipline, nursing requires a breadth and depth of knowledge from human, aesthetic, and scientific domains. As a profession, nursing requires standards, ethics, and accountability to the public as a social contract and covenant. It is this imperative that compels nursing leaders to act in advancing caring within health care systems and practice settings. An increase in magnetism and caring would fulfill a promise to the public and create practice environments that permit "caring as the central and unique focus of nursing" (Leininger, 1981, Foreword) to flourish.

A story for reflection:

> A leader committed to caring as a principle of care in her organization created a book with reflections and pictures and helped the team to ask questions such as:
>
> How might we empower our patients to maintain and regain control over their well-being and recuperation?
>
> How might we offer our patients a variety of ways to be comfortable, to be calmed, to relax, and to be in a better frame of mind?
>
> How might we create comfort and connection through relationships?
>
> How might we make it possible for the patient to pass with dignity, grace, and love? (Boller, 2005)

Readiness: Questions for Self-Reflection

Here are questions that health care leaders can ask themselves as part of consolidating readiness to contribute to transforming their health care system through living the model, Dance of Caring Persons.

> What are your beliefs about caring in your discipline (nursing, medicine, finance, and so on)?
>
> Where are you situated within the organization?
>
> Who else can you dialogue with about your ideas?
>
> Who can you enlist in discerning the importance of caring within your organization?
>
> How big, how small do you want to start?
>
> What energy will help you to succeed in bringing awareness to the organization?
>
> What is your sphere of influence? How might you grow it?
>
> What will you do with outspoken opposition to caring?

MOVING FROM STORY TO ACTION

To Raise Awareness, Build Knowledge, and Articulate Expectations

What might we consider as means to raise awareness about the substantive and significant nature of caring within health care organizations? The stories shared showed different ways to enter the work of transforming practice environments to focus on explicit valuing of caring. An essential step for large system change is to engage the leaders who manage the resources as committed champions to transforming the organization. Engaging the executive leaders is necessary but not sufficient. To be successful, caring must be integrated in all aspects of the system and practitioners must have the tools and resources to do their work of caring effectively.

Assessment of Current State and Future State Within an Organization

From the story-telling process within the boardroom and at the bedside, it might emerge that there is a difference between how caring is currently lived within the organization and how possibilities for living it differently might be created.

> Determining the scope and methods for engaging in change is essential. What will be the scope of the work moving forward and how will the work get done, by whom, and in what time frame with what resources?

Will the commitment to caring transformation happen throughout the organization at once? Or will it start in a smaller venue and then have lessons learned spread throughout?

How is decision making and communication conducted within the organization now? What aspects of those current systems can further the work? What else might be needed? Do new structures or processes need to be developed?

These are important questions to consider so that resources can be properly aligned to move the work forward. Though the results of the caring transformation process will be incorporated into daily work moving forward, the process of change takes dedicated time and resources to make adoption possible. What resources are available?

Starting the Process of Change: Different Organizational Entry Points

1. Engage all senior leaders and have each commit their time, talent, and budget to moving the change throughout their functional areas. Cascade the engagement of the next level of managers within each functional area, to the level of the direct caregiver. Coordination within each functional area occurs vertically within the functional area and coordination happens at the top. This is often called siloed communication, the loyalty and measures of success are within a narrow area of expertise rather than across functions. The integration across functions happens with the leaders of those areas—not across each level of the organization.
2. From the beginning, appoint a steering committee that has representatives from across functional areas and across levels of responsibility—from direct care responsibility to executive-level sponsorship. Each representative then becomes the champion for their peer group. This is often referred to as integrated or horizontal organizational structure, which is a beautiful fit with Dance of Caring Persons.
3. Consider a hybrid model, which has both vertical and horizontal representation in multiple task forces that report to a large cross-sectional steering committee.
4. The champions for the change have to determine what the processes are within their organization, and whether or not this project can use those communication and decision-making bodies or if a new structure is called for.

WHERE TO START?

Aspects to Consider in the Assessment Process

How is the organization currently structured related to decision making, priority setting, and reward systems? This requires an assessment of the current structure, processes, decision-making forums, and communication methods.

A vision for the future that is understandable to all within the organization helps to secure leadership and staff commitment. What is the reason for the change from current practice, what is the personal motivation for changing, and why now? Review the organizational chart, patterns of communication, formal and informal network of opinion leaders as historical data to inform how work currently gets done within the organization. Is there a strong hierarchical model, a distributed model of decision making, shared decision making, shared governance, unit-based council structures? Where can you generate energy for the ideas of caring practice?

Every organization has its own culture, history, and norms. Within your organization what are the "rules" for success, what are the things that are "not done here"? How has your organization dealt with ideas related to humanizing the practice environment? What about those efforts that went well? What about those efforts that became problematic? What can you learn from that history?

The success of prior change efforts will have a direct effect on the willingness of sponsors and staff to engage in a new change effort. If many ideas were tried and it is perceived that "they didn't work" or were a "waste of time," the likelihood for engagement and adoption of this initiative will experience more challenges. Conversely, if the organization has experienced success, then understanding what contributed to that success can aid the planning for this initiative. Setting clear areas of focus (priorities) will help structure this effort for success. Setting up forums for sponsors of the work and those most affected by the change process on a daily basis need to be held to review progression of the efforts. These forums help to sustain engagement and foster expectations about how to stay "on track" with the desired outcomes for this project.

Within any organization there are limited time and resources for carrying out the work. There are always competing priorities. So how might competing priorities for time and resources become reconciled?

STORY ABOUT INTEGRATING PRIORITIES TO MOVE FORWARD WITH A SHARED VISION

The patient care department of a hospital wanted to move forward with pursuit of Magnet status designation. The executive leader believed that caring could serve as a theoretical foundation for the work. Several patient care leaders within that unit also agreed with that point of view and moved forward with inviting participation into a Magnet planning group from the nursing bedside staff. The hospital organization was also very engaged with broader initiatives related to patient safety, interprofessional team communication, clinical documentation system adoption, accreditation requirements, and service delivery improvements. How might these be reconciled? For the staff at the bedside, if caring was seen as "one more thing" and "the flavor of the month," the initiative would not reach its intended purpose, which was to provide a substantive body of knowledge as the foundation of patient care interactions within the hospital. A steering committee was formed with the executive leader as the sponsor of the group. Champions for the initiative included leaders who held different roles (staff nurse, manager, director, aide, physician, financial manager, and others). Over the course of several meetings all of the existing initiatives were mapped and cross-referenced to the Magnet hospital expectations. Once this "cross-walk" was completed, a visual model was developed that helped to "show" the integration. Unit-level discussions were held with the staff responsible for direct patient care (nurses, pharmacists, and others) to ascertain what mattered most to the staff relative to interactions with patients. This helped the "story" emerge about caring. The next step was to link the lived experiences of the nurse/patient story with substantive knowledge about caring science. The requirements for Magnet and the operational expectations related to other initiatives were then aligned. For each initiative a story could be told about what mattered most to a patient and how the many initiatives were linked in order to improve the patient care experience for the patient and the family and for those providing the care.

For initiatives related to hand washing, fall risk prevention, discharge planning, continuity of care, and pain management, it was determined that what mattered most to patients when in the hospital is that they are safe and that they become known as person.

Leah Curtin, former editor of the *American Journal of Nursing*, used to talk about "marketing at the bedside"—that is, the nurse would practice out loud to inform the patient about the nursing role. A similar practicing out loud can occur to convey caring practice.

Good morning, Mrs. Smith, I see that this is your first day after surgery for kidney stones. I am your nurse for the next 8 hours, my job is to detect and monitor subtle changes in your condition important to your recovery, provide for your medications and treatment, coordinate your care with other members of the team, assure your comfort and safety, and help you to become ready to return home. I'm interested in understanding what is most important to you today. As you anticipate the day, what matters most to you today? With your permission, I am going to write this on your communication board so that all staff members can understand your goal for the day.

There will be several members of the team working with me today, their names are listed here; you reach us by pressing this call button. We are all committed to your health—that's why we wash our hands when we come into and out of the room, and why we urge you to use the call bell for any needs that you have. Your well-being is essential and we are vigilant about making sure that you don't experience a fall by getting up unassisted. Keeping you comfortable and pain free is our goal, so we will be offering you pain medication regularly and please don't hesitate to tell us about your pain, should it increase.

This illustration is not meant to be a script. It is an example of intentions that are present when with the patient and that convey knowledge while providing direct care. It is "caring out loud" and could help to build an authentic presence with the patient. Likely such explicit articulation of intent and expectations took no more time than could have been used while performing a task without conversation or with a less purposeful intentional interaction. Professional vigilance by the nurse conveys who the nurse is, what is known, and how that is expressed in nursing situations with the well-being of the patient in mind.

As part of the Magnet program, clinical rounds were focused on knowing "this patient's story." The staff submitted these stories as exemplars of their practice. The stories were then shared and celebrated in various forums.

Establishment of a Steering Committee

Each organizational culture has its own processes for moving work across and through the organization. For some organizations there are established methods for obtaining an executive sponsor for a change, identifying key stakeholders, having identified champions for the change, agents/ambassadors for the change, and the frontline adopters of the expected change.

It is recommended that the structure in which the work of the project will occur be identified in advance. For example, is there to be a cross-sectional steering committee that represents different functions within the organization and people working at different levels in the organization?

Where does decision-making authority lie—for what parts of the project?

The *Collaboration Handbook: Creating, Sustaining and Enjoying the Journey* published by the Amherst Wilder Foundation (Winer & Ray, 1994) helps groups forming for collective work to discern if it is coordination, cooperation, or collaboration in which the group is engaged. The distinction is the degree to which each party is letting go of its "own" exclusive point of view and entering into a shared vision and plan of action. Though this handbook is directed toward community collaboration, the principles and flow of relationship are illustrative of the work of teams in complex organizations seeking guidance and insight for working together for collective change:

Step 1: Envision results by working Individual to Individual—enhancing trust, confirming the vision, and specifying desired results is the work.
Step 2: Empower ourselves by working Individual to Organization—the work in this phase is to confirm organization roles, resolve conflicts, organize the effort, and support the members.

Step 3: Ensure results by working organization to organization—the work in this phase is to manage the work, create and join systems, appraise the results, and renew the effort.

Step 4: Endow continuity by working collaboration to community—the work is to create visibility, involve the community, change the system.

The Role of Sponsors

The sponsor is the person within the organization who has the authority to say "yes" to changes within the unit of interest. The sponsor helps to focus attention. There are many distracters and much "extraneous" noise within an organization. If the sponsor keeps attention on what matters most related to caring, practice will gain momentum. The sponsor along with other members of the steering committee sets the direction and steps for action. They create energy to move toward the desired state in the future, appraising success of milestones along the way. If it is a single unit, then the manager of the unit can be the sponsor of a change. If the unit is across the whole enterprise (multiple units), then the sponsor has to have the authority across the units of concern. Each level of the organization has to have a representative sponsor. For a single unit change, a clinical leader would also need to be part of moving the initiative forward. The sponsors have to be committed to shepherding the process. If caring practice is a "good idea" with no follow-through, then it will neither grow nor be sustained. The sponsor may voice a belief that caring is important and then expect each practitioner to go "live it." Without reinforcement it will not live in the organization. It might live within individuals but not be evident as a substantive commitment to how practice is lived. There are critical moments in the phases of a change process. One example of this would be when a key sponsor leaves. If there had been a strong network built at all levels across the organization, that vacancy may be managed. If not, the project might need to be defined and moved to a smaller unit of service within the organization that can sustain the intentions of the project. If an organization-wide initiative cannot be sustained, perhaps focusing on the medical/surgical units can be sustained because of the network of support. Sometimes people within the direct-care positions have so much commitment to caring practices that they help keep the energy and commitment strong even during times of changing leadership.

Here are suggestions for helping the organization build its capacity for change:

Dialogue about the desired state together and identify your own point of view and what you imagine might be others' points of view that could affect moving forward. Look for serendipity—are there others who are committed to a similar path and could join with your efforts to move the initiative further faster? For example, is there a patient advisory council within the organization that could be part of designing actions for the future. Can you reinforce each other's beliefs and intentions for the future? What about personalized medical care—are there members of the medical staff for whom caring and connection have added value? Each member of the steering committee has a specific and defined role, be clear with one another about what is expected, and in what timeline.

Clinician leaders are essential for any practice change process to be adopted. Identifying the informal opinion leaders is critical to having others see that the desired change could be a "good thing." Someone who has the respect of peers and can communicate ideas and a vision for the future helps to capture the imagination and spirit of others. These clinician leaders can often speak about "both/and" tensions present when moving toward something new. They are the persons who simultaneously speak the truth of hard work and the reward for attempting something new.

Each person experiences and commits to a personal change process. It is in the end a personal commitment. So determining what matters to the person(s) you are trying to enlist in a change process is essential. It is not about what you believe and your efforts to convince others to believe as you do. It is about what another believes and how those beliefs intersect around a common commitment. Any individual will have an internal monitor and a historical record of his or her experience with change processes. It will show up, and it is part of the process. Open discussion about this between people committing to a change together can build trust and energy to work together.

Steering Committee Charter

Formalizing the work of the steering committee through a charter will help to organize the effort and formalize roles, responsibilities, and timelines. This is also where the initial steps and directions of the project are developed and the necessary budget determined. The charter represents the agreement between the larger organization and this committee relative to its purpose and plan. Issues and questions addressed at the steering committee level include the following:

> Purpose of group: Mission
>> Scope of work: Boundaries
>> Expected products: Deliverables
>> Membership
>> Designated leadership roles (chair, alternate chair, minute taker, and so on)
>> Required processes for reviews and approvals
>> Authority for staffing and spending for project
>> Criteria for success—how will it be measured, required reports
>> Monitoring progress toward defined activities, who, how, when, timeline
>> Linkages with other communication decision groups within the organization (how, how often)
>> Valuing and appraising success:
>>> If this initiative is a success, how do staff feel, think, or act differently today than before
>>> If this initiative is a success, how does it affect current measurements related to cost, quality, and satisfaction for the organization as a whole (Martin & Tate, 1997)

Initial Work of the Steering Committee

There are many ways to approach the initial work of the steering committee. Wesorick (2002) outlined her approach for the essential elements to consider in the development of professional practice that is substantively based on principles of caring:

> Shared purpose (vision/engagement)
> Dialogue (team communications)
> Partnering (team interactions)
> Network councils (engagement infrastructure)
> Individual competency (practice, workflow, outcomes)
> Integrated competency (practice, workflow, outcomes)
> Evidence-based (practice, outcomes, tools)
> Scope of practice (roles, workflow, integration)
> Clinical tools, paper/technology (practice, workflow)

Wesorick (2002) and colleagues through the Clinical Practice Model Resource Center (CPMRC, 2012), developed a complete consultation practice that helped organizations assess their current work environment and clinical tools that documented patient care interactions and then systematically moved the organization forward to a state of interprofessional practice ready to adopt electronic tools for clinical documentation (Hanson, 2011; Mason & Wesorick, 2011; Wesorick et al., 1998; Wesorick & Fairfield, 2009; Westmoreland, Wesorick, Hanson, & Wyngard, 2004). The process first involved having interprofessional teams understand and appreciate disciplinary scope of practice, dialogue about that across disciplines, and then apply insights gained to redesign patient care in a way to more fully reflect the kind of care the team desired to provide and the care patients and families expect to receive. The coaching for this transformational process was quite extensive and involved engagement with staff throughout the organization to build capacity for understanding and adopting new practice patterns. This work has now transitioned to the CPM Framework™ and an International Consortium that shares experiences gained in the application of the model in sustainable health care transformation. Within the framework core beliefs, principles, and theories inform six models: health and healing care, partnership culture, interdisciplinary integration, health informatics, and applied evidence-based practice. At the core is the patient, family, community, and caregiver. The CPM Framework has been developed and refined since 1983 and represents an integrated approach to transformational change based on caring (retrieved October 6, 2012, www.CPMRC.com/framework/overview).

Examples from outside of health care are offered by the the Drucker Foundation for nonprofit organizations (1999). They provide a framework for assessment of readiness through asking the following questions:

1. What is our mission?
2. What are our challenges?
3. What are our opportunities?
4. Do we need to revisit the mission?
5. Who is our primary customer?
6. Who are our supporting customers?
7. How will our customer change?
8. What do we believe our primary and supporting customers value?
9. What knowledge do we need to gain from our customer?
10. How will I participate in gaining this knowledge?
11. What are our results?
12. How do we define results?
13. Are we successful?
14. How should we define results?
15. What must we strengthen or abandon?
16. What is our plan?

These questions are asked so that members of the steering committee can be attentive to what matters most. What in the end do we want to be remembered for? The mission transcends today and yet informs what needs to be done today. Answering these questions provides a framework for setting goals and mobilizing resources to get the right things done. Setting the scope of the project emphasizes the importance of knowledge, analysis, courage, experience, and intuition. Planning "doesn't substitute facts for judgment nor science for leadership" (Drucker, 1999, p. 52). Leadership is what makes planning effective. The Drucker Foundation lists elements of effective plans as follows:

1. Abandonment—if we were not in this today, would we choose to do this?
2. Concentration—strengthening what *does* work—what you pay attention to.

3. Innovation—diversity that stirs the imagination—what would the innovation require? Is it what our customers value? How can we make a difference?
4. Risk taking—short-term/long-term reasoned risk—bold risk benefits and costs.
5. Analysis—what don't we know—how might we get information to inform us about what we don't know about 1 to 4 above.
6. Appraisal—how we know that results have been achieved.

A plan begins with a mission and ends with action steps and budget. Action steps establish accountability for objectives—who will do what, by when. Action steps are developed by the people who will carry them out—those closest to the action. The more people are involved and understand the direction, the more committed they are to act.

Throughout the work of the steering committee, facilitative leadership styles help to move the work forward through tapping the power of participation: Principles of facilitative leadership as defined by Interaction Associates (1997) include the following:

1. Sharing an inspiring vision
2. Celebrate accomplishment
3. Coach for performance
4. Facilitate agreement
5. Design pathways to action
6. Seek maximum appropriate involvement
7. Focus on the result through both process and relationship

These concepts are echoed by Plsek (2003, p. 12) related to change and innovation in complex health care organizations. He notes five key elements within an organizational context impact receptivity for change:

1. The nature of relationships—how they are built and maintained
2. The nature of decision making—how it is done and by whom
3. The nature of power and how it is acquired and used
4. The nature of conflicts: How do they arise and what are the common forms of dealing with them
5. The importance placed on individual or collective learning

The facilitative leadership process and innovative change are consistent with caring leadership and moving the work forward.

Resources for Getting Ready

One component of building awareness could involve providing the steering committee with literature about caring science. Review of the organizational chart, patterns of communication, and formal and informal networks of opinion leaders also provides valuable information. Other resources available to help with this assessment process include websites and consulting companies. A list of resources to facilitate the process of readiness is provided in the Resources section of this book. This list should not be considered exhaustive, but it will help you get started in building knowledge needed to support the transformation of your health care system based on the Dance of Caring Persons model. Whatever is decided will take preparation, commitment, effort, and resources. Intentional change requires stewardship.

REFERENCES

American Nurses Credentialing Center. (2012). *Forces of magnetism.* Retrieved from http://nursecredentialing.org/Magnet/ProgramOverview/ForcesofMagnetism.aspx

Boller, J. (2005). *Daily miracles.* Author.

Boykin, A., & Schoenhofer, S. O. (2001). *Nursing as caring: A model for transforming practice* (2nd ed.). Sudbury, MA: Jones & Bartlett.

Campbell, J., Moyers, B. D., & Flowers, B. S. (Eds.). (1988). The *power of myth.* New York, NY: Doubleday.

CPMRC. (2012). *CPM framework.* Grand Rapids, MI: Author. Retrieved from http://www.CPMRC.com

Creative Health Care Management. (2012). *Phases of transformational change: "I2E2."* Retrieved October 2012 from http://chcm.com

D'Alfonso, J. (2012). Caring science and complexity science guiding the practice of hospital and nursing administration practice. In A. Davidson, M. A. Ray, & M. C. Turkel (Eds.), *Nursing, caring, and complexity science: For human environment well-being* (pp. 186–198). New York, NY: Springer Publishing Company.

Davidson, A. W., Ray, M. A., & Turkel, M. C. (2011). *Nursing, caring, and complexity science: For human-environment well-being.* New York, NY: Springer Publishing Company.

Drucker, P. (1999). *The Drucker Foundation self-assessment tool: Participant workbook.* New York, NY: Jossey-Bass. The Drucker Foundation. Retrieved from http://www.pfdf.org

Glouberman, S., & Zimmerman, B. J. (2002). Complicated and complex systems: What would successful reform to Medicare look like? Discussion paper #8, *Commission on the Future of Healthcare in Canada.* July 2002.

Hanson, D. (2011). Evidence-based practice and technology. In M. J. Ball et al. (Eds.). *Nursing informatics: Where caring and technology meet* (4th ed.). New York, NY: Springer Publishing Company.

Hiatt, J. (2006). *ADKAR: A model for change in business, government and our community.* Prosci retrieved from http://www.change-management.com/adkar-book.htm dkar-ISBN-10: 1930885504

Implementation Management Associates. (2010). *Leading people through business changes: Fundamentals of the Accelerating Implementation Methodology (AIM).* Retrieved October 6, 2012, from http://www.imaworldwide.com/Portals/135807/docs/leadingpeoplethrough businesschanges0210_v3.pdf

Interaction Associates. (1997). *Facilitative leadership: Tapping the power of participation.* Boston, MA: Author.

Joint Commission. (n.d.). *Sentinel event data: Root causes by event type. 2004–Third Quarter 2011.* Author. Retrieved from http://www.jointcommission.org/assets/1/18/root_causes_event_type_2004–3q2011.pdf

Kelley, T., Littman, J., & Peters, T. (2001). *The art of innovation: Lessons in creativity from IDEO, America's leading design firm.* New York, NY: Doubleday Business.

Kingston, M. B., & Turkel, M. B. (2012). Caring science and complexity science guiding the practice of hospital and nursing administration practice. In A. W. Davidson, M. A. Ray, & M. C. Turkel (Eds.), *Nursing, caring, and complexity science: For human-environment wellbeing* (pp. 169–198). New York, NY: Springer Publishing Company.

Leininger, M. M. (1981). *Caring, an essential human need. Proceedings of the three national caring conferences.* Detroit, MI: Wayne State University Press.

Martin, P., & Tate, K. (1997). *Project management memory jogger.* GOAL/QPC Salem, NH.

Mason, J., &Wesorick, B. (2011). Successful transformation of a nursing culture. *Nurse Leader, 9*(2), 31–36.

O'Rourke, M. (2003). Rebuilding a professional practice model: The return of role-based accountability. *Nursing Administration Quartelry, 27*(2), 95–105.

O'Rourke, M., & White, A. (2011). Professional role clarity and competency in health care staffing—the missing pieces. *Nursing Economics, 29*(4), 183–184.

O'Rourke, M. W. (2006). Beyond rhetoric to role accountability: A practical and professional model of practice. *Nurse Leader, 4*(3), 28–33.

Patel, E., Nutt, S. L., Qureshi, I., Lister, S., Panesar, S. S., & Carson-Stevens, A. (2012). Leading change in health-care quality with the Institute for Healthcare Improvement Open School. *British Journal of Hospital Medicine, 73*(7), 397–400.

Plsek, P. (1997). *Creativity, innovation and quality.* Milwaukee, WI: Quality Press.

Plsek, P. (2003). *Complexity and the adoption of innovation in health care.* Paper presented January 27–28, National Institute for Health Care Management Foundation, Washington, DC.

Ray, M. A. (1981). A philosophical analysis of caring within nursing. In M. M. Leininger (Ed.), *Caring, an essential human need* (pp. 25–36). New York, NY: National League for Nursing.

Ray, M. A. (1984). The development of a classification system of institutional caring. In M. M. Leininger (Ed.), *Caring, the essence of nursing and health* (pp. 95–112). New York, NY: National League for Nursing.

Ray, M. A. (1989). The theory of bureaucratic caring for nursing practice in the organizational culture. *Nursing Administration Quarterly, 13*(2), 31–42.

Roach, M. S. (1992). *The human act of caring: A blueprint for the health professions* (Rev. ed.). Ottawa, ON: Canadian Hospital Assn.

Rogers, E. M. (2003). *Diffusion of innovations* (5th ed.). New York, NY: Free Press.

Rutherford, P., Philips, J., Coughlan, P., Lee, B., Moen, R., Peck, C., & Taylor, J. (2008). *Transforming care at the bedside how-to guide: Engaging front-line staff in innovation and quality improvement.* Cambridge, MA: Institute for Healthcare Improvement. Retrieved from http://www.IHI.org

Sherwood, G. (1991). Expressions of nurses' caring: The role of the compassionate healer. In D. A. Gaut & M. M. Leininger (Ed.), *Caring, the compassionate healer* (pp. 79–88). New York, NY: National League for Nursing.

Valentine, K. (1988). History, analysis and application of the carative tradition in health and nursing. *Journal of the New York State Nursing Association, 19*(4), 2–8.

Valentine, K. (1989). Caring is more than kindness: Modeling its complexities. *Journal of Nursing Administration, 19*(11), 28–35.

Valentine, K. (1991). Nurse/patient caring: Challenging our conventional wisdom. In D. A. Gaut (Ed.), *Caring: The compassionate healer* (pp. 99–113). New York, NY: National League for Nursing.

Valentine, K. (1995). Values, vision, and action: Creating a care-focused nursing practice environment. In M. Leininger (Ed.), *Power, politics, public policy: A matter of caring* (pp. 99–115). New York, NY: National League for Nursing.

Wesorick, B. (1991). Creating an environment in the hospital setting that supports caring via a Clinical Practice Model (CPM). In D. A. Gaut & M. M. Leininger (Eds.), *Caring, the compassionate healer* (pp. 135–160). New York, NY: National League for Nursing.

Wesorick, B. (2002). 21st century leadership challenge: Creating and sustaining healthy, healing work cultures and integrated service at the point of care. *Nursing Administration Quarterly, 26*(5), 18–32.

Wesorick, B. (2004). A leadership story about caring. *Nursing Administration Quarterly, 28*(4), 271–275.

Wesorick, B., & Fairfield, C. (2009). Leading implementation of technology to transform practice at the point-of-care. In N. Rollins Gantz (Ed.), *101 global leadership lessons for nurses: Shared legacies from leaders and their mentors.* Indianapolis, IN: Sigma Theta Tau International.

Wesorick, B., Shiparski, L., Wyngarden, K., & Troseth, M. (1998). *Partnership council field book: Strategies and tools for co-creating a healthy work place.* Grand Rapids, MI: Practice Field Publishing.

Westmoreland, D., Wesorick, B., Hanson, D., & Wyngarden, K. (2000). Consensual validation of clinical practice model practice guidelines. *Journal of Nursing Care Quality, 14*(4), 16–27.

Wheatley, M. (2006). *Leadership and the new science: Learning about organizations from an orderly universe* (3rd ed.). San Francisco, CA: Berrett-Koehler.

Winer, M. B., & Ray, K. (1994). *Collaboration handbook: Creating, sustaining and enjoying the journey.* St. Paul, MN: Amherst H. Wilder Foundation.

Wolf, Z. R., Miller, M., & Freshwater, D. (2003). A standard of care for caring: A Delphi study. *International Journal for Human Caring, 7*(1), 34–42.

Zimmerman, B., Lindberg, C., & Plsek, P. (1998). *Edgeware: Insights from complexity science for health-care leaders.* Irving, TX: VHA.

Response to Chapter 4

Nancy Hilton, MN, RN, NEA-BC
Chief Nursing Officer
St. Lucie Medical Center

*I*n reading this chapter of getting ready to embark on a large health care transformation, there are so many memories from the past 6 years that jump out at me. I believe I was invited to write the response to this chapter because I lived this exact transformation of enculturating an organization into a caring-based practice. Only several times during one's professional career do all the stars align to set the stage for an almost perfect transformation. I was lucky enough to have the lead role in the following story.

The first question I want to answer is whether it is valuable to frame the practice of nursing around the theory "Nursing as Caring." Six years later, the answer is an emphatic Yes! In 2006, our Nursing Professional Practice Council was charged with selecting a nursing theory for our Magnet journey. There was a definite advantage to selecting the Nursing as Caring theory: (a) we were a "caring" nursing organization; (b) Dr. Anne Boykin practically lived in our backyard; and (c) we had many Florida Atlantic University RNs and nursing students working in our hospital. Once the decision was made, Dr. Boykin started working with the nursing leaders and the staff nurses through her *caring dialogues,* teaching us how to care for self and using direct invitation to hear the "calls for nursing." Over the next year, we developed our nursing philosophy and principles, modified nursing orientation, and shared our exquisite stories utilizing the eight ingredients of caring. I was asked to present the practical side of this theory at the International Association of Human Caring Conference with Dr. Boykin and later pursued a research study utilizing the Nursing as Caring theory.

The second question centers on the approach of spreading this theory hospital-wide. "How do you take a theory focused on nursing and engage the other executives?" I knew from experience that nursing alone could not execute this hospital-wide transformation. In 2008, Hospital Consumer Assessment of Health Providers and Systems (HCAHPS) was a hot topic, and I believe we were three steps ahead of most hospitals because we selected the right theoretical framework. The problem was, how do you entice other ancillary departments to embrace a theory with the word nursing in it? The other staff didn't feel connected, yet they wanted to be a part of this strong movement.

The section in this chapter outlining the seven steps for a nurse leader to make caring visible within an organization is a very pertinent strategy for this transformation. In order to get the chief executive officer (CEO) and other executives involved, I orchestrated a meeting with Dr. Boykin. She quickly reeled them in, and the executives were soon writing their own caring stories. During a regularly scheduled director meeting, the management team shared its stories. The most impactful story was told by the newly hired chief financial officer (CFO). The gossip started spreading that if a "bean counter" could display his caring for the family of a dying patient, so could everyone else. The third step was to design details for the general pattern of the Dance of Caring Persons. This was accomplished on May 8, 2008. The emergency department director had a vision of how we could explain the dance to employees, physicians, volunteers, patients, families, and our community. He wanted an eternal image on the minds of all long after the event had actually occurred. Imagine over 600 people, a fire truck, and an ambulance connected and holding hands while circling the hospital. With Dr. Boykin on my right hand and my family on my left, a helicopter approached at 4:30 p.m. to forever capture the perfect Dance of Caring Persons.

The last steps of establishing broad structures and processes have been accomplished through bedside shift report, intentional hourly rounding, and the use of care boards. We selected these nursing processes because they have a significant impact on promoting a strong caring relationship between the nurse and the patient. It is critical to have your organization grounded in a caring theory or philosophy. Many organizations look to scripting to be the answer to improving the patient experience. This strategy will only work if the staff members know how to care for self and for their patients. We also value caring by sharing caring moment stories at the beginning of every meeting. There is no doubt that the last step is the most difficult and the least energizing—sustaining the caring commitment.

As the authors state, a critical step to getting ready for this transformation is engaging in activities to enhance knowing self as caring person. This is not an easy concept to wrap your arms around. We started to build this knowledge with the nurses. They were involved in caring dialogues. During Nurses Week in 2008, our Nursing Professional Development Council utilized our Nursing as Caring theory as our theme for all the activities. A classroom was turned into a place to care for the nurses for a week. Also that year, nurses were nominated as best demonstrating the eight ingredients of caring. They were recognized at a red-carpet ceremony.

Next, we were ready to share our newfound knowledge with the ancillary departments. Several clinicians such as a respiratory therapist and a dietitian were asked to share one of their caring stories, and the stories were captured on a DVD along with the nursing situations. By utilizing the eight ingredients of caring to share our stories with all of the staff, the Dance of Caring Persons became more real. The decision was made that nursing would utilize the Nursing as Caring theory and hospital-wide we coined the phrase *Culture of Caring* to refer to all of the caregivers. It really worked for us.

In the section labeled Caring and Leadership, there are several concepts that resonated for me. Because this caring journey is not easy, I had to look for partners along the way to build on these concepts. In 2010, I had the opportunity to build on our culture of caring with the Institute for Healthcare Improvement (IHI). We established a year-long project focused on enhancing the patient experience. Through the experts at IHI, we were able to combine the art of caring with the science of evidence-based practices. For example, we selected the process of bedside shift report. I teach bedside shift report in Nursing Orientation because I am so passionate about this process. The IHI was also instrumental in laying the foundation for establishing our Patient/Family Advisory Council (PFAC). I highly recommend every nursing leader research the feasibility of utilizing a group like the PFAC to guide your ongoing journey of commitment to caring.

In the section titled Moving from Story to Action, I want to highlight several concepts that I believe are critical to this type of large-scale transformation. First of all, the chief nursing officer (CNO), in my opinion, has to be the sponsor for this type of change process at a hospital. Enculturating an organization in Nursing as Caring has to start with the chief caregiver, and that is the CNO. This is one task that cannot be delegated. There needs to be other key stakeholders, but I guarantee this transformation will die on the vine if not led by the top nurse leader. Along with the sponsor, there needs to be a steering committee to lay the foundation of this transformation. We invited all four executives to be a part of our steering committee. We all had assignments. There was no freeloading allowed. Next, we selected six key directors, nursing and ancillary, to be part of the steering committee. This group needs to develop a charter and then outline key strategies and action items with deadlines and responsible parties. One thing the CEO and I knew from experience is that you have to have a significant transformation aligned with your vision. The two of us had developed the vision in 1999, and all major changes must be aligned or it quickly becomes a flavor of the month for the staff. In order to build the capacity for change, we established a multidisciplinary team of champions. Every clinical department in the hospital was represented. This group met monthly. In every change process, you need a tipping point and this group of champions allowed us to reach this point as well as represent the Dance of Caring Persons every time we had a meeting because the chairs formed a circle.

There is one statement in this chapter that probably resonates with me more than any other single sentence. "Clinician leaders are essential for any practice change process to be adopted." In addition to Dr. Boykin being the Dean at Florida Atlantic University (FAU), I had partnered with the university to develop the role of the Clinical Nurse Leader (CNL) at my hospital. These CNLs had been immersed in Nursing as Caring for 2 years. The CNLs were the nurse clinician leaders setting the stage for these nursing process changes. Two of the CNLs developed bedside shift report for their capstone project including the use of Nursing as Caring as the framework. I could not have asked for better partners than the CNLs.

Toward the end of the chapter, there is a reference to the Drucker Foundation and the elements of effective plans. As a leadership team, it is crucial that you return to your plans every 6 months, and take an honest look at how you are doing. Are we reaching our intended goals or are we off track? I knew we were not going to abandon our journey so the next step is to ascertain how we strengthen what does work. I was asked by our corporate leadership to describe to other hospitals how we strategized this transformation. One of the keys at all levels of our organization is rounding. After a year, we developed a diagram for every employee to visualize his or her involvement in rounding. Once again, I was able to tie this image to our Dance of Caring Persons. I had to allow for innovation within this model. Our ICU staff performs hospitality rounds the next day after patients are transferred to another department. Our Orthopedic and Spine Institute staff initiated afternoon-tea rounding. Every department was charged with how we can make a difference to our patients and families. Every quarter, the steering committee analyzes our HCAHPS data, our verbatim comments, and feedback from our rounding audits. Then there is cause for celebration. Recognition needs to be both spontaneous and strategic.

I want to summarize by addressing a question raised in the text that I hear all day long: We don't have enough time and resources to implement this transformation, or there are too many conflicting priorities…My response is, you won't have a hospital in the future if you don't implement a transition focusing on caring. Everyone has to be invited to the Dance of Caring Persons. I had to make a personal commitment 6 years ago, and I still make that commitment every day. Intentional change of this magnitude does require stewardship from the CNO and the entire nursing management team.

Chapter 5

Gathering and Applying Resources:
Action Toward Practice Change

*T*he purpose of this chapter is to assist leaders located throughout organizational functions to understand how to move the vision of caring-based cultures forward. In Chapter 4, the focus was on raising awareness for the desire to develop a culture substantively based on human caring as well as to enlist leadership sponsors throughout the organization. In this chapter, we focus on the "how" of taking action within organizations and at the unit level—the "getting set" phase of planning and resource acquisition.

The fundamental question in this chapter is how do we do this work together to intentionally actualize a vision for a health care system grounded in caring? How do we structure ourselves for achieving and sustaining success in a way that matters most to those we care for and that is lifegiving to those providing care? What processes and structures do we put in place to develop and guide our behavior, knowledge, and actions based on the values explicit in the Dance of Caring Persons? The spirit evident at the end of "getting set" is widespread confidence that there are resources and support for moving forward with the commitment to an intentional change process.

Earlier, we outlined five phases in a change process. The first two phases are about "getting ready" to embark on the journey of moving the culture toward caring as a dominant value. The last three phases are about "getting set" and "going." This chapter focuses on preparing persons to adopt the change, creating a culture that reinforces and motivates persons toward sustaining that change and continually providing the opportunity to grow in caring.

As detailed in Chapter 4, we have organized the phases of this change process as follows:

1. Create awareness
2. Build knowledge and articulate expectations
3. Prepare the first adopters, increase the desire for change
4. Enable and motivate all users
5. Build proficiency and reinforce skill

IMPLEMENTING CHANGE

When considering how to move forward, we need to be clear on the dimension of the change process that is the immediate focus, to whom it is directed, the purpose for the particular phase of the change process, the period of time needed, and an understanding of the tools and resources needed and the source of them. This is the "alternating rhythm" between broad goals and focus within the organization and specific unit-level goals. The work of this phase of change can be related to Swanson's (2010) Level III domain of caring, conditions that enhance or diminish the likelihood that caring will occur. The information and insight gained through considering these issues about actualizing the desired change will determine how to organize department-level councils for action.

The work of these department-level councils is to lead the action steps at the unit level. In order to do that, roles and responsibilities for carrying out agreed-upon activities will need to be determined and defined. Clarity of responsibility helps to grow the confidence of unit members to take risks and tolerate ambiguity as new behaviors and actions are tried. This phase of the process relates to Roach's (2002) attributes of caring, competence, and confidence, and to Swanson's (2010) Level IV caring actions. How do we as a unit-level council carry out our work to enhance caring actions? During this phase, tools and resources need to be provided to the councils to learn basic project management, meeting skills, communication basics, and resources for leading change. In addition, the members need to explore tools and processes for breakthrough thinking, creativity, and innovation.

Consequences of this change process need to be valued and prized, corresponding with Swanson's (2010) Level V domain of caring. How many persons have been prepared to meet these new expectations? How do we know that? What are the persons describing that is different from their descriptions before the change process was initiated? What is the visible evidence that a culture of caring is growing? What are staff members, patients, and families saying, thinking, or feeling? Within the customary measures of success in the organization, what do measures of productivity, cost, satisfaction, or quality indicate related to desired changes?

MAKING THE COMMITMENT ACTIONABLE

Making the commitment actionable requires a number of preparatory actions.

1. Identifying the "first adopters" or ambassadors for change—who will help lead this phase peer to peer throughout the organization?

This involves selecting trusted opinion leaders from among the peer groups (charge nurse, patient care assistants, physicians, unit clerk, pharmacist, and so on) who are willing to engage in the process and serve as leaders of the effort.

2. Preparing the ambassadors with focused training, resources, and ongoing coaching.

Training involves both engagement of the spirit of creativity and meaning as well as analytic skills and change management processes. All the ways of knowing about and growing in caring are open to development, including ethical, empirical, aesthetic, personal, and practical knowing (Carper, 1978). Using the whole brain through both creative and analytic work processes adds momentum and energy to the progress of the initiative.

3. Translating these new perspectives into operational practices in a sustained fashion.

How does this new perspective link with existing initiatives and yet fundamentally change them to reflect a commitment to a culture of caring? What communication, symbols, rituals, and celebrations need to be present to signal an adoption of these principles?

Let us explore each of these three ideas and provide guidelines for moving the work forward.

IDENTIFYING AND SELECTING AMBASSADORS FOR CHANGE

We will proceed from the assumption that the change processes related to building a culture substantively based on caring practice spans multiple units of service within the organization. It may not span the entire organization, yet within the chosen span of influence, the thought leaders and sponsors have the authority to act within the unit. Though any one individual may choose to change the way he or she practices (and individual change will make a difference), our focus is on collective action across more than one unit of service. The principles can be applied to larger units of service or smaller ones. Our focus, for purposes of illustration, is an interprofessional patient care service within a hospital setting.

Our example involves a multiunit, interprofessional group interested in substantively increasing caring within the practices of the organization in this case, we are assuming a hospital. It could be any organization.

Inviting Participation: Identifying First Adopters

We assume that the sponsor group (described in Chapter 4) has determined that this is an initiative worthy of attention and support. In order to convey the commitment the organization is making to caring, who within that group will "tell the story," through what methods, to what audiences, over what period of time?

Within organizations, there is often a communication department whose staff is skilled in helping to answer those questions and craft messages that will inspire the hearts and minds of staff and invite them to engage in the journey. How this initiative appeals to logic, values, and emotions will help to connect with the relevance of this initiative to the daily work of the staff and will help to motivate and persuade engagement in the journey.

Ambassadors for Change

The group that will be the ambassadors of change will be guided by the sponsor group identified in Chapter 4. These ambassadors are closest to the work of patient care, they are trusted by their colleagues to represent the authentic concerns and aspirations of the day-to-day professional and to practice interactions with each other and with families and patients.

The ambassadors need not be the most "agreeable" to the proposed initiative, as healthy skepticism and constructive feedback helps to strengthen the ambassador group. Otherwise the effort could be viewed as a proxy for "management's latest new idea," and seen as inauthentic.

Inviting participation is both an invitation to specific persons and an open invitation to the entire staff. So the champion for the change, let us say this is the director of nursing, would talk with those who report directly, asking for the key opinion leaders within various roles and shifts within the affected units to be nominated. Then the champion would reach out personally to each of those persons and explain what the initiative is. The conversation might be something like this:

> Thank you, Mary, for making time to meet with me today. Robert, your manager, tells me that you make wonderful contributions to patient care within your unit. It seems that your coworkers listen to your ideas about how to get things done and enjoy working with you. That is leadership and I want to let you know how much I appreciate what you do every day to make a difference in the lives of our patients and families.
>
> As you know, health care is constantly changing, there are many different demands on our time and attention. We never want to lose focus on the caring relationship as core to the work that we do. To that end, a group from across the organization has become intrigued with how to make caring practices more visible within our day-to-day care for patients in a way that matters to patients and staff. We think that this is important because human-to-human interaction is the core of healing and health. We want to do whatever we can to enhance the caring quality of patient care experiences because it has been shown to make a difference in patients' well-being and satisfaction, and reduce complications that lead to rehospitalization. Now we want to extend that thinking and have a group of bedside providers help to strengthen or transform the possibility for caring to be more evident and substantive in our day-to-day work. It is the staff persons at the bedside who are experts in knowing what might be done.
>
> What are your thoughts about this? What, if anything, have you noticed about our way of being with patients and families? When we're at our best at Lincoln Hospital, what does it look and feel like? When we're not at our best, relative to caring, what does it look like and feel like?
>
> Our intention is to gather caring ambassadors from across different units, shifts, and roles to serve as thought partners, leaders, and champions to move this project forward. This is high priority for the senior leadership team and we will be providing time for you to meet with us about this work once a month for 2 hours. You'll be paid and your shift will be covered.
>
> We'll start out with a 2-day educational retreat together, to better clarify expectations, explain what resources are available, and offer coaching and support to help structure this initiative for success. We are starting this with a 1-year commitment, reviewing and refining our progress regularly. You are so important to the success of this initiative; might we count on you to join? Please think it over and get back to me within the week.

Department Council

The members selected through invitation, as illustrated above, can also be joined by members solicited at large through an announced invitation for members to join the Department Council. Open invitation combined with solicited membership can both grow diversity of viewpoints and tap the strength of acknowledged care-staff leadership.

The role of the Department Council is to provide consistency across unit-level work and serve as a forum to focus collective work plans, assess need for and secure access to organizational resources, define measures of success, identify opportunities for development, celebration, and methods for integrating the work of this council into ongoing operational initiatives.

Many units within hospitals have "dashboards" for cost, safety, quality, and satisfaction that are monitored on a monthly or quarterly basis and provide feedback to staff about core measures. This Department Council might identify ways that substantive changes related to caring practices could become a focus in those broader initiatives. For example, the "caring out loud" example detailed in Chapter 4 might be trialed by each of the units and feedback on the dashboard measures might be used to track any changes.

Perhaps there would be new measures that would be put on the dashboard—for example, communication boards (identifying staff, patients' goals for the day, discharge plan, contacts consistently accurate and up to date). The work of the Department Council involves identifying and integrating the caring initiative within current task forces, operations groups, committees, and so on, so that the work that is ongoing within the organization might be informed by how it relates to the primacy of caring.

Unit-Level Council

Essentially, all staff members on the unit are members of the unit-level council. Each has a voice in determining the progress toward the initiatives, issues, concerns, actions. Shared decision making happens within the department or cross-unit council. Each person on the unit needs to have a two-way mechanism for knowing about and contributing to the work of the Department Council. This can happen through multiple means of communication, such as phone-trees, listservs, or a buddy system for sharing information.

The idea is to make certain that each person on the unit is engaged in the work of the caring initiative. Simply posting minutes of Department Council meetings does not engender the two-way conversation, idea generation, or critique necessary to truly make changes that each person adopts within the unit. Authentic listening to each person's point of view is a key principle in creating a culture for caring.

Preparing the Ambassadors With Focused Training, Resources, and Ongoing Coaching: The Focus of Work

Caring includes who we are, what we know, and how we put that into action in interactions with others toward enhancing their well-being. The quality of that interaction has implications for cost, quality, and satisfaction. The degree to which caring is experienced is affected by structural aspects of the environment (resources available, technology, staff), and philosophical beliefs related to spirituality, ethics, and trust (Valentine, 1989, 2013). The attributes of the nurse (or care provider)—professional vigilance, knowledge (affective and cognitive)—make a difference in the caring relationship with patients and families. The focus of substantive changes in caring relationships might occur at different places in different organizations—it depends on the "call" toward what matters most.

Creating a Culture of Continuous Learning

The Institute of Medicine report, *Best Care at Lower Cost: The Path to Continuously Learning Health Care in America* (Smith, Saunders, Stuckhardt, & McGinnis, 2012), addresses the complexities of health care today and their impact on culture. The vision expressed in this report focuses on "achieving a learning health care system—one in which science and informatics, patient–clinician partnerships, incentives, and culture are aligned to promote and enable continuous and real-time improvement in both the effectiveness and efficiency of care" (p. S-11). It calls for a culture of teamwork, collaboration, and adaptability in support of continuous learning.

Consider these questions:

- How do we currently promote a culture of continuous learning within our organization?
- In what ways can caring science become paired with that current structure or process?
- How might we:
  - Transform our beliefs about persons and hierarchies
  - Examine the whole versus parts
  - Value knowledge and expertise as lived by individual persons
  - Inspire the internal striving to care

○ Connect person to person
○ See abundance versus scarcity
○ Value caring as essential
○ Experience a sense of commitment to caring ideals and values

Pink (2006) authored *A Whole New Mind: Why Right-Brainers Will Rule the Future*. In it he makes the case that the machine metaphor for work within systems is outdated. Linear, sequential problem solving is necessary, but not sufficient for our societies to grow and advance as human beings. "The future belongs to a very different kind of person with a very different kind of mind-creators, empathizers, pattern recognizers, and meaning makers" (p. 1). Pink believes that we are moving toward a "Conceptual Age" that focuses on the big picture in inventive and empathic ways. In his point of view there are six aptitudes or "six senses" that are important to recognize and develop. These are design, story, symphony, empathy, play, and meaning:

Design—involves function, beauty, and emotional connection
Story—the ability to fashion a compelling narrative
Symphony—synthesis of parts into a whole
Empathy—understanding others from their point of view, relationships, and
    caring
Play—humor, games, lightheartedness, laughter
Meaning—purpose, transcendence, and spiritual fulfillment (pp. 65–67)

These aptitudes are linked to "high concept" (create beauty, detect patterns and opportunities, craft narrative, and combine seemingly unrelated ideas into a new invention; Pink, 2006). "High touch" fields of study and work—such as health care—involve the ability to empathize and engage in the subtle processes of human interaction. Then Pink discusses neuroscience, the structure of the brain and skills that can be employed to more fully develop right-hemisphere thinking combined with analytic skills.

These ideas are applied within nursing through the American Nurses Credentialing Center's Magnet Recognition Program that has resources and examples of developing professional practice environments (http://www.nursecredentialing.org/Magnet.aspx). The Magnet program focuses on the following:

• Transformational leadership
• Structural empowerment
• Exemplary professional practice
• New knowledge, innovation, and improvements
• Empirical quality improvements

Principles versus rules help create patterns that shape caring cultures and cultures of safety. Magnet hospital evaluation processes are pattern versus rule based, that is, excellence is discerned from patterns aggregated from individual practitioners rather than from prescriptive criteria. Magnet hospital evaluation processes are consistent with reframing the view of hospitals as complex adaptive systems and those designated as a Magnet hospital meet consumer expectations for quality, safety, and care. Caring science is based on multidimensional complex patterns aggregated from the lived experience of the nurse and we have research-based criteria for the practice work environment that shows measurably better patient outcomes (Aiken, Clarke, & Sloan, 2002) as well as improved staff recruitment and retention. It can be said that Magnet-designated hospitals and those based in caring share similar patterns of excellence and, therefore, an increase in Magnet hospitals will also increase caring in health care systems because it promotes living the vision of the actualized nurse authentically. Caring within nursing situations is accomplished through decentralization to the autonomous nurse and guided by principles, with patients at the center of the circle of concern. It helps promote "Nurturing of persons living caring and growing in caring...whole and complete in the moment" (Boykin & Schoenhofer, 2001, p. 11).

What follows is a story about the transformative process of a hospital, now a Magnet-designated hospital, during its early years of coming to a commitment to caring-based professional practice (Valentine, 1992). The dynamics of caring directly impact patient care. Over time, the leadership group, and then the staff came to articulate and value what it means to be human at a vulnerable moment wholly dependent on the trust of health care providers. The story is one in which intentional caring leadership helped to create a practice environment that staff and patients value. This is a glimpse into building a culture of caring that is sustained over time.

STORY OF PROFESSIONAL PRACTICE MODEL DEVELOPMENT WITH ONGOING TRAINING

A hospital in a rural area experienced a sudden and profound nursing shortage that caused the closure of beds for the first time in its history due to a lack of qualified staff. Experienced staff sought advantages for professional growth in more urban areas with better access to education and promotional opportunities. The replacement staff was inexperienced and lacked the mentoring and guidance necessary to develop expert clinical skills. The executive leadership team determined that major changes were in order to create a professional practice environment that would recruit and retain nursing and other patient care staff. A strategic plan with tactical actions, deadlines, and deliverables was developed and put into action. Caring served as a theoretical framework guiding nursing leadership toward a professional practice model. There were multiple dimensions to the plan:

1. Bring education degree-completion programs on site for place-bound staff.
2. Hire clinical nurse specialists to partner with unit-level nurse managers to serve as clinical mentors and to develop and guide standards of care.
3. Attract doctoral-level faculty to assist in mentoring staff and managers, offer continuing education programs that were marketed regionally to reattract experienced staff to the hospital. Engage in practice-based research.
4. Enlistment of physician staff as champions versus critics for novice nursing staff.
5. Human resource efforts to recruit and retain staff based on enriched market-based packages.

Throughout the timeline of this transformational change process, the nursing management team engaged in personal and professional development that helped them to lead the efforts guided by a lens of substantive caring. They wanted to know themselves more fully as caring persons and create the possibility for staff to do the same. They used a series of aesthetic, empirical, ethical, and personal ways of knowing to achieve this goal.

Vision. The education and management leaders gathered for a half-day retreat to consider the vision of the patient care services for the future. They were asked to visually create what they wanted the future of the organization to look like, feel like, be seen as, and known for by others. Using painting, drawing, and collage, two-person teams constructed 3-dimensional visions of the future. The story of these visions was then shared with other "creators of the future." A shared sense of knowing self and other and shared hopes and dreams helped to form a foundation of trust and commitment to articulate and move toward this vision. The aesthetically represented vision was then translated into words, shared throughout the organization and became a guiding document for the transformative work.

Over the course of a 4-year journey toward professional practice, the leadership team themselves grew in knowing themselves and each other as caring leaders. The team used both analytic and metaphorical tools to help articulate, value, and guide the next steps in building a professional practice environment based on caring, in which the staffing issue was resolved, expert mentors were in place, education was brought on site, and unit-level staff work related to practice and research was unfolding.

Early Work. Early work to transform the environment for professional practice addressed the situation characterized by the large RN vacancy rate, a sense that nursing was not valued within the larger organization. The metaphor for this view was one of invisibility, and "us versus them." Actions taken in this early stage included values clarification and empiric data collection for strategic plan that was collaborative. The caring phase focused on the expressed experience that staff wanted to be cared for and about by others, guided by the question: Who cares about us?

Emerging leadership development was achieved with a new director experienced in facilitative leadership, and shared decision making set expectations for collaboration and broad-scale involvement combined with practice accountability. The metaphor for this aspect of the change process was "Leaving 'traditional' authoritarian ways, moving toward an orchestra with each person having an assigned role as part of the whole." Actions undertaken in the emerging leadership focus included skill acquisition for facilitative leadership, personality inventory, listening, and appreciative inquiry, and empirical data collection from staff about work environment. The caring phase revolved around the theme that helping staff do their work well is our duty as caring manager. The question that guided this aspect of the work was: How can we take cares (worries) away from staff? How can we create the possibilities for caring to occur?

Mid-Term Work. Mid-term work involved differentiating roles and responsibilities, norming and storming phase of new team. The metaphor for this aspect was a jazz band versus orchestra, improvisation can be beautiful. Actions included using analogous thinking to explore concepts of power and empowerment, situational leadership delegation and empowerment, and total quality management analytic skills. The caring phase involved the questions of what is the scope of our responsibility to take care of/not take care of the organization as a whole? And is it our right to claim caring as unique to us?

Late-Term Work. Late-term work focused on coming to confidence about different ways of being as a choice—performing the role of the leader with skill. The metaphor reflecting this aspect was: cycle of life, caring rituals of gathering, and letting go. Actions in the constancy of change "chaos" focused on the idea that principles and ethics ground our decision making, and on understanding alternating rhythms of shared leadership. Authentic presence with staff and patients was promoted through coaching for commitment versus compliance. The caring phase of this aspect was guided by the questions: How can I help myself to be and become more fully caring? How might I help others? What do our patients think caring is, that's what matters most.

Transferable Observations From This Story

The ambassador group made a long-term commitment for transformational leadership and the alternating rhythm between local and broader focus within the organization. The work of the group stayed focused on executing the strategic plan and used personal exploration, story, symphony, meaning, empathy, and play in the design of their high-touch culture creating the patient care experience based on caring.

Ideas for innovation and creativity, pattern seeking, and synthesis as relationships grow characterized by empathy and play are emerging in unlikely places. The 2012 State of the Science Congress in Washington, DC, hosted by the Council for the Advancement of Nursing Science, focused on Discovery through Innovation. There was an encouragement to lend *New Eyes for Old Problems: Accelerating Pathways to Innovation in Nursing Science* (Mooney, 2012). Other speakers talked about moving innovation forward. The final keynote speaker, Roberta Kraus, PhD, discussed the need for "Boundary Spanning

Leadership," a vision advocated by the Center for Creative Leadership (www.ccl.org; Yip, Ernst, & Campbell, 2011).

Senior executives who led organizations with at least 500 people contributed their perspectives about the necessity of creating spans across boundaries that serve a higher vision or goal through creating a new direction, alignment, and commitment. They offer that working across boundaries is essential for innovation—executives rate innovation as having the most important impact on their organizations going forward. In order to foster that innovation, employees need to collaborate across functions, employees at all levels need to feel empowered, and the organization as a whole needs to commit to learning.

Awareness of the interconnectedness within the organization across functions and roles affects success. Crossing boundaries includes vertical boundaries across levels of hierarchy and horizontal boundaries across functions and expertise, including relationships with stakeholders beyond the boundaries of the organization. Demographic (across diverse groups, gender, race, nationality) and geographic (across regional and locality) considerations are also important (Yip et al., 2011). The main message is to see boundaries as an opportunity to bridge to new ideas rather than as barriers.

With a recognition of the need for innovation and collaborative work, what resources does the ambassador group need to have available in order to perform well as a group and advance the development of a culture of caring? Listed here are the types of training and resources that need to be available to the ambassador group:

Basic Tools for Working Together as a Team

1. Commit to become a member.
2. Develop team norms, ground rules, mutual agreements about how the work will get done.
3. Determine meeting guidelines—how the meetings will be managed, conducted, and structured.
4. Set the agenda and time associated; assign meeting roles, facilitator, recorder, meeting times, and place, communication of minutes, assignment of responsible person for determined action items, and accountability for follow-through back to the group.

Determine the Charter for This Ambassador Group

1. Write an overview of the scope of the work.
2. Determine a start and end date and the circle of influence that the group has. What is expected along the way to show progress?
3. What needs to be evident to indicate that this team is succeeding?
4. Who must approve or review the work of this group?
5. What are milestones along the way that have reports and evidence of progress?
6. What limits are there on spending or number of staff who can be involved and paid?
7. Who needs to be kept informed of the work of this group, how often, and through what communication methods?
8. What else is happening within the organization that might derail or delay this initiative?
9. Have the charter approved by the sponsor group, clarify expectations (Martin & Tate, 1997).

Convene and Progress With Work

1. Conduct meetings.
2. Develop overall plan.
3. Determine decisions and actions and track progress.
4. Identify educational needs for ambassadors for continuing work. For example:
    a. Innovation and creativity skills
    b. Caring for self
    c. Competency–scope of practice
    d. Evaluation, valuing outcomes
    e. Scholarly readings and research related to caring
    f. Processes for decision making (voting, consensus, unilateral)
5. Reaffirm commitment as an ambassador.

Tools for Creativity, Innovation and Prototyping, and Organizing Information for Decision Making

1. Tools for generating and grouping ideas include brainstorming, affinity and interrelationship diagrams, cause-and-effect fishbone, force-field analysis
2. Storytelling, observation in the field, analogous thinking. Story boards combined with plan, do check, (study), act
3. Tools for narrowing and deciding among choices include nominal group technique, prioritization
4. Tools for tracking implementation progress flowchart, such as a Gantt Matrix (Brossard & Ritter, 1994)

Edward de Bono was the 2009 European Union Ambassador for Creativity. He takes the mystery out of creative thinking and helps to develop tools, programs, and processes for lateral thinking. He opened the first-ever Pentagon meeting on creativity. In the book, *The Mechanism of the Mind* (de Bono, 1969), he proposed that creativity is a necessary mechanism in a self-organizing information systems, viewing asymmetric patterns as the basis of perception. He asserts that constructive and creative thinking includes the following:

1. Acknowledges thinking as a skill
2. Develops the skill of practical thinking
3. Encourages others to look at their own thinking and the thinking of others

There are many resources for creativity including www.Corthinking.com and www.GoCreate.com.

The Institute for Healthcare Improvement (IHI) and the Robert Wood Johnson Foundation partnered in increasing the capacity of staff at the bedside to transform care through innovation and quality improvement (Rutherford et al., 2008). Ten hospitals received technical support for five major areas:

1. Transformational leadership
2. Safe and reliable care
3. Vitality and team work
4. Value-added care processes
5. Patient-centered care

This partnership resulted in the production of a toolkit for others to learn from and use the processes tested in these hospitals. The IHI currently holds many webinars, conferences, and learning communities that further develop processes for innovation and quality improvement (http://www.ihi.org/programs/strategicinitiatives/TransformingCareAtTheBedside). Other sources for learning about initiatives for patient-centered care and healing environments are the Institute for Patient- and Family-Centered Care (http://www.familycenteredcare.org and the Planetree Model http://www.planetree.org).

In summary, the work of the ambassador group committed to growing a substantive and significant culture of caring requires ongoing opportunities reflective of an organization committed to continuous learning. The resources available within the larger organization related to leadership and skill development need to be integrated into the work of this Department Council.

SPECIAL TOPICS RELEVANT TO CREATING PROFESSIONAL PRACTICE ENVIRONMENTS GROUNDED IN CARING

Health care organizations have a public trust to uphold related to safety, competence, and caring. Persons who have entered the healing arts and are licensed to practice have made a commitment to practice to the full breadth and depth of their theoretical and applied knowledge. An individual practitioner cannot choose to fulfill only a portion of the licensure requirements. The commitment is for the full scope of practice. Traditionally, there have been hierarchical relationships between health care professionals that influence power relationships and scope of practice. Let us consider scope of practice and power within cultures of caring.

Because health care settings are populated by many different licensed personnel, it is important that each professional understands the scope of practice of the other. This is rarely done in a systematic manner within health care organizations, yet it is vital to understanding the public trust that each licensed professional has committed to uphold. Each professional should practice to the full scope of their license in order to fulfill that promise to the public.

Scope of practice is critical to explore when transforming the practice work environment because it is the foundation for assuring patient safety, quality satisfaction, regulatory compliance, legal practice standards, and reimbursement for the scope of services provided. Scope of practice is the set of legally sanctioned clinical functions that authorizes a health care practitioner to provide care. State laws are the primary source defining what each discipline may claim as its scope of practice. Professional accreditation standards and federal law such as Medicare guidelines also influence scope of practice.

Any given agency or organization can make a decision to narrow the scope of practice through policies, but organizations are not authorized to expand the scope of practice to accommodate their needs or expectations. As more organizations convert to electronic medical records, each documented note is stamped and signed by the professional who wrote it. Therefore, if practitioners are operating outside of their legal scope, it becomes transparent to any legal or audit processes. This makes it compelling for practitioners to discuss their scope of practice within the team. This can become a topic for the Departmental Council. It is a part of coming to know each other as caring person.

In short, how I choose to show up for work each day is influenced by my expectations for the contributions that I am obligated to provide to those in my care. If other team members are not aware of those obligations, it may affect our communication, our relationship, and our collective care to patients and families. As nursing philosopher–scientists Roach (2002) and Locsin (2007) have clearly explained, competence is core to caring.

Within the scope of practice are core competencies. Execution of core competencies leads to the patient plan of care provided by each member of the care team. O'Rourke's

(2003) nine steps for professional role accountability and professional practice competencies are as follows:

1. Data collection and data assessment
2. Comprehensive assessment of the patient condition with diagnosis
3. Planning and outcome identification
4. Implementation
5. Evaluation
6. Teaching
7. Dynamic integration of steps 1 to 6 based on critical thinking
8. Determination of the stability of the patient condition, breadth and depth of clinical knowledge, and experience with the patient condition and patient population
9. Dynamic integration of previous eight steps based on critical thinking, substantial scientific knowledge, theory (general and specific), research findings, determination of appropriate supervision for delegation or assignment of care tasks, and care coordination

Each professional, within the relevant role, uses these steps in the same fashion. So how do professionals begin to understand what to expect from one another while caring for patients as members of the team? The scope of practice for each member of the team can be shared and a discussion can follow to clarifying any uncertainties. Here are some questions that could guide that discussion:

What is common across each of the disciplines? What is unique? In common areas of practice, how do we actualize our role now? How might each of us actualize our role differently? In what way might that enhance or detract from the caring relationship between staff and patient/family? Discuss implications for operations, workflow, and education based on insights about the scope of practice.

The design of care delivery within a unit must stem from the scope of practice and yet where there are shared accountabilities, what opportunities might be explored? For example, if the scope of practice for physical therapy (PT) is to diagnose and treat conditions related to strength, flexibility, and mobility, how might that relate to the nurses' plan for ambulation for the patient? Within interprofessional practice, the goal is to have coordinated care focused on the patient's progression toward recovery, identification and prevention of complications, and promotion of well-being. Coordination of care is the role of the RN. Many different professionals may have similar skill competence (both PT and RN can ambulate a patient). Yet role competence defines the accountability for the specific assessment and intervention defined by licensure, knowledge, and education. Role competence is about authority and accountability to act in improving the health of the patient; skill competence is about the quality of that action.

The goal is to ensure that each professional's talent is recognized and used to the fullest. Regulatory requirements are dynamic and create changes in practice opportunities that then require further dialogue. Conversations about the scope of practice may reveal new insights about the expectations of one's peers; it can create tension as well as collaboration. It is essential to understanding how to best work together as a team for the betterment of the patient. It is the responsibility of each professional to understand and be able to articulate the specific requirements of the scope of practice for that discipline and its related standards of practice.

The Process of Interacting During Department Meetings

Scope of practice helps to define expectations for each person's role. An equally important competence is the ability to communicate effectively with one another and to attend to the relationship among team members. Strong cultures result from "consistent, visible role modeling and leadership, consistent feedback on performance—positive and negative—constant communication about what is important in the organization and sharing stories of how the organization's culture played a critical role in patients, staff or visitor experience" (Schein, 1990, p. 35). Basing all decisions and actions in the values prioritized by the organization and effectively communicating these beliefs to all in the organization have been found to be essential to success.

A Practical Strategy to Promote Being Present: A Key Skill in Collaboration for Change

Many times we rush to a meeting still focused on our own work or some other activity outside of the purpose of the meeting. One way to get centered and become present to be with and listen to each other is the process of "check in" (Wheeler & Chinn, 1989). Check in is a brief statement by each person present—it centers the group on the shared purpose for being together and what each hopes to gain by being present.

Imagine if you started your departmental council check in by each person briefly reflecting about the meaning of assumptions related to the Dance of Caring Persons. Each person speaks briefly. It serves to get the members connected to the present and to reaffirm the underlying assumptions of the work of moving toward a culture of caring. It serves as a ritual, signaling something is different about this work.

Assumptions of the Dance of Caring Persons
- No person is better than another; each is respected and valued as person
- All persons are committed to knowing other as caring; all are committed to the one seeking to be cared for
- There are different ways of knowing; and the expertise of each person is valued for his or her unique contribution
- Persons are committed because the care that all persons are called to live and grow is valued
- Decisions reflect "what ought to be"
- Caring is our gift; our way of living
- Persons are nurtured in caring relationships

Another way to focus the conversation about caring within the committee meeting and challenge assumptions is suggested by Dr. Madeleine Leininger's (1989) forecast regarding the future knowledge about care and caring:

- Ethos of caring in practice and education is pervasive
- Transcultural-based care by 2010
- Demand for care knowledge and skills, new models of care delivery
- Engagement in public agendas and advocacy for healthy lifestyles, wellness, care maintenance practices, and other modalities
- Qualitative research contributes to substantive knowledge base of caring

In what ways do you think these projections have become a reality . . . or do you think they have not become a reality? How might they become more evident within a culture of caring? What actions might it suggest for us within our department? Dr. Leininger offered these future forecasts during a conference in which the tone of the meeting was about overcoming duality. That is, it was thought that one had to choose either caring or technology; quantitative or qualitative, humanistic or objective. To what degree do you believe we still hold that duality? To what degree do we see that we have moved to a "both/and" perspective?

Assuming a "both/and" perspective, we can frame questions differently and focus on exploring the dynamics as:

- How might we use technology to personalize care for individuals through relationship-based care?
- How might we assure accountability through measurement of relevant variables and have expressive narrative that powerfully conveys meaningful care experiences?
- How might we advance substantive knowledge in caring science and accelerate its adoption into education, practice, and research?
- How might we advance policy makers' substantive value of caring through advocating for both virtue and knowledge attributes of the nurse?

POWER

We often harbor certain assumptions about power as "good" or "bad." Power is a neutral term meaning "to be able," to be able—to act. Power from within is to be able to use inner strength and conviction to act. Power over is power to dominate with others or in an external environment. Wheeler and Chin (1989) provide a much expanded perspective on power:

Power of Process
Power of Letting Go
Power of the Whole
Power of Collectivity
Power of Unity
Power of Sharing
Power of Integration
Power of Nurturing
Power of Distribution
Power of Intuition
Power of Consciousness
Power of Diversity
Power of Responsibility

One exercise that helps to create dialogue about assumptions of power is to use analogous thinking such as:
Power is like a...flower
Power is like a...fire

Each person chooses an analogy and then draws a picture of power as that analogy. Dialogue follows and insights about the meaning of power for this group can emerge. This can stimulate conversations about how the group members want to address power within the group, how to deal with differences, how to deal with conflict, how to inspire collaboration with differentiated roles and talents.

A Story From Practice

Envisioning the Future: Growing in Caring While Expanding Services

An interprofessional team worked to provide a comprehensive memory assessment for persons concerned with memory loss. In the same location, an adult day center was operating for persons with mild and moderate cognitive impairment. Anticipating an expansion of services, the entire team went on retreat for one day to understand and articulate what is working well and if the center were to expand what would need to continue to be evident and in place. There were two components of the retreat, one was about teamwork, the second was about current and future design of programs.

One exercise was used in advance of the retreat asking each person what he or she would want our team to Stop Doing, Start Doing, or Keep Doing as we work together. These were compiled in advance and at the retreat members of the team read from each list. They did not read their own. In this way the team was able to "hear" from the entire group. A debriefing allowed the group to discuss common themes in each category and then to prioritize actions based on the discussion.

Second, the team engaged in a process called "World Café." In this process, tables were set up that focused on particular program areas that we wanted to examine and potentially redesign with the anticipation of expansion. A playful atmosphere was set up with different continents designated for different sets of questions. Team members moved to different continents and topics to create the most diversity of opinion. At each "continent" a recorder stayed behind to capture the overall conversation at each table. The whole group debriefed hearing the ideas generated for each topic. Discussion followed. Then each continent recorder posted the recommendations suggested for each topic. All team members were then able to indicate across all of the topics that they thought were the highest priority to act upon in the short term, near term, and long term.

The overall focus for the day was how to create the best caring experience for patients and families as they used the services of the center. Many action steps were generated and acted upon. Here are a few of them:

1. To have the persons coming for diagnostic services have a different entrance and view than for those participants already in the day program. Persons coming for diagnosis fear a deterioration and seeing participants requiring that level of care fueled fear.
2. A marketing plan to build awareness of the center in preparation for expansion, emphasizing the unique features of the program and the academic club atmosphere found as part of a university campus.
3. Providing greater privacy and focused attention for intake information.
4. Providing a "live voice" receptionist and operator so that persons with memory disorder could speak to a real person.
5. Staff development focused on theories and practices of caring.
6. Interprofessional rounds led by an advanced practice nurse practitioner and caring scholar to reinforce theoretical depth and breadth of knowledge for practice.

Translating These New Perspectives Into Operational Practices in a Sustained Fashion

The fundamental questions in this phase are how does this new caring perspective link with existing initiatives and yet fundamentally change them to reflect a commitment to a culture of caring? What communication, symbols, rituals, and celebrations need to be present to signal an adoption of these principles?

We learned in Chapter 3 that there are five primary and five secondary ways leaders of organizations embed their views into organizations (Schein, 1990). The primary ways that views are embedded are as follows:

- What leaders pay attention to, measure, and control
- How leaders react to critical incidents and organizational crises

- Deliberate role modeling and coaching
- Operational criteria for the allocation of rewards and status
- Operational criteria for recruitment, selection, promotion, retirement, and excommunications

The secondary ways include the following:

- The organization's design and structure
- Organizational systems and procedures
- The design of physical space, facades, and buildings
- Stories, legends, myths, and symbols
- Formal statements of organizational philosophy

Strategies in this chapter suggest ways that leaders throughout the organization, from bedside through boardroom, might clearly identify what they pay attention to related to caring practices:

1. What is newly measured or measured in a different way?
2. What new patterns of behavior serve to role model articulated expectations?
3. What coaching is available to individuals or groups to strengthen caring practices?
4. How are caring practices embedded within feedback related to performance and advancement?

As we appraise our progress within our work environments:

1. Is there anything related to how we gather together to decide the direction of the organization that has changed?
2. Do we do anything differently related to procedures or systems of operations?
3. Does our physical space reflect our values and beliefs about patient and staff well-being and comfort?
4. Who are we celebrating as a hero or heroine, what stories are we telling with pride about our work?
5. How do we present ourselves to others related to our philosophy and actions?

One example of a board-level focus is the Hospital Consumer Assessment of Health Providers and Systems (HCAHPS). This survey focuses on understanding health care quality by the consumers' experience. This report is essentially about a person's health care encounter. Questions asked of patients are as follows:

- During this hospital stay, how often did nurses treat you with courtesy and respect?
- During this hospital stay, how often did nurses listen carefully to you?
- During this hospital stay, how often did the nurses explain things in a way you could understand?
- During this hospital stay, after you pressed the call button, how often did you get help as soon as you wanted it?
- During this hospital stay, how often did doctors listen carefully to you?
- During this hospital stay, how often did doctors explain things in a way you could understand?

During the work of the department-level meetings, these questions could become the focus for increasing the culture of caring within the organization; for example, there could be dialogue among the committee members about each of these areas. Following the dialogue, the members could dialogue about what might be done to move actions more closely toward what is believed. Data could be collected through observation or survey about what the current experience is for staff. A plan could be developed to increase the sense of courtesy and respect, and then it could be appraised within each unit and eventually staff could see if it was reflected in any positive changes in the HCAHPS scores. In this way the work of the board and the work of the bedside are aligned toward common values. Examples of questions that might be considered include the following:

- When we consider courtesy and respect from the patient's experience—what does it look like, what is happening, what interactions occur?
- When this goes well for us, what conditions are present?
- What might we do to ensure that those conditions are present more often?
- What actions does this suggest?
- How might we test out these actions in a small test of change?
- When we consider the patient's experience of being listened to carefully—what is observed, experienced by the staff and the patient? How might we create more opportunities for that to occur?
- When patients experience having things explained to them in a way that they can understand, what is observed, experienced, related between the staff member and the patient?
- From the patient's experience with the call button, what might we observe about response times, interaction, conversation, and engagement with staff and the patient?

This same kind of conversion from high-level organizational goals to the lived experience of caring at the bedside can help to align values and vision together and ensure that structural changes are made within the organization to sustain those changes.

REFERENCES

Aiken, L. H., Clarke, S. P., & Sloan, D. M. (2002). Hospital staffing, organization, and quality of care: Cross-national findings. *International Journal for Quality in Health Care, 14*(1), 5–14.

Boykin, A., & Schoenhofer, S. O. (2001). *Nursing as caring: A model for transforming practice.* Sudbury, MA: Jones & Bartlett.

Brossard, M., & Ritter, M. (1994). *The Memory Jogger II: A pocket guide of tools for continuous improvement and effective planning.* Salem, NH: Goal/QPC.

Carper, B. A. (1978). Fundamental patterns of knowing in nursing. *Advances in Nursing Science, 1*(1), 13–23.

de Bono, E. (1969). *The mechanism of the mind.* New York, NY: Simon & Schuster.

Leininger, M. M. (1989). Assumptions about knowledge of care and caring. In J. S. Stevenson & T. Tripp-Reimer (Eds.), *Knowledge about care and caring: State of the art and future developments: Proceedings of a Wingspread Conference, February 1–3, 1989, Wingspread Conference Center, Racine, Wisconsin.* Washington, DC: American Academy of Nursing.

Locsin, R. C. (2007). Machine technologies and caring in nursing. *Journal of Nursing Scholarship, 27*(3), 201–203.

Martin, P., & Tate, K. (1997). *Project Management Memory Jogger: A desktop guide for project teams.* Salem, NH: Goal/QPC.

Mooney, K. (2012). *New eyes for old problems: Accelerating pathways to innovation in nursing science.* Paper presented at Discovery through Innovation, 2012 State of the Science Congress on Nursing Research, Council for the Advancement of Nursing Science, Discovery and Innovation, Washington DC, September 13–15, 2012.

O'Rourke, M. (2003). Rebuilding a professional practice model: The return of role-based accountability. *Nursing Administration Quarterly, 27*(2), 95–105.

Pink, D. H. (2006). *A whole new mind: Why right-brainers will rule the future.* New York, NY: The Berkeley Group.

Roach, M. S. (2002). *Caring, the human mode of being: A blueprint for the health professions* (2nd ed.). Ottawa, ON: CHA.

Schein, E. H. (1990). Organizational culture. *American Psychologist, 45*(2), 109–119. doi:10.1037/0003-066X.45.2.109

Smith, M., Saunders, S., Stuckhardt, J., & McGinnis, M. (Eds.). (2012). *Best care at lower cost: The path to continuously learning health care in America (Institute of Medicine).* Washington, DC: The National Academies Press.

Swanson, K. M. (2010). Kristen Swanson's theory of caring. In M. E. Parker & M. C. Smith (Eds.), *Nursing theories and nursing practice* (3rd ed., pp. 428–438). Philadelphia: F. A. Davis.

Valentine, K. (1989). Caring is more than kindness: Modeling its complexities. *Journal of Nursing Administration, 19*(11), 28–35.

Valentine, K. (1992). Strategic planning for professional practice. *Journal of Nursing Care Quality, 6*(3), 1–12.

Valentine, K. (2013). Exploration of the relationship between caring and cost. In M. C. Smith, M. C. Turkel, & Z. Wolf (Eds.), *Caring in nursing classics: An essential resource* (pp. 497–506). New York, NY: Springer. Reprinted from *Holistic Nursing Practice,* 1997, *11*(4), 71–81.

Wheeler, C., & Chinn, P. (1989). *Peace and power. A handbook of feminist process* (2nd ed.). New York, NY: National League for Nursing.

Yip, J., Ernst, C., & Campbell, M. (2011). *Boundary-spanning leadership: Mission critical perspectives from the executive suite.* Center for Creative Leadership Organizational Leadership White Paper Series. Retrieved from http://www.ccl.org

Response to Chapter 5

Valerie Fong, MSN, RN
Chief Nursing Information Officer
Providence Health & Services

*T*he health care delivery system in the United States is in chaos. This is not news. As a result of general systemic disarray, health care organizations across the country are engaged in a seemingly endless continuum of process improvement initiatives to change the lives and health of our populations—individuals, families, and communities—for the best possible outcomes. Successful transformational work in health care requires more than strategy. The authors outline very clear steps for building, preparing, and enabling resources and action toward practice change. To bring these ideas to fruition, leader awareness is needed on the point that successful transformation is not the result of merely gathering together a group of individuals and performing multiple transactions without engaging those individuals from a caring-based perspective.

As patient care becomes increasingly complex, the work necessary to create the organizational leadership and infrastructure to support that complexity multiplies at least 10-fold. In many ways, health care transformation is made even more difficult because it is the people, and not the processes, that need to be kept front and center. After all, it is easier work to create one-dimensional processes than it is to deal with more challenging three-dimensional personnel problems. However, caring is also what keeps the health care industry so very high-touch.

A caring-based perspective is urgently needed to progress a bigger vision in the complex work of health care transformation. Execution of that vision involves organization, collaboration, harnessing energy and expertise, and, most importantly, paying utmost attention to and trusting the people that are doing the work. In my experience, the latter is the vital component that needs to be in place in order to bring the ideas presented in the chapter to sustainable reality. Maintaining a large-picture perspective of successful transformation outcomes through deliberate connections with people as individuals has the power to provide some semblance of order to the chaos of health care and requires patience, understanding, and stamina. At its core, successfully transforming health care depends on more than simply changing a few processes, or introducing some new innovative tools. It requires a caring-based perspective with specific attention to those that perform the work, and an acknowledgment of the views from their vantage point.

It is not atypical for the people resources involved in any one initiative to get pulled into other parallel high-priority work creating a hyper-frenzy of activity, effort, and tenacity to get things done during limited hours in the day. This is very challenging to sustain, and is the reality of what health care organizations everywhere experience today. The initiative overload tends to leave limited expertise and energy to draw from and results in more transactional versus transformational change—one where people become focused on *just barely getting by* as they check off one thing after another on some grand checklist of "to do's." In this environment, a caring-based perspective for health care transformation is essential; its value priceless. Does overreliance on the crisis of the moment overshadow a caring-based perspective?

The authors focus on establishing clarity of responsibility to grow confidence of department unit members within the clinical practice arena. As they point out, the principles of their approach to moving the vision of caring-based cultures forward can (and should) span more than one unit of service. One unit of service I provide is comprised of a team of individuals in the nontraditional health care role of clinical informatics. As I reflect on the chapter components and my work with this team of informatics specialists, it has become clear to me that more emphasis on a caring-based perspective is needed in the practice-technology space in order to successfully advance health care transformation.

Recently, I have had the privilege of hiring and onboarding this brand new team of highly intelligent and motivated individuals into nondirect patient care roles as one of many components in a larger organizational transformation toward having a shared information service across an integrated organization that spans five states. This clinical informatics role is new to the organization and has primary focus on providing elbow-to-elbow support for clinicians and providers throughout the pre- and post-implementation activities of an organizational-wide transition to information technologies in the clinical practice space such as the electronic health record (EHR). At the same time that this team is forming, the organization is undergoing massive changes with the consolidation of human resources, supply chain, information systems, and financial services, and the standardization of local and regional operational practices and policies into larger organizational shared service pillars. Many members of the team have been transferred from decades-long service in previous clinical roles in the organization. Fifty percent of the team has a clinical background. It has been difficult for many of the individuals to make the connections between the *new* work they are now engaged in away from direct patient care and the alignment with the larger organizational transformation efforts that are under way. In a situation where direct patient care is not being provided, it is easy to lose sight of where a caring-based perspective has a place. "What's my role? Where do I belong?" are some of the laments voiced from many on the team in addition to the other frustrations that they are experiencing as part of being a new team caught in the midst of such big changes. It does not help that there is a perception from the former clinical practice peers of the individual team members that by moving to the *dark side* of technology, they have relinquished the caring-based connotation and perspective that is so much more easily linked in the acts of providing direct patient care. Although they are no longer caring for patients directly, I find myself spending a great deal of time with the team engaged in what can be described as a *caring service* recovery effort. Their journey of transformation away from direct patient care has required that I lead them through being open to exploring new ways of doing things; new views of what it means to provide care. They appear hungry for my reminders to them that they are still in the caring business as care extenders—caring for the caregivers that are closest to the patient. I wonder at what point in the larger transformation journey will it become commonly accepted and acknowledged that there is an authentic expression of caring that exists in this type of role. Although the role provides an opportunity for growth in understanding what caring means beyond the more obvious direct patient care venue, a change in perceptions amidst organizational ambiguity and uncertainty about the expectations of the role is compounding the efforts needed for the usual new team forming and norming stages.

I have intentionally overcommunicated the vision for how this role plays into the larger organizational transformation, and I have articulated the expectations for the individuals for flexibility and preparedness for dealing with great ambiguity. Initially, I understood the immediate contribution to the larger organizational transformation into a fast-paced practice-technology world to be that of planning, creating, preparing, and developing a new team empowered to assist those that are closest to the patients. Like many leaders, I tackled this with great enthusiasm and wanted to be able to move faster with less for the mere desire to move on to the next pieces of work. I provided for basic structure needs, such as physical home-based work locations, hardware and software resources, schedules, and guiding principles of the role, not too unlike those things outlined by the authors in the section of the chapter on *Making the Commitment Actionable*. Soon, however, many of the team members began experiencing a great degree of angst and frustration about the unexpected and were getting caught up in the sheer turmoil of the other organizational changes occurring around them. I tried to *fix* these anxieties using a standard project management and process-oriented methodology by providing more and more written communications and process clarifications, resources, and team structures—things that only quieted the anxieties for a few days at a time. Finally, in trying to uncover the root of the frustrations and discontent, I pulled myself away from my own day-to-day fires of the moment and met casually with several of the individuals on a one-on-one basis. I soon found that listening, treating them as individuals versus a team-at-large, and being open to changing course in response to the view of things as seen from their vantage point was the most effective in alleviating the unrest—something I had neglected to do, as I was getting caught up in my own initiative frenzy. I realized that although I could not control the chaos of all the rest of the moving parts in the organizational transformation, the one thing within my control was allowing some time away from the crisis of the moment for a caring-based perspective to reemerge. It takes heart and courage to allow for a few steps backward before making the bigger stride.

I want to establish a sense of urgency that we simply cannot afford to disenfranchise those that are executing the work. Health care transformation is a team sport. Although we can bulldoze our way through checking off initiative completion one after another, we risk moving so quickly that we lose sight of what's important. A caring-based perspective is foundational in clearing the chaos and navigating through ambiguity and uncertainty. A caring-based perspective is neither going to stop things from moving so quickly nor remove the pandemonium of health care transformation. However, people are vital to successful health care transformation outcomes, and a caring-based perspective refocuses us on the fact people are the ones that matter the most. The authors hit the mark right on target about the need and strategies for "coming to know each other as a caring person."

Strategies for Creating a Transformational Culture of Caring in Health Care Systems

Charting a course for grounding the transformation of a health care system so that caring becomes the guiding principle of the organization requires the kinds of "getting ready" and "getting set" thinking, planning, and practices we presented in Chapters 4 and 5. In Section III, we turn to the task of detailing specific strategies organized around certain key system focal points. Chapter 6 discusses strategies for formalizing and implementing the mission and supporting documents and processes, including human resources (HR). Chapter 7 addresses aspects of leadership from the Dance of Caring Persons perspective, while Chapter 8 focuses on communication processes from the same perspective. Chapter 9 offers a new way of approaches, outcomes, assessment, and performance evaluation.

Chapter 6

Transforming the Organizational Mission

Specific strategies for achieving shared understanding of purpose in an integrated way—a way that values the person as person and as participant, as well as valuing the system as a human system—will be the focus of our attention in this chapter. In particular, we address the development of major guiding documents and human resource functions to ensure that they reflect and support the unity of purpose expressed in the Dance of Caring Persons model. Core values of the model point to strategies that emphasize respect for persons, meaningful participation, and consensus building.

From this grounding, dialogic structures and processes will be suggested to ensure opportunities for participation within work groups and throughout the organization, both laterally and horizontally. Recognition will also be given to those members of the Dance of Caring Persons whose roles, although importantly connected to the process, are at a distance from the day-to-day enterprise—groups from the community, for example, and even stockholders in corporate health care systems. It is recognized that active involvement in transforming the organizational mission will include input into the nature of the transformation, design, and redesign of methods for translating a renewed shared mission into action plans for various functional units, and ongoing ratification of the institutional mission.

MISSION STATEMENT: WHY, WHAT, HOW

Experts on the topic of mission statements in health care systems concluded in a 2008 study that organizations need to invest in "redesigning a work environment that stresses the importance of the organizational mission statement and provides detailed information on the ways that individual organizational members can contribute in realizing the mission statement" (Desmidt, Prinzie, & Heene, 2008, p. 1433). Transforming a health care system to create a culture of caring is a system-wide process that responds to the challenge of making the mission statement relevant by transforming the workplace environment. Nurses and associated direct-care staff have often felt a disconnect between their institution's stated value priorities (espoused values) and the structures and culture of the workplace (expressed values). It has been acknowledged in the professional literature and in private conversations that creating vibrant, reflective mission statements is either just another fad that will pass out of favor when the next one comes along, or a tool of administrative control. Faculty members in schools of nursing, medicine, allied health, and other disciplines tend to avoid the process of updating or transforming mission statements and other values-based guiding program documents, largely because it *is* a process, a human process, a human dialogic process that involves creating explicit value priorities, if it is carried out in a way that results in added value to the organization as in the following example:

> The mission of the Christine E. Lynn College of Nursing at Florida Atlantic University is to create and live a caring-based program. A program in which caring directs not only the study of nursing but all aspects of the program. The program is grounded in the belief that all persons are caring and that caring is an essential domain of nursing knowledge. The commitment to caring directs all actions. It obligates us to know each other as caring; to support the sharing of knowledge, values, and beliefs; to understand other's views; to search for new solutions to problems from a caring perspective; to share responsibility and authority; and to always treat each other in a manner reflective of the specialness of person. The role of the administrator is to "nurture ideas…model living and growing in caring, co-create a culture in which the study of nursing can be achieved freely and fully, ground all actions in a commitment to caring as a way of living, and treat others with the same care, concern and understanding as those entrusted to our care. (Boykin, 1994, p. 17)

In a 2005 study that found no content differences between for-profit and nonprofit hospital mission statements, Bolon asserted that despite mission statements being a highly regarded management tool, "the hospital industry lags far behind other sectors in the design, development, and use of mission statements" (Boykin, 1994, p. 8). Bolon's advice for hospital executives on this matter was that they "must not view mission statement development as busywork or an academic exercise…[but] need to realize that a well-constructed mission statement provides the foundation for the hospital's future success" (Boykin, 1994, p. 8).

In the study of Finnish nurses' use of organizational mission statements, Desmidt, Prinzie, and Heene (2008) found that the nurses who were more likely to actually use the mission statement to guide their functioning were those:

> (1) who have a positive attitude towards the mission statement, (2) who perceive pressure from superiors and colleagues to use the mission statement, (3) who feel they are in control of performing such behavior, and (4) who are formally involved in the mission statement communication processes. (Desmidt et al., 2008, p. 1433)

Experience indicates that these findings hold true for health care workers in other disciplines as well. The Dance of Caring Persons model facilitates this outcome—internalized alignment of mission statement and work-related activities within the system—because of the emphasis on valuing persons as persons, and valuing the contributions of all, with full acknowledgment that all stakeholders are actively engaged in the "dance" that is the health care system.

The organizational mission statement is often called a "planning document," and that is an accurate description. However, it is only a useful description when the approach to planning recognizes it as an ongoing process and not a one-time or an occasional activity. Planning is recognized as a temporary resting place in a continuous path in organizations whose leaders and members realize the need to be a learning organization. The term "continuous quality improvement" helps us to move our thinking from planning as a somewhat static activity to a more dynamic and complex view, one that is an all-embracing process to keep today's complex dynamic systems growing and changing in response to multidimensional pressures and opportunities for life-sustaining innovation. In Chapter 9 of this book, we focus on specific strategies regarding the process of outcome assessment from the perspective of the Dance of Caring Persons—and of course, outcome assessment begins with the formalization of a clear articulation of mission.

We have seen in Chapters 4 and 5 some of the early work that leads up to formalization of a mission statement and all that flows from it. The professional organizational development literature offers a rich informational field for the design and dissemination of major value-based guiding documents like mission and vision statements. One rather straightforward approach to understanding what should be expressed in a mission statement is offered by Radtke (1998). She suggests that the written mission statement should clearly answer three questions:

1. What are the opportunities or needs that we are to address (organization's purpose)?
2. What are we doing to address those needs (organization's business)?
3. What beliefs or principles guide our work (organization's core values)?

Most authorities advise that mission statements should be short, clear, and free of jargon—written in a language that can be easily understood by all stakeholder groups. In our model, we might say that those who are "core dancers" are the persons who are providing care services and immediate support to that service provision, and those who are "dancing at a distance," such as corporate stockholders and/or the community, are the ones who are providing the sociopolitical context for the organization. Another suggestion frequently made is that mission statements should language the uniqueness of the organization, distinguishing it from others in its category. Health care systems grounded in a culture of caring would most likely make that very explicit in their mission statement.

We have briefly addressed the "why" and the "what" of a mission statement, and those aspects are important. What we want to emphasize here, though, is the process—how to go about the process of developing a mission statement for a health care system that takes its core values from the Dance of Caring Persons, and infusing every organizational function and activity with that visible value. It is in the action strategies where, as the saying goes, the "rubber meets the road," where the real transformation must take place, and it is most difficult to accomplish when the transformation sought is a complete cultural transformation. One online source suggests that "the mission development process involves envisioning the future, creating a task force to develop the mission statement, formulating a draft mission statement, communicating the final mission statement to the entire organization, and implementing the statement" (Stone, 1996). However, we think that Desmidt, Prinzie, and Heene (2008) offer a more helpful broad look at the process of developing and activating the mission statement as the guiding document in a health care system:

> …hospitals should develop a carefully crafted implementation and communication plan in order to promote the organizational mission statement.…such an implementation and communication plan should consist of a balanced combination of formal and informal measures…managers should increase the accessibility and relevance of the formal mission statement by weaving use of the mission statement into the hour-by-hour activities of the organization. Aligning organizational procedures, such as performance appraisals and assessments, with the values expressed in the mission statement and clarifying their mutual connection to the organization's members will increase the visibility and practical relevance of the mission statement. (Desmidt et al., 2008, p. 1443)

It should be noted that the creation of a shared vision of the mission of a health care system grounded in the Dance of Caring Persons model and the formalization of that vision into an institutional statement of mission are two related, though different, dimensions of the overall process. As members of a health care system share meaningful stories of caring in their roles, not only is a shared vision being created but the language of the mission statement is being developed as well. Similarly, in the formal process of writing a mission statement, the understanding of the mission deepens as it becomes crystallized in the formal statement of that mission. This being the case, it will be important to institute strategies for managing the synergistic feedback process. Adamson and Bailie (2012) cited Mezirow and other authorities on transformational learning in recommending that groups "ideally should allow for affect, critically reflect, limit the influence of disruptive members, and have equal opportunity to challenge and generalize learning" (Adamson & Bailie, 2012, p. 140). One research approach that could be adapted as a participative strategy is called group phenomenology (Schoenhofer, 2002).

STRATEGY: PARTICIPATIVE GENERATIVE–SYNTHESIS PROCESS

In small work groups, horizontal and vertical, members of the system, including patients and families, and leaders from the surrounding community as well as persons employed within the system, persons would be invited to tell personal stories of meaningful health care experiences—stories that epitomize the "ideal" health care experience. Those stories could come from experiences of receiving personally meaningful health care as well as from experiences of having been the providers of personally meaningful health care. We have found that the guidelines for the storytelling are important for focus and relevance to the task at hand. For example, persons might be invited to "tell a story of your best experience with health care (provider or recipient), one that stands out for you as the way health care should be, that expresses the kind of care you would want for yourself and those closest to you. Recall that experience, in detail—the sights, sounds, smells, who was there, what were the surroundings; try to relive that experience. When you have reconnected with the experience fully, write the story of the experience—a story of the 'best health care ever.' When you are finished writing the story, add one sentence, a sentence that flows directly from inside the story itself (rather than being from an 'outside view'). Finish the sentence that begins with the words: The essence of health care is . . . "

When everyone has finished writing their stories, including the final sentence, invite them to read their stories aloud. (When time is unlimited, stories can be recounted verbally, but we have found that relevance, focus, and fairness are maximized when stories are written and then read.) Allowing the stories to be shared and savored is all that is needed; analysis seems to dilute the power of connectedness created in the experience.

A final step is synthesis—the creating of shared meaning as illuminated in the one-sentence statement about the essence of the health care situation shared in the story. This step can be taken at another time, but is more productive if it immediately follows the sharing of stories. Here is an approach to synthesis that strengthens the connectedness created in the sharing and that clarifies shared meaning—we might call it a process of creating shared meaning. Each of the final sentences is written on a whiteboard or butcher paper or other mechanism useful for group work. The sentences can be compiled in an electronic document and displayed on each person's laptop or smartphone screen, but it is useful to have the sentences also displayed in a common format. The next step is to begin to delete words that are not meaning-laden, words like "the," "and," "through," "goes," and so on, leaving only the nouns and if desired, key verbs and adjectives. The next step in this synthesis process is to identify words that are synonyms, retaining those that most richly convey the sense of the similar terms. Both of these steps are done by consensus; one of the most valuable aspects of the entire strategy is the dialogue that occurs in achieving consensus in these phases—it is here that shared meaning is co-created. At this point, the remaining words may be recorded for later synthesis work by a group that integrates these terms. Better yet, the original group would continue this process to the next step—using the remaining terms to develop a one- or two-sentence statement that conveys the shared meaning expressed through the stories; those sentences would "distill the essence" of stories shared in the group. The sentences could then be taken to a group that has representation from all the groups participating in the strategy, preferably all the members of the organization, but at least includes members selected by their own constituent groups. At the next level of synthesis, a similar process would take place, until ultimately, a proposed mission statement would be shared for comment by members of the system or their constituent representatives, and a final statement approved.

Obviously, a select group could take the results of several collections of stories and derive a mission statement that reflects a shared view of the institutional mission. However, from the perspective of the Dance of Caring Persons, two strengths are likely to be waived by a "select group" approach. One strength is "buy in," a genuine sense of participation and ownership that serves as a significant pillar of the success of a system-wide transformation. The other strength of the "inclusiveness" approach over the "select" approach is the creative wisdom that emerges from valuing the contributions of all. If a "select group" approach is taken, buy in and connectedness could be facilitated by creating a table that shows linkages between phrases in the mission statement and verbatim quotes from a range of stories.

Other guiding documents, in addition to the mission statement, need to be included in strategic design. For example, in unit or department direct-care practice patterns, there has been a trend in the 21st century toward the use of clinical paths to standardize care in order to achieve safety, effectiveness, and cost-saving outcomes. One of the most desired features of clinical paths is standardization. In thinking about unique missions of various health care systems, there is a balance to be sought between standardization and uniqueness. For example, not all health care systems will be grounded in the explicit values of the Dance of Caring Persons and thus clinical paths may not directly address nuances of "caring" as a lived core value and "care" as a general designator synonymous with technical health-related activities. Clinical paths in health care systems grounded in the Dance of Caring Persons will necessarily reflect important caring science-based processes that may or may not be recognized in other systems.

Clinical paths are one example, and there are many other aspects in health care system management where a balance between standardization and creativity is a difficult though necessary consideration. Health records and health care recording and communicating processes are generally purchased in a standardized design format and most commercial health record systems allow for system-specific tailoring. However, when the health care system is grounded in caring, specific functional system designers/modifiers will most likely face a learning curve in terms of creating recording options and recording language that serve the purposes of a health care system grounded in an explicit value of caring. As was noted in the Response in Chapter 2, "care" has become a term largely synonymous with "activity" and generally does not convey the full sense expressed in "caring." Other commercially developed health care system management tools for outcome evaluation, public relations, recruitment, and continuing education would also need to be carefully selected to be congruent with the Dance of Caring Persons, and then most likely would need to be modified to some extent. The next section of this chapter will explore the broad role of the HR function in a health care system grounded in caring.

THE ROLE OF HUMAN RESOURCES

Many of us have experienced the HR area from a traditional perspective, a perspective focused on tasks and managing, policing, and controlling employee behavior often through rigid policies. Traditional HR management practices were designed for industrial organizations where the key functions of hiring, firing, and training were mechanical.

They were not designed for health care organizations where the focus is providing caring service to those seeking care. As a result, practices of HR are often designed to improve the performance of the organization rather than to promote the well-being of employees and the system as a whole.

Opinions vary on the readiness of HR management to support transformation. The image of HR managers is that of people managers or change agents. Yet, they have in the past often been powerless to enact personnel management of the workforce. This is because their role is viewed as supportive, but not central to the organization; and/or the implementation of policies falls to line-managers (Guest & Woodrow, 2012). Macfarlane et al. (2011) believe that HR today has successfully modernized complex health organizations. This includes recruiting staff with skills in service transformation; developing the workforce; redesigning and creating new roles; linking staff development to service needs; supporting workforce planning; and creating opportunities for sharing, learning, and the exchange of knowledge.

Guest and Woodrow (2012) point out that the current issue is not the absence of working-life HR practices, but rather the extent to which policies and practices can be effectively implemented. They cite a four-stage implementation process proposed by Guest and Bos-Nehles:

- Deciding to introduce or amend an HR practice
- Determining the quality of the policy and associated practices
- Implementing the practices on the ground
- Assessing the quality of the implementation (Guest & Woodrow, 2012)

A strong HR system must meet certain conditions to be successful. The policies and practices need to be distinctive so that they are easily recognized; their purpose must be understood; they need to be communicated clearly and consistently throughout the organization; and there should be a transparent means–end association (Bowen & Ostroff, 2004).

Buchan (2004) asserts that "getting HR policy and management 'right' has to be at the core of any sustainable solution to health system performance" (para. 1). He cites multiple studies that show the positive and cumulative relationship between people management and business performance. Highlighted are the successes of Magnet hospitals. His key message is the importance of bundling HR strategies. Bundling is the development of focused strategies that, when taken together, synergistically instill trust and foster commitment among employees and facilitate organizational change. Strategic HR management is central to successful organizational change because it aligns HR functions not only to each other, but also to the overall organizational strategy. Transformation is sustained by implementing bundled HR interventions that *fit* with the organizational mission and priorities: supporting autonomous working by nurses; enabling participation in decision making; facilitating career development; and enabling high-level skills to be deployed effectively sustain transformation. Underscored is the importance of a *fit* between the HR approach and the characteristics, context, and priorities of the organization; and acknowledgment that *bundles* versus single uncoordinated interventions will better sustain change in organizations.

The future success of health care organizations calls for a new approach to HR that is conceptually clear on that which guides its strategies—an approach guided by the mission of the organization that holds employees, the health care system, and those served and their well-being as the focus. HR represents the most precious resource of organizations—the entire workforce—persons—*all* persons in *all* roles. It is the voice for the whole. HR is about "managing" this precious resource.

Transformation of health care systems requires a new perspective from which HR policies and practices are created and implemented. The Dance of Caring Persons is the philosophical grounding for this change. From a person perspective it conveys that each person is respected, valued, and treated fairly and equitably; and from a system perspective it conveys the importance of focusing on the values of the *whole*. It is the organizational mission and vision that provide employees with a sense of purpose and make clear the values held dear. Health care organizations often lack a clear understanding of their strategic intent and as a result HR initiatives lack coherence and focus (Khatri, 2006). The Dance of Caring Persons is a unifying framework for a health care system grounded in caring. Each person is recognized as living caring and having knowledge essential to the success of the organization. The Dance creates a culture in which individuals believe that who they are and what they know is important, valued, and of benefit to the whole. From this perspective, persons view themselves as partners in the organization and see their contributions as essential to the organization's overall success.

HR capability is built around the mission of the organization. HR management leadership plays a key role in building HR capability but overall, developing the capabilities of HR is an important organizational responsibility. All HR personnel must demonstrate a *buy in* of the mission and vision. Organizational transformation includes a commitment to organizational learning that is essential in order to create a new culture. In health care systems it is the values, beliefs, and norms that provide the context for meaning. These influence how and what is deemed important and what one learns.

Change in cultures occurs as individuals accept and live fundamental values of the organization and, therefore, engage in relationships in new ways. HR personnel will need to clearly understand the mission and vision of the organization and be able to answer these necessary questions: What is a caring-based culture? Why is a caring-based culture central to the health care system? What is the value of caring to employees, patients, families, and all stakeholders? How is such a culture created and evaluated? What is the direct link of the role of HR personnel to systems outcomes?

Understanding that the mission of the health care organization is to foster the creation of a culture of caring enables HR to focus on the outcomes HR is seeking to achieve rather than on isolated tasks. This clarity of focus drives all actions and strategies. With the aim of creating a culture of caring, an initial step in the transformation process might be to review existing policies and processes to determine the fit with the mission, then co-create with others in the organization strategies to imbed the culture in caring values. Ultimately, the success of HR strategies is determined by outcomes achieved. Examples of key outcomes achieved through the integration of caring values are improved quality of care; increased patient and employee satisfaction; improved safety; and decreased costs. (A further discussion of outcomes is in Chapter 9.)

HR staff persons in collaboration with others in the organization will need to develop structures, processes, and management tools from a caring perspective. Although this may initially seem like an overwhelming task, it will be quickly realized that the Dance of Caring Persons offers the organization a definite competitive edge. The model is unique and valuable. It fosters employee and patient satisfaction and consequently makes the health care system an *employer of choice*. Developing one's own management tools or choosing to enhance those already in existence with caring content increases the competitive edge by demonstrating the uniqueness of their system. Some examples of processes that fit the organizational mission of creating a culture of caring might be helpful here. Let us look at recruitment, orientation, retention, appraisal, and training and development processes.

Recruitment and selection of employees begins the process of socialization in the organization. Recruitment and retention of employees is important to service and operational excellence. Obviously, it is essential that persons being recruited are assessed for the requisite knowledge and skills needed for a particular role. In addition, they will be expected to hold values congruent with those of the organization. The bigger question in recruitment is *who is the person seeking to join our caring-based community?* Coming to know person as person and person as caring is an important focus of the interview process—both for the applicant and the employer. One of the initial aspects of the process is attracting persons who hold values similar to the core values of the organization. Thus, the languaging of the recruitment materials is important. When seeking to know the person being considered for a position as one who is "right" for the explicitly caring-based organization, the process might include the following:

- Inviting persons to share a story in which they lived caring; or ways in which they see themselves as expressing caring at work (may be a verbal or written part of the process)
- Sharing with the applicant one's own story of living caring
- Engaging in dialogue on how caring was uniquely lived in the stories shared

This approach makes clear the values of the organization and expectations of what it means to be a member of this health care organization.

The orientation process should also reflect the values of the organization. The use of an interprofessional video as one way of conveying examples of living caring in various roles is described in Chapter 9. This video, based on Mayeroff's caring ingredients, could be shown and discussed at all orientations. Orientees could be invited to share their story of living caring. They might reflect on and perhaps offer a written response to the question "How do I live my patience, knowing, trust, alternating rhythms, humility, hope, and courage in the ordinariness of life?" These stories would then be shared with others in the group. Such an exercise calls one to reflect on the meaning of caring and to appreciate the unique ways caring is expressed. It begins to frame the experience of being in a caring-based culture.

Studer (2004) suggests that five-pillar leadership focused on people, service, quality, finance, and growth ensures a retained workforce. It is the focus on people that results in increased engagement, satisfaction, retention, and ultimately gains in all other pillars.

Retention of employees is a major challenge in health care. Retention is important for many reasons, including continuity and excellence in care, advancing the institutional mission, and decreasing costs to the organization. After having invested in strategies for recruitment and selection, it makes sense that a health care system carry that investment through to retention. Having made efforts to recruit employees who share core values epitomized in the Dance of Caring Persons, retention of those persons in the workforce will depend on employees experiencing a high level of congruence between those values that are espoused and those that are actually and consistently expressed in everyday organizational practices. Here is an example of what we mean:

> Research at a for-profit hospital focused on transforming a practice setting through caring values highlights the importance of leaders being able to translate values into action in order to retain staff (Boykin, Schoenhofer, Smith, St. Jean, & Aleman, 2003). The first step of the research process focused on coming-to-know values, ideas, and activities that mattered to both direct and indirect care providers as well as patients and families. Themes emerging from this coming-to-know process were:
>
> - Commitment
> - Being there out of concern for the other
> - Truly listening leads to truly knowing and responding to that which matters

- Nurturing the person living and growing in caring through unique expressions of caring
- Value experienced from the mutuality of the experience
- Valuing contributions of other members of the health care team

The next phase of the process centered on creating ways to reflect these values in the practice setting. Examples of strategies identified by staff to support the living of these values included:

- Developing a hallway display with pictures and stories of each staff member. This was a way for employees as well as patients and families to come to know them as person
- Making available for all, articles on caring to support growing in the knowledge of caring
- Creating a bulletin board in the staff lounge using Mayeroff's caring ingredients and inviting staff to post examples of how they lived caring or witnessed others living caring for each of the caring ingredients
- Creating work schedules to support the unique needs of individuals, i.e., increasing flexibility to accommodate family or educational needs
- Inviting administrators to dialogue with them on the unit regarding issues of care (transforming the "we" versus "they" attitude to "us")
- Transforming the practice of nursing from task orientation to person centered
- Creating appraisal systems to mirror the living of caring values
- Creating compensation structures grounded in caring (see Valentine, 1993, for an example)

Successful retention of employees calls for leaders to come to know them as persons; identify what matters to them; create innovative responses; foster their living and growing in caring; and create a sense of community. HR policies and processes need to be flexible and grounded in the value of persons to the organization.

A common and growing issue facing health care today that directly impacts retention is bullying. This issue often falls in the lap of HR but remains unaddressed. Why does bullying continue to be such a problem in health care? It is not that there are no policies in place to deal with this issue. Guest and Woodrow (2012) cite Bauman in noting that although the "policies and practices are in place, there is often an absence of what he termed 'the moral impulse' to ensure that they are implemented fully and consistently" (Guest & Woodrow, 2012, p. 117). Two antecedents of bullying cited by Guest and Woodrow are "lack of perceived organizational support and lack of faith in the HR system to address the issue in a supportive way if a complaint is made" (Guest & Woodrow, 2012, p. 115). The consequences of bullying not only have serious consequences on those being bullied but also the cost of bullying extends to those who are not direct targets, for example, patients.

How would living the values of the Dance of Caring Persons facilitate addressing this issue of bullying? When an organization makes clear its commitment to living caring values, the expectation is that all who choose to join the system are willing to embrace and grow with these values and beliefs. From the perspective of caring, there is only one right way of relating and that is to respect each other as caring person. If after counseling, the offender chooses to continue bullying behavior, the obligation of HR would be to terminate the employee as his or her values do not fit with those of the organization and hinder the growth of the mission. Living the commitment to organizational values in this way is not easy. Removing someone for continuing bullying behavior is a difficult situation as it may be that the offender is an otherwise esteemed person, valued by the institution. It is exactly this strong professional culture in health care that often prevents these situations from being appropriately addressed—addressed with consequences. Yet, a commitment to the values of the organization must guide all actions. Guest and Woodrow (2012) cite Kantian ethics as a fundamental grounding for the relationship between HR and employees. Relevant Kantian maxims include "treat others as you would have them treat you; persons should always be treated as ends in themselves and not as means to an end." These principles are important in all aspects of the organization. They call to question "What ought to be?"

Betty Tsarnas, an NP, shared a story from the early days of her practice as an RN. This is an example of bullying and how one nurse leader responded in a way that had the potential for promoting growth in caring.

> It was the story that I wrote that took place about 25 or so years ago. I worked on the night shift in the ICU unit and was the charge nurse at a large teaching hospital in New York. We had a new cardiothoracic surgeon who was very difficult to work with. He was very demanding and never told us what he wanted but would belittle us if we applied the tape on his patients' post op dressings going in the wrong direction. We kept a record each time he would criticize a nurse so that we knew how to care for his patients. He wanted weights on all his patients every day. On the night shift we bathed the patients and weighed them. One night I accepted one of his patients from the PAC, a very unstable critical patient who had been in the OR for many hours. The patient had a balloon pump, Swan-Ganz catheter and arterial line, monitor, CVP line, chest tube, and about five different IV medications all keeping him alive. During the night several of the other nurses helped me and we gently attempted two times to turn this patient onto the sling to raise him above the bed to get his weight, and then we decided to abort this idea. The patient did well through the night. The surgeon arrived at 5:50 a.m. which he did at the exactly same time each morning and focused only on the weight not being done. I was yelled at, belittled, and there was no chance to discuss or reason with him. I went home and was called several hours later by the Director of Nursing of this 1,000-bed hospital, who put the surgeon on the phone to apologize to me. (I wish I could remember her name but it was a long time ago and she was a wonderful nursing leader who always stood up for her nurses.) It was a wonderful hospital to work at because the nursing department supported us, trained us— I had a 2-month orientation to the critical care unit. We had a 12-bed unit and worked each night with six nurses. We were well trained, and we were well respected by the physicians as a whole. The cardiac surgeon was the only physician with whom I ever had a difficulty.

Approaches to training and development of employees further convey values held by the organization. Rather than limiting development programs to a predetermined prescribed set of offerings—those determined by others as essential—it would also be important to ascertain from employees their hopes and dreams for learning and growing. Continuing to grow in a culture of caring requires time for critical reflection. Critical reflection is defined by Mezirow as "questioning and perhaps challenging existing values, beliefs, and assumptions" (Adamson & Baile, 2012, p. 144). Providing employees the opportunity to reflect and dialogue with each other, formally or informally, supports the value of coming to know other, sharing knowledge, and creating community.

In summary, a range of strategies for achieving a transformation in the organizational mission have been suggested. The strategies identified here are examples of ways to accomplish development, diffusion, and uptake of a transformed mission. Every sector of the organization needs to be involved in creating a statement that translates a vision of core values into the foundation for action planning. Sample approaches to the development of the institutional mission statement include the use of stories that exemplify individual contributions to the living of the envisioned mission, and a group process for gathering ideas and achieving a shared understanding of the purpose of the organization, the business of the organization, and the core values of the organization. The broad HR function, guided by the HR department, brings the mission into every facet of the organization, offering guidelines for effective engagement of all persons who are members of the system. Once the members of the health care system are well grounded in a substantive knowledge of caring, creative strategies can be devised from all quarters of the system. The strategies we are offering as exemplars are intended to stimulate the development of a visible, functional culture of caring that is inclusive and dynamic.

REFERENCES

Adamson, C. W., & Baile, J. W. (2012). Education versus learning: Restorative practices in higher education. *Journal of Transformative Education, 10*(3), 139–156. doi:10.1177/1541344612463265

Bowen, D. E., & Ostroff, C. (2004). Understanding HRM-firm performance linkages: The role of the "strength" of the HRM system. *Academy of Management Review, 29*, 203–221.

Boykin, A. (1994). Creating a caring environment for nursing education. In A. Boykin (Ed.), *Living a caring-based program.* New York, NY: National League for Nursing.

Boykin, A., Schoenhofer, S. O., Smith, N., St. Jean, J., & Aleman, D. (2003). Transforming practice using a caring-based nursing model. *Nursing Administration Quarterly, 27*(3), 223–230.

Buchan, J. (2004). What difference does ("good") HRM make? *Human Resources for Health, 2*(6). doi:10:1186/1478-4491-2-6. Retrieved from http://www.human-resources-health.com/content/2/1/6

Desmidt, S., Prinzie, A., & Heene, A. (2008). The level and determinants of mission statement use: A questionnaire survey. *International Journal of Nursing Studies, 45*(10), 1433–1441.

Guest, D., & Woodrow, C. (2012). Exploring the boundaries of human resource managers' responsibilities. *Journal of Business Ethics, 111,* 109–119. doi:10.1007/s10551-012-1438-8.

Khatri, N. (2006). Building HR capacity in health care organizations. *Health Care Management Review, 31*(1), 45–54.

Macfarlane, F., Greenhalgh, T., Humphrey, C., Hughes, J., Butler, C., & Pawson, R. (2011). A few workforce in the making? A case study of strategic human resource management in a whole-system change effort in healthcare. *Journal of Health and Organizational Management, 25*(1), 55–72.

Radtke, J. M. (1998). How to write a mission statement. *The Grantsmanship Center Magazine, 68*(1).

Schoenhofer, S. O. (2002). Philosophical underpinnings of an emergent methodology for nursing as caring inquiry. *Nursing Science Quarterly, 15*(4), 275–280.

Stone, R. A. (1996). Mission statements revisited. *SAM Advanced Management Journal, 61*(1). Retrieved from http://www.freepatentsonline.com/article/SAM-Advanced-Management-Journal/18446696.html

Studer, Q. (2004). The value of employee retention. *Healthcare Financial Management, 58*(1), 52–57.

Valentine, K. (1993). Utilization of research on caring in the development of a nurse compensation system. In D. A. Gaut (Ed.), *Caring: A global agenda* (Ch. 22). New York, NY: National League for Nursing.

Response to Chapter 6

Janet Y. Harris, DNP
Chief Nursing Executive and
Chief Nursing Officer–Adult
University of Mississippi Medical Center Hospitals

*T*his chapter provides an excellent framework for leaders. The caring philosophy must be embedded in the mission with the thread of caring underpinning all of the work of the organization. Often, in organizations, there are so many competing priorities that focus can be easily lost. Unification of documents, plans, and communications should include the consistent message of caring. This work cannot be carried out by a single individual; leaders at all levels of the organization must clearly articulate and live the mission. Most important, the commitment must come from the highest level of the organization. This individual must also understand the language of caring, speak the language, and demonstrate it at all times. Signing of a contract that outlines the mission, vision, and values of the organization can help to solidify the commitment and provide an ongoing visual reminder to all in the workplace. Documents should be displayed in prominent places throughout the organization. All members of the organization should hold their peers accountable to the mission and values.

To assist in the endeavor, as stated in this chapter, potential recruits must be evaluated to assure "fit" with the organizational mission and culture of caring. Testing for characteristics and fit can offer valuable insights and assist in hiring the "right" person up front—rather than having to remove them out once hired. Perhaps a particular group, in addition to human resources (HR) staff, could be assigned the responsibility to serve as continuity advocates and assist in monitoring publications, policies, and new initiatives. The basic question should always be "Does this activity or action support the mission of the organization?" Only with the consistent and constant messaging from all leaders in an organization will the shared understanding be lived in the dance.

Ultimately, through sharing the stories of the caregivers and patients who can articulate and describe the caring relationship and their personal experiences, the caring behaviors will become the foundation of the organizational culture. Valuing, prizing, and recognizing caregivers will ultimately drive and sustain the caring mission.

As a leader in a large organization, it is important to personally demonstrate these values to staff. Although time and resources are barriers in today's health care environments, priorities must be set within a weekly schedule to allow for these activities. A few processes have worked effectively in our organization. First, all of the senior administrative staff members now make weekly patient rounds. This gives administrators immediate access to patient feedback, demonstrates caring for patients, and allows, in some cases, for immediate operational improvements.

A program called "Where in the U" allows senior executives to spend time or "shadow" selected frontline staff members. This is accomplished from a random drawing of frontline staff each month. After the experience, both the frontline staff and senior staff report on what was learned from the experience. For example, time spent by the nurse executive in the ICU allowed hands on care for patients—side by side with the staff. A third process implemented is called "Sip and Say." In this 1-hour, one-on-one conversation, the nurse executive gets to know new managers and educators more personally—discussing career goals, personal goals, and how they enjoy spending their spare time. Relationships are developed that allow for open and comfortable exchange going forward. Lastly, the DAISY Award program highlights the accomplishments of nurses that go above and beyond in caring for patients. A ceremony on the nurse's home unit allows for a public celebration and recognition for caring behaviors.

Chapter 7

Transforming Leadership Structures and Processes

*F*or the past decade, literature on the type of leadership needed to transform health care systems focused primarily on either transactional or transformational models. Understandably, health care organizations choose a leadership style based on the values and beliefs of the culture that are important to them. The literature has made clear that leadership and management styles of leaders in health care directly influence retention, patient and employee satisfaction, and overall success of the organization. Transactional leadership is described as identifying the expectations of followers and responding to them, thereby establishing a close link between effort and reward (Popper, 2000). Transformational leadership has four dimensions: charisma, inspirational motivation, intellectual stimulation, and individualized consideration (Bass & Avolio, 1990). Through this approach, leaders empower others, foster creativity, instill respect, and generate commitment to the mission of the organization. More recently, the concept of strengths-based leadership has been proposed as another paradigm for transforming systems of care. The focus of this type of leadership is "recognizing, mobilizing, capitalizing and developing a person's strengths to promote health and facilitate healing" (Gottlieb, Gottlieb, & Shamian, 2012, p. 39).

The concept of transformational leadership was first described by Burns (1978) in a book called *Leadership*. Since that time, there has been considerable exploration of the concept, and general agreement about its characteristics, even if specific language and emphasis might differ across authors. Transformational leadership is required to navigate within complex adaptive systems within today's health care environment. In this chapter, it is not our intention to provide an exhaustive review of the nature of transformational leadership, but rather to sample a few salient ideas related to leadership from the 1990s, as those leaders imagined the challenges in the 21st century. As the largest single group of health care providers, nursing leaders took aspects of transformational leadership to heart, focusing on leadership development for both frontline staff and those in formal leadership positions. The commitment to transformational leadership is codified within the Magnet hospital designation recognition program offered through the American Nurses Credentialing Center (ANCC). Additionally, the Institute for Healthcare Improvement (IHI), as an international, interprofessional organization committed to safe and effective health care systems, also emphasizes the importance of transformational change and transformational leadership. In the Transforming Care at the Bedside (TCAB) initiative (Viney, Batcheller, Houston, & Belcik, 2006), transformational leadership is one of the five key dimensions that help to improve performance within hospitals. These dimensions are as follows:

- Transformational leadership
- Safe and reliable care
- Vitality and teamwork
- Patient-centered care
- Value-added care processes

In follow-up studies conducted across 12 health care systems (Lukas et al., 2007), mixed methods evaluation identified characteristics present in successful transformation of patient care:

1. Impetus to transform
2. Leadership commitment to quality
3. Improvement initiatives
4. Alignment of resources and actions at all levels of the organization to achieve consistent goals
5. Integration to bridge boundaries across components within the system

The Safety Net Medical Home Initiative's (SNMHI, 2010) Implementation Guide for community-based medical home initiatives also highlights engaged leadership as a key strategy along with continuous and team-based healing relationships, patient-centered interactions, quality, access, care coordination, and evidence-based care.

In summary, leadership is a key success factor in transforming practice environments regardless of whether the setting is hospital or community based or whether the focus is a particular discipline (ANCC Magnet) or interprofessional (IHI). Though we will be presenting a particular perspective from the experience of working primarily with the nursing leaders, these principles translate to each discipline within the organization and each health care leader.

ANCC'S MAGNET RECOGNITION PROGRAM AND A CULTURE OF CARING

As an example of a discipline's commitment to transformational leadership, the ANCC Magnet Model Components identified one of its core factors for success as "Transformational Leadership" (ANCC, 2012). What this includes is the ability of leaders to thrive within an ever-changing environment and ensure that values, beliefs, and behaviors are consistently aligned for the well-being of those served and the staff who provide those services. The transformational leader must have an eye to the future and help each staff member move toward that future with competence and confidence. Emphasis is placed on listening, collaborating across departments, and articulating a vision that can be actualized and sustained within complex adaptive systems that help "birth new ideas and innovations" (ANCC Magnet Model, retrieved November 2012, www.nursecredentialing.org).

Complementary components of the Magnet model give further foundation to caring leadership in health care systems. In addition to transformational leadership, the other key components of the model are structural empowerment, exemplary professional practice, and new knowledge, innovation, and improvements, all functioning within a global perspective and focused on delivering empirical outcomes. Structural empowerment involves an emphasis on strong professional practice and partnership formation within an organization and with the community it serves to achieve outcomes that matter to each. For Magnet-designated hospitals, it matters how professional practice is developed and sustained to ensure that the substantive knowledge of the discipline of nursing is practiced in collaboration with other interdisciplinary professionals for each to achieve exemplary care processes and outcomes for those served. Contributions to new knowledge generation, innovation, and improvements are part of the ethical imperative of being a member of a professional discipline pledged to uphold the public trust in the enactment of that role. Monitoring and measuring results to show what difference has been made in practice is an area of increasing emphasis within the program.

Bennis and Nanus, in their seminal 1985 work on leadership, list core activities for transformational leaders:

1. Create attention through vision
2. Create meaning through communication
3. Create trust through positioning
4. Deploy oneself effectively

These ideas might inspire leaders to reflect on the following:

- How effectively do I convey my vision to others in the organization and create the experience of a shared purpose?
- In what ways do I invite dialogue on ideas to enhance shared understanding and create meaning?
- How does my way of being instill trust? Do I truly listen, hear, and respond to that which matters?

Leadership is essential in every organization. This chapter offers an innovative paradigm for transforming leadership in health care systems. This paradigm—Dance of Caring Persons—has caring as its core value. The attributes of caring described by Roach (2002)—competence, compassion, confidence, commitment, conscience, and comportment—are used as a framework for discussion of leadership in health care. Roach presented these attributes in relationship to caring and nursing in particular as she questioned: "What is a nurse doing when she or he is caring?" and "What obligations are entailed in caring?" (p. 45) It is apparent to us that these same questions reframed can and should be asked of all persons in health care. Caring should be the locus for rules, principles, and norms governing practice in health care systems.

In this chapter, we will invite you to consider the meaning of each of Roach's caring attributes in relationship to leadership in the organization as well as strategies for bringing these attributes to life. Although the content in this chapter is relevant to leaders throughout the organization, the focus will be on those in designated leadership positions by nature of their role and responsibilities, particularly nurse leaders. This framework of Roach's 6Cs of caring is a useful approach to a discussion of the qualities required to lead in the transformation of health care in your setting as well.

COMPETENCE

Competence, a multifaceted concept, is required of all leaders in health care organizations. Competence is described as "having the knowledge, judgment, skills, energy, experience and motivation required to respond adequately to the demands of one's professional responsibilities" (Roach, 2002, p. 54). When speaking of competence, she states that caring demands a competence of the highest order. In whatever one's job, position, or level of responsibility, expertise is understood as a norm of caring. One of Mayeroff's (1971) expressions of caring, knowing, further elaborates on competence. He says caring includes knowledge that is explicit and implicit; and direct and indirect as well as knowing "that" and knowing "how." Knowing explicitly is being able to relate what one knows; knowing implicitly is not being able to articulate all that one knows (e.g., about a friend); knowing "that" refers to the abstract knowing of something but not being necessarily able to apply it; knowing "how" refers to doing something; direct knowing is encountering or experiencing whereas indirect knowing is knowledge about something. Mayeroff makes clear that caring involves a depth of knowledge.

The competencies needed by leaders to transform health care systems can seem overwhelming and the list of demands for requisite knowledge competencies continues to grow. Obviously, there are many competency expectations of nurse leaders. Some, in particular, are communication and relationship management, leadership, knowledge of the health care environment, business skills and principles, and professionalism (American Association of Critical-Care Nurses [AACN], 2005). These are in addition to the expectation that nurse leaders design models of patient care delivery, advance the profession, serve as stewards of nursing, participate in political advocacy for patient care and the profession, as well as leverage new technologies (Swick, Doulaveris, & Christensen, 2012). The Center for Nursing Leadership (1990) described aspects of nursing leadership that are broad enough to apply to all leaders in health care. These realms of leadership are holding the truth, intellectual and emotional self, discovery of potential, quest for the adventure toward knowing, diversity as a vehicle to wholeness, appreciation of ambiguity, knowing something of life, holding multiple perspectives without judgment, and keeping commitments to oneself. It is not the intent of this section to discuss all of the competencies needed to effectively lead but rather to offer a broad view of competencies through the lens of caring.

Strategies for Growing in Competency in Caring

Knowing Self as Caring Person

There are numerous ways for leaders to grow in and build competence in caring. One of the first and the most significant strategies is to focus on coming to know self as caring person. This is an essential part of the self-knowledge that is basic to leadership grounded in caring. It calls for humility, courage, trust, and a continual openness to knowing self through one's daily encounters.

An effective and practical strategy for coming to know self directly as caring person is through reflection. Recall a story or experience of caring you hold dear. Ask yourself the following questions:

- How did I live my knowing, patience, alternating rhythm, courage, hope, trust, honesty, and humility?
- Has my understanding of self as caring changed how I live my life?
- How might I grow in my caring competency?
- Am I open to truly knowing self as caring?
- Does not each day present me with the opportunity to further knowing of self as caring?
- What insights and appreciations of myself as caring person surfaced in this reflection?

Understanding one's personal expressions of caring enhances the knowing of other as caring. Conversely, knowing other as caring helps one to continue to grow in knowing self as caring. Through a focus on coming to know self, one can begin to appreciate the many unique ways caring is lived and what it means to be human, what it means to be caring. Reflection creates an understanding of how one's story connects to that of others—creating a sense of shared humanity. Personal knowing is necessary for engaging in authentic relationships. One is authentic in being for another if it results in freedom of others and inauthentic if permeated by dominance and depersonalization (Roach, 2002). Other characteristics of authentic leaders include the ability to understand their own purpose, practice solid values, establish enduring relationships, lead with a heart, and practice self-discipline (George, 2003).

O'Connor (2008) uses the Center for Nursing Leadership's description of intellectual and emotional intelligence as another way of knowing self. In addition to intellectual competencies needed, she speaks of strategies to develop emotional competencies such as:

- Self-awareness—knowing self and how we come across to others
- Regulation of moods and emotions—ability not to react to situations
- Motivation—having a passion for nursing [*or one's own discipline*]
- Empathy—ability of the leader to understand and identify with others
  Empathy calls for really hearing, understanding, and responding with sensitivity
- Social skill—the ability to build and cultivate relationships and other essential caring competencies

Knowing self is integral to the practice of caring-based nursing administration. It is through a continual focus on knowing self as caring that one grows in the knowledge and skills to know and affirm caring in others. It is this understanding that frees leaders to nurture and support others. It is this understanding that enables nurse leaders to infuse health care organizations with an understanding of what it means to live caring. A nurse leader in an emergency department shared this reflection:

> It is crucial that the leader first knows self as caring person and identifies personal ways of living and growing in caring. Through this knowing, one can more easily *see* others (both professionally and personally) as living caring and honor their unique expressions. Commitment to knowing myself as a caring person opened for me the opportunity to know staff as caring persons and to realize how important my role was to nurturing their living and growing in caring. I had to let go and trust staff and not exert my positional authority. I had to see myself as one of the performers in the dance of caring persons but not as preeminent. (Boykin, Schoenhofer, Bulfin, Baldwin, & McCarthy, 2005)

Knowing Self and Other as Caring Person

One hospital that launched an initiative to introduce a culture of caring created a videotape depicting staff members' unique living of caring in their role. This was an effective strategy to help illuminate what it means for all persons in the system to live caring. Mayeroff's expressions of caring were used as a guide in creating a video in which the following examples of living caring were shared.

- *Knowing*—a monitor tech related a story of how she noticed an elderly, confused patient sitting near the nurse's station. She heard the patient's call to be noticed and comforted. In a most beautiful response, she took a pillowcase and fashioned a doll out of it and gave it to the patient, who cradled the doll as a mother would her child. The patient became content.

- *Courage*—a physician shared a story of how he lived his courage as he sat with an elderly couple and learned that the elderly husband was abusing his wife. He had to report this situation.
- *Hope*—a nurse shared a story in which a dying patient asked her if she knew her favorite song, "You Are My Sunshine," the song she and her husband first danced to. The nurse sang to the dying woman.
- *Honesty*—two nurses told how they lived out who they were in their care for a dying patient who evidently lived on the street. They provided scented lotion, soft music, and essential oils. They stayed with her following the shift report. The patient smiled at them just before she died.
- *Alternating rhythm*—a nurse shared how prepared she felt to care for a trauma victim as she drew from a broad knowledge base to care competently and compassionately.
- *Patience*—a nurse told how he sat with a family and supported them as they struggled with the decision to place a loved one in hospice.
- *Trust*—a nursing administrator told a story of "letting go" of his positional authority and trusting others.
- *Humility*—a physician's assistant told of how he was about to do a procedure on a patient when a nurse approached him and expressed why she was concerned about his proceeding with this. He described how he learned from this experienced nurse.

The video served several purposes. It was useful as a way to facilitate dialogue on caring at staff meetings. Staff persons, after viewing the tape, were invited to contribute their stories of living caring. The more caring was discussed, the more meaning it had to staff. They began to use the language of caring and talk about how the knowledge of caring directed not only their work life but also their personal life. The staff shared that this understanding was changing their way of being.

The video was also used to orient new staff to caring values. In an orientation manual on caring, designed by caring champions leading the initiative at a community hospital, Mayeroff's (1971) expressions of caring were described. After reflection on these, new employees viewed the video as a way to understand what it means to live caring. They were then invited to reflect on how they live caring day to day. Examples of living caring were written next to each of the expressions and shared. This attention to knowing self as caring was an integral and upfront aspect of orientation. As a result, new employees began to understand why caring was the central value of the organization and how they could participate in living that organizational value through their own role responsibilities.

Caring for Self

The importance of caring for self was discussed in Chapters 3 and 4. We want to again mention the importance of leaders modeling ways to care for self and instilling the importance of work–life balance. The story of the nurse practitioner in Chapter 3 poignantly describes practicing in a survival mode. It points to the need to prioritize self-care. That story detailed the nurse's preoccupation with her personal and complex life world and its impact on her practice. Although physically with her patient in the exam room, the nurse practitioner was unable to be present, to see, to hear, to nurse. Her ability to care was hindered because the work environment failed to notice her struggle. How might her story have been different if someone had heard and responded to her own call to be nurtured and supported in the moment?

Some health care organizations have realized the importance of having a designated safe place for staff to go to reflect and reengage after difficult encounters or difficult decisions. One hospital converted a room into what they called a *sacred place*. The room was painted in soothing earth tones, had relaxing music, massage chairs, and essential oils available. Staff members were supported to leave their area of practice, take a few minutes to "be" and refocus their energies. The recognition by colleagues of their call to be nurtured and supported adds to a strong work culture. A story shared by nurse Beth Olafson from an experience when she was a new nurse illustrates the importance of nurturing and supporting colleagues.

> I recall the first death of a baby for whom I was caring and how my preceptor brought the baby to the family and intentionally took me along to be a part of the ritual of saying good-bye. When thinking about the death of the first child I coded, the caring of my coworkers became vividly apparent. My preceptor quietly, unknown to me, watched from the window. I was given a quiet space to cry and reflect on the situation after the immediate crisis had passed. My patients were cared for by others. The physician took the time to explain what had happened to the baby before it was born that resulted in death. My coworkers including the physician were my support.

Caring requires that leaders in health care organizations attend to personal well-being. In order to truly care for others, one must first care for self and feel in balance in one's own work and personal life. Role modeling the importance of caring for self is a visible and important strategy for leaders. These strategies might be as simple as leaving one's office to eat or using the time to engage in conversation with colleagues; taking a walk; or participating in self-care exercises such as meditation or yoga. Leaders should also be attentive to the needs of their staff and ways they can create a healthy work environment. Even businesses outside of health care are coming to understand the need for leaders to role model how to renew personal energy and to develop "rituals" or habits for health such as taking a walk for a mental breather, or always eating lunch away from the work environment. Tony Schwartz, chief executive officer (CEO) of the Energy Project, notes that "human beings don't operate like computers... people perform at their peak when they alternate between periods of intense focus and intermittent renewal" (Schwartz, 2010, p. 67). Leaders within the organization set the tone and it is important for the leader to provide the environment for cultivating creativity, communicating values, sharing passion, and renewing energy.

Knowledge Development in Caring

In addition to the personal knowing of caring, developed knowledge of caring is paramount for a substantive base for leadership. Personal, empirical, ethical, and aesthetic ways of knowing (Carper, 1978) shape the in-depth understanding of caring. Those in leadership roles must be committed to creating a learning organization grounded in caring.

EMPIRICAL KNOWING OF CARING

The empirical knowledge needed to lead competently is vast. As mentioned earlier, the aim of this chapter is to focus on the knowledge of caring needed to lead transformation in health care settings. In addition to Mayeroff and Roach, there are various perspectives on caring available for study, particularly in the nursing literature. We often read and hear that "caring is the essence of nursing." Although this is accepted as true, it often remains difficult for nurses to articulate exactly what this means. Caring is sometimes understood more as an emotion than as a concept of great depth and meaning—often misconstrued as "being nice." Many nurses graduated at a time when the knowledge base on caring was just emerging and caring, as a concept, wasn't studied. Today, caring should be studied as an essential domain of nursing and health care knowledge both in education and in practice. Studying caring enhances caring capabilities.

Leaders in health care organizations play a key role in advancing the understanding of caring. To meet this responsibility, they must first become grounded in an explicit knowledge of caring. Leaders need to believe in—live a commitment to—the importance of caring knowledge to the organization. Because caring is the very essence of why health care systems exist, growing in the knowledge of caring is important—if not more important—than all other competencies recognized as important to the organization. This commitment is made visible by routinely devoting time to engaging in dialogue on caring.

Mentoring is an important process to facilitate the knowing of caring and growth of the other. Mentorship is a lifelong process in which a person with greater knowledge or experience in an area nurtures the personal and professional development of a person with less experience. "In caring as helping the other grow, I experience what I care for as an extension of myself and at the same time as something separate from me that I respect in its own right" (Mayeroff, 1971, p. 5). A mentor is a "sponsor, encourager, and friend to a less skilled or less experienced person for the purposes of promoting the latter's professional and/or personal development" (Anderson & Shannon, 1988, p. 39). In mentoring, a leader invites others into his or her world and risks being vulnerable as one's humanity is shared. Mentoring calls for coming to know person as person, person as caring, and hopes and dreams for growing in caring. There is mutual growth as the process is grounded in self-reflection. Leaders must live a commitment to the ongoing development of health care professionals grounded in caring values to transform and sustain health care organizations.

The following story exemplifies how nurse leaders often initiate transformational initiatives in health care:

> The nursing division in an acute care setting had decided to implement Nursing as Caring as their practice model. In the process of implementation of this model, the chief nursing officer realized that the core values of this model were not nursing specific but should be the values that ground the whole of the organization. There was the realization that unless there was a "buy in" of the importance of grounding not just nursing, but the entire organization in caring, the culture as a whole would not change.
>
> After a discussion with the chief executive officer, it was agreed that there would be a meeting of all leaders in the organization—everyone from the executive leadership to the director's level—to engage in a beginning discussion of what it would mean to ground their organization in caring values. At this meeting, everyone sat in a circle. Caring was discussed using Mayeroff's expressions. Each person was invited to share a story of how they lived caring in their role. One person, elated with the opportunity to dialogue on caring, said "I am so excited I am screaming inside."
>
> The first person to share his story (as recounted in Chapter 2) was the chief financial officer. An example of another story told by the chief operating officer follows below:
>
> On a Thursday morning after doing rounds, I returned to my office where I had a message from a nursing director who rarely called. I returned the call immediately. The nursing director expressed frustration with being unable to meet a seemingly simple patient's request— answering what time the patient would go to Special Procedures.
>
> After hanging up the phone, I immediately left my office and went to imaging. I asked the nurse if she had heard about the patient on the second floor who was NPO, had her case cancelled the day before, had not heard from her physician, and was anxiously waiting. The nurse explained that an emergency case was taking place and taking longer than expected. I listened to everything she had to say. Then I asked, "When will the patient on the second

floor be able to come down?" She thought maybe in 3 hours. I reminded her the patient had been NPO for many hours.

We shortened the 3 hours into 2 hours and turned the maybe into "the patient will definitely be in the procedure room by 2:30." This was the sort of caring and communication that was needed. It is easy for us to forget the lack of control that is felt by patients when entering the hospital. We see this take place daily and know the system quite well, so we must remember to continually view our service through the perspectives and perceptions of the patients we serve.

I went to the patient's room and apologized for the delay, explained the emergency procedure that accounted for the lack of visibility by her physician and the Special Procedure staff, and assured her she would be in Special Procedures by 2:30. The nursing director was grateful as together we cared for our patient.

Participants proudly articulated how their role connected to those served. Many were eager to tell the stories they held dear. The opportunity to come together with no agenda other than to begin to understand caring and how it could become the unifying, explicit value of the organization was powerful. At the end of this meeting, the CEO asked, "How can one sustain a culture of caring?" Strategies to advance the infusion of caring values were discussed. The strategies determined by the group included the formation of major committees. The committees were (a) vision, culture, customer care standards; (b) Nursing as Caring theory as a guide, nursing practice, and patient rounding; and (c) environment of care and physician involvement. Each committee, with representation from the executive suite as well as all other areas of the hospital, developed strategies to ground the organization in caring. Because leaders throughout the organization were involved in the unfolding of this new vision, ways of being with staff also began to change. The result was that the employees believed this effort to be "real."

Strategies for enhancing the explicit knowing of caring within the organization include the following:

- Having reading materials on caring available in areas accessible to all employees
- Dialoguing with interprofessional team members on what appear to be paradoxes in caring (i.e., caring and economics, caring and politics, caring and curing)
- Designating certain materials to be read by all employees and discussing them at staff meetings
- Requesting that all councils, staff meetings, and so on begin with a story of living caring, and spend time reflecting and dialoguing on how caring was lived
- Supporting staff to attend and present at conferences focused on advancing caring knowledge such as the International Association for Human Caring; colloquia of the Anne Boykin Institute for the Advancement of Caring in Nursing at the Christine E. Lynn College of Nursing at Florida Atlantic University; and Watson's Caring Science Institute
- Exploring with those being mentored the nature of one's discipline and evolving new understandings and innovative ideas
- Establishing formal programs to build caring knowledge
- Living a commitment to ongoing informal mentoring
- Cultivating leadership grounding in caring at all levels
- Helping others understand situations from the context of the organization
- Assisting colleagues to identify their patterns of caring and hopes for growing in caring competency
- Honoring mentoring meetings; being honest
- Supporting a culture for ongoing learning of caring

ETHICAL KNOWING OF CARING

Roach (2002) states that caring is the locus of nursing ethics and that caring is living in the context of relational responsibilities to self and to others. The nurses' responsibility in caring for others is to "recognize their need for meaning and purpose in life, the importance of their existing relationships, and our responsibility to help them make meaningful decisions about their lives" (Porter, 2011, p. 107). As health care professionals, we are obligated to give care that reflects the values of person as person and person as caring. Fulfilling this obligation calls for the ability to be intentionally present to those cared for in every moment of an encounter. Lack of time is not a reason not to "be present." Caring is not an add-on, it is what we uniquely offer through the preparation that we have as health care professionals. Within the profession of nursing, nurses are educated to be moral agents of care; practitioners of other health care disciplines are similarly educated. It is understood that health care is a moral enterprise and health care organizations are obligated to support direct care through organizational processes (Porter, 2011). The ethical knowing inherent in caring challenges leaders to clarify their own beliefs and values and to consider the moral and ethical basis of all actions. Strategies leaders may consider related to their moral obligations are discussed under the heading "conscience."

AESTHETIC KNOWING IN CARING

Aesthetic knowing is the integration of personal, empirical, and ethical knowing as lived uniquely in health care situations. The aesthetic dimension of caring focuses on the art and the creativity of our practice as centered on knowing person as caring. Aesthetic knowing enhances one's understanding of the connectedness between and among persons and objects (Boykin, Parker, & Schoenhofer, 1994). The artistry of aesthetic knowing calls for trust, patience, and courage. Each person in health care is called to live every moment fully—to bring to their role hopes and dreams—and to create the best for those cared for. Strategies for bringing forth this knowing are addressed under the heading "compassion."

Roach (2002) describes how competence is humanized by compassion. "While competence without compassion can be brutal and inhumane, compassion without competence may be no more than a meaningless, if not harmful, intrusion into the life of a person or persons needing help" (p. 54). This powerful observation by Roach reminds us that there is a close connection between competence and compassion. We have suggested the complex multidimensional nature of competence as an expression of caring in health care and will now explore the ethical and practical meaning of another caring attribute, compassion.

COMPASSION

We have our own definition and experiences of compassion. Some would say that compassion is *the* manifestation of caring. There are other more formal definitions. Compassion is:

> a way of living born out of an awareness of one's relationship to all living creatures; engendering a response of participation in the experience of another; a sensitivity to the pain and brokenness of the other; a quality of presence which allows one to share with and make room for the other. (Roach, 2002, p. 50)

Historically, nurses were taught to be empathic, but remain detached from those nursed. There was an assumption that if a nurse became too close to a patient, care may be ineffective. Basically, nurses, physicians, and other health care professionals were taught not to become involved, not to be compassionate. Compassion implies a level of participation in the world of another. "Compassion…works from a strength born of awareness of shared weakness, and not from someone else's weakness…and from the awareness of the mutuality of us all" (Fox, 1990, p. 2). Fox elaborates that compassion operates at the same level as celebration, as what matters is being one with another. It is this sense of togetherness that allows us to rejoice in another's joy and grieve at another's sorrow.

Compassion implies vulnerability. We are vulnerable from the day we are born; physically, socially, we can't make it without others. There is also a vulnerability in health care professions between the one providing care and the one to be cared for. One can choose to be in *power with* or *power over* relationships. *Power over* is generally understood "as the ability to dominate another person or group…[and] usually comes from force or threat" (Conflict Research Consortium, 1998, para. 1). In contrast, *power with* relationships maintain the integrity of power, the ability to accomplish something while maintaining an equality of authority and advantage (Daniel, 1998). In these *power with* relationships there is a mutual knowing of other as a caring person. There is a sense of connectedness as their stories resonate with our own. "By recognizing vulnerability and choosing to engage in it with others, nurses are true to the discipline that has caring as its central premise" (p. 192). The caring that is nursing "must be a lived experience of caring, communicated intentionally, and in authentic presence through a person-with-person interconnectedness, a sense of oneness with self and other" (Boykin & Schoenhofer, 2001a, p. 25). The caring that is unique within other health care professions must also be intentional and authentic, through person-with-person interconnectedness. James Finley is a psychologist and former Trappist monk and student of Thomas Merton. Finley's work helps healers reconnect with their own healing core so that each might fully engage in the healing process with those who seek our care. He explores the ability to treat the whole person through becoming a contemplative clinician, engaging in seven phases of healing that allow the clinician to be in the moment that transcends suffering, while in the midst of suffering (Finley, 2012). Caring and presence are not unique to nursing, but they are uniquely experienced through nursing, just as they would be uniquely experienced though the lens of any discipline that adopts substantive caring knowledge as core to its discipline. Finley's work provides an excellent example from psychology, a discipline complementary to nursing and medicine, of articulating the authentic person-to-person presence in a caring moment.

To live the connectedness implicit in the Dance of Caring Persons, leaders in health care organizations must demonstrate competency in compassion. How can leaders convey the valuing of compassion? It begins with a valuing of person, valuing a life with dignity. Another fundamental way to become more compassionate is to make time daily for reflection:

- How often in our lives have we been touched because we were the recipients of another's compassion for us or because we witnessed extraordinary compassion? Reflect on a recent experience of being touched by compassion.
- Consider how one's role is lived out with others. What is modeled, *power with* or *power over*? Are some people basically lost or invisible in your role?
- Does one's role actually inflict pain and suffering?
- How is the valuing of humanity expressed?
- How do we both celebrate and suffer with those in the organization?

It is inspiring to imagine leaders in health care organizations considering the importance of compassion to organizational well-being—yet how distant is this imagined reality from what is known in today's competitive, detached, and entrenched culture of "care."

The transformation we are advocating calls for courage and drastically different ways of being with and for each other. It requires leaders to be intentionally present to help others grow in caring; it calls for a recognition and celebration of the connectedness we share.

Health care leaders have the opportunity to live compassion by entering the world of those who seek care and through the stories of colleagues. Sharing health/nursing situations is one way to foster compassion, advance the understanding of caring, and to communicate with others in the organization. Nursing situations are "shared lived experiences in which the caring between the nurse and one nursed enhances personhood" (Boykin & Schoenhofer, 2001a, p. 13). Such health care situations, moments of clinical connection, are the focus of the work of practice of each health care profession (e.g., medicine, nursing, social work, physical therapy, pharmacy, pastoral counseling, and others). For nursing, it is in the nursing situation that one comes to know the other as caring, attends to calls for caring, and creates caring responses that nurtures personhood. In the two stories that follow, a chief nursing officer, Nancy Hilton, and a directory of a telemetry area, Joe St. Jean, relate their living of compassion.

> Never, ever lose sight of the patient. What I do best is to utilize the art of storytelling to translate nursing into the language of the boardroom. The ability to convince the "C Suite" why we need to make transformative changes can often best be depicted through a simple nursing situation. The following story describes the need to honor, respect, and celebrate what matters most to the patient. I received a frantic phone call one morning from a family member who also happens to be one of our ED nurses. Her grandfather was a patient in our hospital and his father had died just 2 days prior. What mattered most was for her grandfather to attend his father's funeral. The physician had not been willing to write orders to release him for 6 hours due to his condition. If the patient left against medical advice, he would be charged 100% of the hospital bill. After several phone calls to the attending and consulting physicians, I was able to convince them that the granddaughter would be able to care for him with the use of a hospital wheelchair and by taking his medications with him. I could not imagine missing my own father's funeral. I know that through my authentic presence, I made a difference in this family's life.

> She had been on the unit for several weeks now. This is a long stay for our patients. She had been transferred to us from the intensive care unit following a major stroke. Her left side was without movement and her speech was very often difficult to understand. However, the nursing staff had soon come to appreciate her quick wit and delightful sense of humor. To be so positive after all she has been through is really a gift, we thought. A change became evident in the last several days. She was less witty and increasingly withdrawn. She continued working diligently with physical therapy and was making great strides. We learned she was a concert pianist who lived in an assisted care facility with her husband of 60 years. What was important to this lady? What really mattered to her? She shared with us that what she so enjoyed and what mattered to her was to return to her husband and play the piano for him...his one pleasure. "Show tunes," that is what she liked to play best.
>
> Hearing her call for hope in the moment, the director and another nurse, knowing there was a piano in one of the conference rooms, decided to bring it to her. As the piano was wheeled into the room, the patient's eyes lit up. She was brought over to the piano and to the delight of the patient and the nursing staff, she played a beautiful rendition of "Heart and Soul." (Boykin, Schoenhofer, Smith, St. Jean, & Aleman, 2003, p. 228)

Both of these stories illustrate the commitment of leaders to act based on their beliefs and values. Both leaders demonstrated aesthetic knowing—the creative processes of engaging, interpreting, and envisioning (Chinn & Kramer, 1991). This knowing was expressed in the artistry of the moment. Both leaders affirmed to staff the importance of compassionate care. When nursing staff witness nurse leaders living out their devotion to those nursed, it frees them to be authentic in their practice. The same would be true as practitioners of other disciplines model such authentic presence in practice.

Georges (2011) offers a powerful perspective of compassion and nursing:

> The day we stop valuing compassion as an essential of nursing practice or resisting the creation of biotoxic, compassionless environments, we cease to be "nurses," but we will have become something qualitatively different. And the possibility of what that different entity could become has frightening implications for nursing. (p. 134)

Strategies for the continual development of compassion in health care leaders include the following:

- Reflecting on one's own personal experiences of compassion
- Being open and willing to disclose your own vulnerability and humanity
- Caring for self in order to deal with the pain and suffering in health care systems and not become burned out
- Knowing stories of those with whom one works
- Engaging with unit managers as well as staff to hear directly issues and concerns that impact practice
- Creating opportunities for colleagues to reflect on their practice and create aesthetic expressions
- Taking risks to create new ways to practice that brings out the connectedness to others
- Infusing dignity and self-respect in all interactions
- Engaging coworkers in shared meaning of vision for practice
- Recognizing and affirming those who share stories of taking risks to live compassionate care

CONFIDENCE

What makes confidence so important in our lives is that often we do not have—or did not have—the surety that is basic to our living, personally and professionally. We have witnessed the lack of self-esteem in others who were dominated by overbearing parents, teachers, friends, and lovers. We also may feel rejected by those people most important in our lives. It is precisely this feeling, this experience of being made to feel alone that makes confidence so necessary. Confidence is the quality that fosters trusting relationships (Roach, 2002). How does a leader build trust among staff? Leaders must have that sense of self, that knowing of self that is the foundation for self-confidence. Leaders who are anxious about their own security, about being accepted by others, or obtaining personal rewards will find it difficult to have the energy and the time to address concerns of others (Nyberg, 1989). Nyberg further points out that these feelings of inadequacy often result in administrators having favorites who maintain the nurse leader's power by not questioning or challenging him or her. This way of being stifles creativity and growth of the other because the other is seen as competitive and threatening to the leader. Nyberg's comments again illustrate that the knowing of self as caring person is a priority in the role of a leader.

The confidence of the leader in turn influences the leadership style and the ability of the leader to know other as caring. Porter-O'Grady and Malloch (2002) have observed that less than confident leaders may "work diligently to preserve the status quo, avoiding tinkering with current processes for fear of making mistakes" (p. 157); when that occurs, opportunities for learning and for creativity are passed over, and frequently employees are paralyzed to the point of "retiring on the job" for fear of making an error or of retribution for mistakes. The confident leader holds expectations "based on a mindset that recognizes human fallibility and uncertainty, rather than on being right all the time" (p. 158). Being a confident leader who inspires confidence in colleagues involves compassion for self and for others while valuing competence as the norm.

A physician interested in learning what gave his patients confidence conducted an informal survey of patients, hospital workers, and fellow physicians. Three qualities were paramount in his study: caring, communication (listening and explaining), and competence (Stone, 2006). Patients emphasized the importance of health care providers sitting down, listening, explaining, and talking directly and honestly with them. Aren't these some of the same hoped-for qualities that staff persons look for in leaders? Do these same qualities not instill confidence in the staff?

Strategies for growing confidence in health care leaders include the following:

- Being visible with staff and listening
- Working out difficult situations with colleagues—giving each person his or her say
- Following through on commitments
- Involving staff in decision making
- Being the spokesperson for caring in the health care system
- Being open, listening, and accepting the views of others
- Establishing an environment of mutual respect

COMMITMENT

Leaders in health care organizations are charged with multiple levels of commitment. There is a commitment to oneself as leader, to the discipline and profession, and to the role within the organization. Commitment is defined as a "complex affective response characterized by a convergence between one's desires and one's obligations, and by a deliberate choice to act in accordance with them" (Roach, 2002, p. 62). She believes that commitment is evident when that to which one is committed is synonymous with what one prefers to do. Caring is living in the context of these relational responsibilities.

Commitments reflect one's view of the nature of being human. They determine the manner of being with self and others. When one accepts the belief that all persons are caring, also accepted are the obligations that rest with it. Any relationship between people or groups carries with it mutual expectations. From the perspective of caring, the expectation is belief in the dignity and worth of person.

COMMITMENT TO SELF

It is said that charity begins at home—in other words our first obligation is to self. For the leader of health care, the first level of relational responsibility is to oneself. As discussed earlier, the core commitment is related to the belief that all persons are caring. Knowing self as caring is essential to all other levels of relational responsibility. Commitment to caring is binding and choices are based on a devotion to this commitment.

Leaders hold a vision—an "ideal picture of how a leader would like things to be" (Gurka, 1995, p. 169)—that flows from one's beliefs and values. For nurse leaders this vision must be linked to an understanding of nursing as a discipline of knowledge and professional practice. For other disciplines, an understanding of the discipline's substantive knowledge and professional practice is also essential. This perspective is key to effectively articulating and advocating for the work of each discipline in service to those who seek our care. Remaining steadfast to one's vision, beliefs, and values is one of the most important and difficult aspects of any leader's role. At times commitment calls for extraordinary courage and trust. As one commits self to the values and beliefs held dear, the passion to live one's vision becomes even more firmly grounded. The challenge is to bring the vision to life and to remain authentic to self in the process—to choose "to be who we are." Said another way, the challenge is to act in accordance with beliefs and values. The leader's responsibility is to convey the vision to others in the organization as clearly as possible in order to inspire hope and support—creating a shared purpose.

Just as knowing self as caring is a prerequisite to knowing others as caring, so too is personal empowerment necessary in order to support the empowerment of others. The philosophy of self-empowerment is rooted in the perspective that each person has inherent worth. The process of self-empowerment is one of self-discovery (Hotter, 1992). Another significant aspect of this description is that self-empowerment is an ongoing process—a process, rather than merely a program to be taught and implemented.

COMMITMENT TO THE DISCIPLINE AND PROFESSION

Nursing is the largest single group of health care providers represented across the continuum of care. As such, nursing as a practice discipline is presented as an illustrative example applicable in whole or part to other interprofessional disciplines, depending on the scope of practice taught and embraced by each profession.

Because we are nurses, we can speak with greater depth about how nurse leaders accept responsibility for leading the discipline of nursing in practice by virtue of accepting their role. The quality of nursing leadership is one of the Forces of Magnetism (ANCC, 2004). It refers to the importance of a nurse leader having a clear conceptualization of nursing. It also refers to a leader who is strong in supporting the staff. As indicated by the term "nurse" in nurse leader, the focus of nursing leadership is on those receiving nursing care as well as those providing nursing care. Because nursing is charged with leadership for those receiving nursing care, interprofessional care coordination is part of the role of nursing leadership. Leading the discipline implies that the nurse leader has an explicit conception of nursing and that the focus of nursing is clear. A well-developed framework for nursing is foundational to grounding *nursing* service and communicating *nursing's* unique contribution to the health care team. Nurse leaders practicing from a nursing framework ground all activities in relation to those nursed. All activities are aimed at creating, maintaining, and supporting an environment in which calls for nursing are heard and nurturing responses offered. The nurse leader

> supports colleagues as caring persons, nurtures that which matters for excellence in practice, secures resources, communicates the nature of the discipline, models living and growing in caring, and co-creates a culture in which the practice of nursing makes visible the value of caring. (Boykin & Schoenhofer, 2001b, p. 6)

Because caring is a substantive domain of theoretical knowledge and professional practice for the nursing discipline, nurse leaders must be clear in their conception of nursing in order to communicate to others the focus and value of caring.

From the perspective of the theory of Nursing as Caring, the focus of nursing involves the nurturing of persons living caring and growing in caring (Boykin & Schoenhofer, 2001a). Nurse leaders live a commitment to grow in the knowledge of what it means to be human, to be caring. A significant way of discovering this knowledge is through engaging in nursing situations either personally or through the stories of colleagues. The degree to which the theory of Nursing as Caring is resonant with other health care disciplines is discovered through dialogue and testing of the principles within interprofessional practice. The principles are likely to apply in each discipline, though each will be reflected through the practice lens unique to that discipline. This connectedness and unity of diversity is what contributes to the richness of the care experience for all involved.

The practice of nursing is directly linked to an understanding of the discipline. Nursing practice grounded in a theoretical perspective of nursing provides nurses the language needed to talk about the nature of nursing; and to make clear what it is that nurses do. These same principles apply to each health care discipline, that is, substantive knowledge of each discipline communicates the language and meaning specific to the focus of that discipline's work. It is critical for each health care leader to co-create and support environments of care where each discipline can practice, reflect, and build knowledge from a discipline-specific framework as well as the shared framework of collaborative practice. The professional identity for each discipline evolves from an understanding of the nature of that discipline in communion with the disciplinary perspectives of related disciplines. All health care leaders are instrumental in supporting staff to ground their practice in the beliefs and values they hold dear.

Our covenant with society requires that we respond to the trust placed in us as health care workers. The relationship to the patient is primary. Health care professionals must have the responsibility, authority, and autonomy to practice consistent with professional standards of the relevant discipline. Empowering colleagues is an important part of a leader's commitment to colleagues and to those served. Some outcomes of empowerment are changes in self-confidence and self-esteem; changes in relationship with others—both patients and other health care providers; and changes in behavior of patients as they became more empowered (Falk-Rafael, 2001). The literature reveals that the empowerment of nurses results in their increased engagement in the health care setting, increased nurse satisfaction, and increased patient satisfaction (Bargagliotti, 2012; Fasoli, 2010; Gifford, 2002). Empowerment encourages authentic and innovative practice promoting the fullness of being, as well as to advocate for those seeking care—to commit to what ought to be. It is the role of the nurse leader to ensure such freedom exists in the practice of nursing and to collaborate with other disciplines toward the same freedom.

COMMITMENT TO THE ORGANIZATION

Traditionally, the commitment of the nurse leader was centered on protecting the organization from legal, reputational, ethical, and/or financial risk (Cole, 2010). The same might be said for any leader in health care. It is not an apt description of a nurse leader's commitment to the organization. The obligations inherent in all leadership roles of the organization must be centered in the persons cared for. Health care leaders must be committed to living caring with all persons in the health care organization and to creating a work environment that is healthy for those cared for as well as for those providing care. Nursing literature is replete with evidence of unhealthy environments in which some nurses practice (Kramer, 2010; Ray, Turkel, & Marino, 2002; Wesorick, 2002). The common factors of an unhealthy work environment are related to environmental stressors. Among the nurses' experience are increased workload, decreased staff, poor communications, work conflicts, interpersonal conflicts, and perception of nonsupportive leadership.

In recognition of the impact of work environment on quality care and patient outcomes, nursing organizations have developed standards for a healthy and healthful work environment. The AACN (2005) endorsed six standards to promote a healthy work environment: (a) skilled communication, (b) true collaboration between nurses and among nurses and colleagues, (c) effective decision making both in patient care and at the organizational level, (d) appropriate staffing levels, (e) meaningful recognition of the value that individuals and nursing bring to patient care and the organization, and (f) authentic leadership.

The Nursing Organizations Alliance (2004) developed nine elements essential to a healthful practice work environment. These are (a) a collaborative practice culture, (b) communication-rich culture, (c) a culture of accountability, (d) the presence of adequate number of qualified nurses, (e) the presence of expert, competent, credible, visible leadership, (f) shared decision making at all levels, (g) the encouragement of professional practice and continued growth/development, (h) recognition of the value of nursing's contribution, and (i) recognition by nurses for their meaningful contribution to practice (2004).

Both sets of criteria express the important role of nurse leaders in creating caring environments, inspiring a vision, taking risks, and supporting colleagues—through a culture of interpersonal valuing, mutual respect, and personal empowerment (Porter-O'Grady & Malloch, 2007; Sherman & Pross, 2010). It is through enactment of these key aspects of leadership that those in health care organizations will experience being valued, being supported, and being free to truly nurse.

Strategies for growing in commitment to caring include the following:

- Co-creating an environment in which practice is grounded in disciplinary knowledge and advancement of that knowledge is supported
- Being visible with direct-care providers to hear their stories and to establish a mutual knowing
- Initiating opportunities to listen and share important stories of caring. Stories keep all members of the system connected to those cared for, in touch with what matters, aware of what resources need to be secured and allocated to respond to the needs of those seeking care
- Coming to know those within the system as caring person. Beginning this process of knowing with those who report directly to them
- Engaging colleagues in dialogues on how to ground work environments in values held dear
- Creating interprofessional opportunities to reflect and dialogue on caring as lived in practice
- Empowering colleagues to practice authentically
- Being open to continuously knowing caring in the moment
- Supporting the hopes and dreams of colleagues related to creating an ideal practice environment
- Projecting an openness and desire to be available and creating ways for this to live
- Designing with colleagues a practice model that is grounded in caring and fosters creativity and responsivity to caring
- Communicating the value and nature of caring throughout the system
- Speaking the language of caring
- Representing nursing as the largest single health care discipline by serving as a member of the governing board

CONSCIENCE

Another foundational attribute of caring is conscience. Conscience is "a state of moral awareness; a compass directing one's behavior according to the moral fitness of things" (Roach, 2002, p. 60). Conscience grows out of a process of valuing self and other.

Commitments drive obligations. Therefore, if one is committed to living the value of caring, it is this commitment that ought to direct all actions, serving as the conscience. Accepting one's commitments is what leads to authentic living. According to Roach, authentic existence is acting in accord with self and conscious awareness. Inauthentic existence is failing to act in accord with this awareness. For example, it is the conflict involved in living authentically that often leads to moral distress in nursing practice. Nurses are often called upon as the moral agent of health care organizations. All aspects of the organization—patients, families, and the organization itself—benefit from the moral courage of nurses. However, on a daily basis, nurses experience conflict when their commitment to the organization is misaligned with their responsibility to the patient (Corley, 2002). Similar conflicts can arise with other members of the health care team. When this happens, the nurse often experiences two phases of moral distress. The first is when the nurse experiences the conflict. The second is when the nurse doesn't act (Cole, 2010). The conflict between what one should but didn't do can result in moral distress. Over time the resultant effects of this can be low self-esteem, self-hate, job dissatisfaction, and horizontal violence as these feelings of anger are directed toward others (Corley, 2002).

What could be more distressing for a nurse or another health care professional than reflecting on one's practice and knowing that one didn't live out one's beliefs and values—to realize you have broken the sacred covenant with those seeking care? All practitioners have undoubtedly had this experience on occasion. But what if this experience was the norm of practice? In a powerful narration, a physician shared his own experience of truth-telling. The situation was one in which Casey, an infant with a congenital heart defect, was losing her tenuous grasp on life, and a decision was made by this physician to attempt a therapeutic intervention that had known risks but was also potentially life-saving. In the process of the intervention, an error was made and the child died; the explanation given to the parents by a colleague omitted the mention of the error. The physician, however, was keenly attuned to his own moral compass and choosing authenticity, realized that his desire to help the child had moved him to overreach. "As they started to go I stopped them. 'Wait,' I said, 'There's more.'" (Boyte, 2001, p. 254). He then told the parents about their child's last moments of life. What gave him the courage to live his authenticity, to act from his conscience? He explained "they had entrusted me with their daughter's life. I owed them the truth" (p. 254).

There can be no more important role for a leader than to be sensitive to signs of moral distress in employees. This means that the leader must know employees and be watchful for changes in performance or engagement that might signal moral distress. Part of being tuned into this possibility would involve being aware of specific patient situations that may place health care professionals in the kind of "damned if you do, damned if you don't" position—of knowing that something needs to be done, but feeling the pressure to avoid rocking the boat. Some potential indicators of moral distress include poor communication, defensiveness, lack of trust resulting in failure to collaborate (AACN, n.d.). The leader must challenge aspects of the system that prevent them and other team members from living their responsibilities to humankind.

Strategies for growing in caring consciousness include the following:

- Discussing with managers the importance of being tuned into changes in staff engagement or performance that might signal moral distress
- Educating staff about moral distress
- Supporting staff who experience moral distress
- Creating forums for interprofessional discussion of ethical concerns
- Coming to know colleagues and supporting their concerns

- Creating policies and procedures that allow for the uniqueness of the situation to be considered
- Originating all actions in caring
- Relating to others respectfully
- Speaking with a common voice on behalf of what ought to be for those cared for
- Appointing staff nurses and other disciplines to ethics committees
- Studying and implementing AACN's 4A's to rise above moral distress: Ask, Affirm, Assess, Act

COMPORTMENT

As a term, comportment is not a common term associated with nursing practice. The concept of comportment was added to Roach's (2002) 5C's to answer the question, "Are nursing dress and language in harmony with professional beliefs regarding respect for person?" She understands comportment as bearing, demeanor, or to be in harmony with. Comportment addresses the importance of maintaining harmony between beliefs about the intrinsic dignity of self and other, and the manner in which a person presents himself or herself as a professional caregiver (p. 131). Dress and language symbolize the values of an organization. They may or may not reflect a caring presence of the nurse or other health care provider especially when we consider "how" we dress and "how" we speak.

Although the term "comportment" may be reminiscent of earlier school days, it is important to consider how we portray the image of the nurse and the health care team. What does the dress and language of health care providers communicate to patients and families? Are dress and language congruent with professional norms? Do they engender respect? The idea of comportment is not to imply a particular way a staff member should dress but rather to dress in a way suitable for both patients and the practice setting (Roach, 2002). Professional dress and language convey not only respect for the profession but also for those with whom one interacts. Comportment as a "caring behavior may be one exemplar of living caring in our intentional practice" (Roach & Maykut, 2010, p. 25).

The Forces of Magnetism (ANCC, 2012) refer to the image of nursing, as how nurses are viewed by the organization. A positive image would convey the integral nature of quality care to the nurse's practice. A positive image would hold nurse leaders as respected and valued colleagues.

We all present an image. Hopefully, the image we present is a real indicator of the ideal that we strive to be. "Caring is the art of nursing, the way of being, the comportment of the nurse in the sacred dance of healing with the client" (Smith, 1999, p. 20). Each discipline comports itself within the dance in a manner that reflects values and beliefs. Strategies for comportment include the following:

- Conveying professional presentation
- Addressing people respectfully
- Discussing with colleagues how emotional reactions to situations may or may not convey caring
- Role-playing ways to remain present with others during difficult encounters

The broad dimensions of leadership that have been presented are extensive and all-encompassing. They are meant to be. They are the ideals leaders must continually strive to meet. This is true for each professional discipline and its leaders. As nurses, we believe in ideals, many of which we have considered in this chapter. It is the living of these ideals that defines who we are and what we believe—from the way we present ourselves in our dress to the depth of our being at one in our caring with those we are privileged to nurse.

LEADERSHIP: QUESTIONS FOR CONSIDERATION

- What attribute of caring do I find most difficult to live in my role as leader? Why? How might I grow in my caring competencies?
- In what ways am I leading the transformation of health care grounded in caring values?
- If I were asked, how would I describe the importance of caring to members of the executive team?
- Do I believe this vision for leadership is possible? How can I best actualize this vision?
- Do my actions consistently reflect my beliefs and values?
- How can I free myself and others to live out one's authentic self?
- How would my leadership style be described by others?

REFERENCES

American Association of Critical-Care Nurses. (2005). *AACN standards for establishing and sustaining healthy work environments: A journey to excellence.* Aliso Viejo, CA: Author.

American Association of Critical-Care Nurses. (n.d.). *The 4A's to rise above moral distress.* Retrieved from http://www.aacn.org/WD/Practice/Docs/4As_to_Rise_Above_Moral_Distress.pdf

American Nurses Credentialing Center. (2004). *Magnet recognition program recognizing excellence in nursing service: Application manual 2005.* Washington, DC: American Nurses.

American Nurses Credentialing Center. (2012). *Forces of magnetism.* Retrieved from http://www.nursecredentialing.org/Magnet/ProgramOverview/HistoryoftheMagnetProgram/ForcesofMagnetism

American Nurses Credentialing Center. (n.d.). *Magnet recognition model.* Retrieved from http://www.nursecredentialing.org/Magnet/ProgramOverview/New-Magnet-Model

Anderson, E. M., & Shannon, A. L. (1988). Toward a conceptualization of mentoring. *Journal of Teacher Education, 39,* 38–42.

Bargagliotti, L., (2012). Work engagement in nursing: A context analysis. *Journal of Advanced Nursing, 68,* 1414–1428.

Bass, B. M., & Avolio, B. J. (1990). The implications of transactional and transformational leadership for individual team and organizational development. In R. W. Woodman & W. A. Passmore (Eds.), *Research in organizational change and development.* Greenwich, CT: JAI Press.

Bennis, W., & Nanus, B. (1985). *Leadership: The strategies for taking charge.* New York, NY: HarperCollins.

Boykin, A., Parker, M., & Schoenhofer, S. O. (1994). Aesthetic knowing grounded in an explicit conception of nursing. *Nursing Science Quarterly, 7*(4), 158–161.

Boykin, A., & Schoenhofer, S. O. (2001a). *Nursing as caring: A model for transforming practice.* Sudbury, MA: Jones & Bartlett.

Boykin, A., & Schoenhofer, S. O. (2001b). The role of nursing leadership in creating caring environments in health care delivery systems. *Nursing Administration Quarterly, 25*(3), 1–7.

Boykin, A., Schoenhofer, S. O., Bulfin, S., Baldwin, J., & McCarthy, D. (2005). Living caring in practice: The transformative power of the theory of nursing as caring. *International Journal for Human Caring, 9*(3), 15–19.

Boykin, A., Schoenhofer, S. O., Smith, N., St. Jean, J., & Aleman, D. (2003). Transforming practice using a caring-based nursing model. *Nursing Administration Quarterly, 27*(3), 223–230.

Boyte, W. R. (2001). Casey's legacy. *Health Affairs, 20,* 250–254. doi:10.1377/hlthaff.20.2.250

Burns, J. M. (1978). *Leadership.* New York: Harper & Row.

Carper, B. A. (1978). Fundamental patterns of knowing in nursing. *Advances in Nursing Science, 1*(1), 13–23.

Center for Nursing Leadership. (1990). *The dimensions of leadership.* Retrieved from http://www.cnl.org/ways_of_leading.htm

Chinn, P. L., & Kramer, M. (1991). *Theory and nursing*. St. Louis, MO: Mosby-Year Book.

Cole, E. (2010). Moral courage and the nurse leader. *Online Journal of Issues in Nursing, 15*(3). Retrieved from http://gm6.nursingworld.org/MainMenuCategories/ANAMarketplace/ANAPeriodicals/OJIN/TableofContents/Vol152010/No3-Sept-2010/Moral-Courage-for-Nurse-Leaders.aspx

Conflict Research Consortium. (1998). *The nature of power*. Retrieved from http://www.colorado.edu/conflict/peace/power.htm

Corley, M. (2002). Nurse moral distress: A proposed theory and research agenda. *Nursing Ethics, 9*(6), 636–650.

Daniel, L. (1998). Vulnerability as a key to authenticity. *Image: Journal of Nursing Scholarship, 30*(2), 191–192.

Falk-Rafael, A. (2001). Empowerment as a process of evolving consciousness: A model of empowering caring. *Advances in Nursing Science, 24*(1), 1–16.

Fasoli, D. (2010). The culture of nursing engagement. *Nursing Administration Quarterly, 34*(1), 18–29.

Finley, J. B. (2012). *Compassion as a path to spiritual awakening and inner peace.* Lecture presented at Florida Atlantic University, October 12, 2012.

Fox, M. (1990). *A spirituality named compassion.* San Francisco, CA: Harper.

George, B. (2003). *Authentic leadership: Rediscovering the secrets to creating lasting change.* San Francisco: Jossey-Bass.

Georges, J. M. (2011). Evidence of the unspeakable. *Advances in Nursing Science, 34*(2), 130–135.

Gifford, B. (2002). The relationship between hospital unit culture and nurses' quality of work life. *Journal of Healthcare Management, 47*(1), 13–25.

Gottlieb, L., Gottlieb, B., & Shamian, J. (2012). Principles of strengths-based nursing leadership for strengths-based nursing care: A new paradigm for nursing and healthcare in the 21st century. *Nursing Leadership, 25*(2), 38–50.

Gurka, A. (1995). Transformational leadership: Qualities and strategies for the CNS. *Clinical Nurse Specialist, 9*(3), 169–174.

Hotter, A. (1992). The clinical nurse specialist and empowerment: Say goodbye to the fairy godmother. *Nursing Administration Quarterly, 16*(3), 50–51.

Kramer, M. (2010). Nine structures and leadership practices essential for a magnetic (healthy) work environment. *Nursing Administration Quarterly, 34*(1), 4–17.

Lukas, C., Holmes, S., Cohen, A., Restuccia, J., Cramer, I., Schwartz, M., & Charns, M. (2007). Transformational change in healthcare systems: An organizational model. *Health Care Management Review, 32*(4), 309–32. doi:10.1097/01.HMR.0000296785.29718.5d

Mayeroff, M. (1971). *On caring.* New York, NY: Harper & Row.

Nursing Organizations Alliance. (2004). *Principles and elements of a healthful practice/work environment.* Lexington, KY: Nursing Organizations Alliance.

Nyberg, J. (1989). The element of caring in nursing administration. *Nursing Administration Quarterly, 13*(3), 9–16.

O'Connor, M. (2008). The dimensions of leadership. *Nursing Administration Quarterly, 32*(1), 21–26.

Popper, M. (2000). The development of charismatic leaders. *Political Psychology, 21*(4), 729–744.

Porter, S. (2011). Bringing values back into evidence-based nursing: The role of patients in resisting empiricism. *Advances in Nursing Science, 34*(2), 106–118.

Porter-O'Grady, T., & Malloch, K. (2007). *Quantum leadership: A textbook of new leadership.* Sudbury, MA: Jones & Bartlett.

Ray, M., Turkel, M., & Marino, F. (2002). The transformative process for nursing in workforce redevelopment. *Nursing Administration Quarterly, 26*(2), 1–14.

Roach, M. S. (2002). *Caring, the human mode of being: A blueprint for the health professionals.* Ottawa, ON: The Canadian Hospital Association Press.

Roach, M. S., & Maykut, C. (2010). Comportment: A caring attribute in the formation of intentional presence. *International Journal for Human Caring, 14*(4), 22–26.

Safety Net Medical Home Initiative. (SNMHI). (2010, November). *Implementation guide: Strategies for guiding PCMH transformation from within.* Retrieved from http://www.improvingchroniccare.org/downloads/engaged_leadership.pdf

Schwartz, T. (2010, June). The productivity paradox: How Sony Pictures gets more out of people by demanding less. *Harvard Business Review*. Retreived from http://hbr.org/2010/06/the-productivity-paradox-how-sony-pictures-gets-more-out-of-people-by-demanding-less/ar/1

Sherman, R. O., & Pross, E. (2010). Growing future nurse leaders to build and sustain healthy work environments at the unit level. *Online Journal of Issues in Nursing, 15*(1), Manuscript 1.

Smith, M. (1999). Caring and the science of unitary human beings. *Advances in Nursing Science, 21*(4), 14–34.

Stone, N. (2006). Clinical confidence and the three C's: Caring, communicating, and competence. *The American Journal of Medicine, 119*, 1–2.

Swick, M., Doulaveris, P., & Christensen, P. (2012). Model of care transformation. *Nursing Administration Quarterly, 36*(4), 314–319.

Viney, M., Batcheller, J., Houston, S., & Belcik, K. (2006). Transforming care at the bedside: Designing new care systems in an age of complexity. *Journal of Nursing Care Quality, 21*(2), 143–150.

Wesorick, B. (2002). 21st century leadership challenge: Creating and sustaining healthy, healing work cultures and integrated service at the point of care. *Nursing Administration Quarterly, 26*(5), 18–32.

Response to Chapter 7

Raymond Barfield, MD, PhD
Associate Professor of Pediatrics and Christian Philosophy
Duke University

*A*t an advanced course on pain management, we were about to be addressed by a world leader in pain, a physician who had been a Rhodes Scholar, who had nearly 200 publications, and who had revolutionized the approach to neonatal pain through his ground-breaking research. His lecture topic was *Advances in Basic Science Research on Pain*. He stood up and clicked to his first slide—a picture of a man in a gray beard who, the physician–scientist said, had taught him a great deal about love. He then spent 10 minutes talking about the importance of love in the care of the patients we treat for pain. After making his points about love as the context for everything we do, he went on to tell us about his most recent basic research in the biology of pain. Admiration for his research would have left us inspired. But the fact that such a famous leader in the field would take time to emphasize the importance of love in the care of those who are ill or suffering left a permanent mark on the participants. When leaders embrace transformative practices in their own lives, the members of their organization are more likely to feel emboldened to do the same, to step out in a direction that may seem risky, but that also has the feel of something right and valuable.

In the United States, one of the most pressing issues shaping the horizon of health care is cost. It is not very controversial to say that health care economics is at a point of genuine crisis. In such a crisis, it is all too easy for the language of economics to usurp the language of care in the clinical setting. And at first glance this makes some sense—if the crisis is with health care costs, then the dominant focus should be on cost and cost cutting. But it is precisely in the middle of such a crisis that transformative leadership can make the greatest impact through creative surprise. When the famous pain researcher began his talk on the most important advances in the field with a 10-minute discussion of the value of love, the audience was surprised, delighted, and moved. When a leader in the health care field says by word and action that in an economic crisis radical transformation is needed, and the most radical transformation is to underscore the value of caring, this is a surprising response. But how can such a response be asserted when we have such an enormous crisis on our hands? Here is a statement that comes to mind: "Resolving this crisis is going to be challenging, but if we stay true to our central value of care, even if we find ourselves with fewer physical resources, we might nonetheless deepen the well of human presence and comfort for the sick, and even relearn lessons that have been lost in the age of high-tech medicine." Or perhaps this: "As we work to resolve the economic crisis, let us never forget to grow in our capacity to care for each other, because caring is the essence of the health care system, and if we lose the gift of caring, we lose our compass, we lose the sense of why we do this, and the economic issues become unsolvable."

The point of statements like these is that even in enormous crisis, our goals are never served by forgetting our deepest priorities. Caring is a primary value, not a derivative value. We do not encourage caring so that patient satisfaction scores go up, causing more patients to come to our hospital, improving our bottom line. Emphasizing a caring-based perspective in health care transformation allows leaders to tap into a rich and permanent reservoir that motivates us to be present to the ill and the suffering, and the dying in a way that nothing else can—and this feeds the humanity both of leaders and those they lead. Making economic goals subservient to the goals of caring is a powerful way of creating sustainable health care systems because it fits human experience in a way that a mere ledger sheet cannot. And so, if economic changes are needed, they are not needed so that we can *meet the budget* or *cut losses* or *improve the bottom line*. If economic changes are needed, they are needed because this is the only way to extend *care* to as many people as possible, for as long as possible. They are needed because the value of *caring* is so great that we cannot let the juggernaut of technology untethered to genuine human goals beyond mere biological duration bankrupt health care and undercut our goals of caring. The theme suggested by this example is a theme of remembering what our ends are, and what the means to our ends are. Transformative leaders will keep this straight in their minds.

The question of means and ends is tremendously important, and ignoring the distinction has led to a lot of bad will toward leaders. Do leaders have a primary obligation to look out for the health care system? Patients? Staff? Their primary obligation determines their *ends*, so is everything else considered a *means*? If, for example, patients are categorized as *consumers* and a leader insists that an institution use the language of *the customer is always right*, the health care workers are degraded because they become mere means to the end of pleasing the customer—they become technology dispensers. The patients likewise are degraded because very few would place the experience of being on the threshold of death in the same category as picking out a suit or a prom dress. But suppose the institution is identified as the primary end. In this case both the patients and the providers might become means for sustaining the institution, and this does not seem right. What is radical about the caring-based perspective on transformative leadership is that it allows the assessment of means and ends to lead us to the conclusion that only the institution can be identified as a "means"—but it is a means that is meant to facilitate the ends that caring persons express, whether as a patient or as a provider.

Building on this point, it is fairly easy to see what it would mean to identify the institutions as the means for reaching the patient's ends or goals. But what about the providers? Transformative leaders do well to take note of the fact that we spend most of our waking life at work. What we do at work shapes the way we live outside of work. Creating an environment for providers is a moral effort that can, if done well, contribute to the character and happiness of the providers, and if done poorly, contribute to their harm.

One last example of how a caring-based perspective can transform health care. Consider the importance of "competence." Caring-based leadership sees competence as an expression of care. Anyone who has taken a multiple-choice test knows that it is possible to fill in the right boxes and get an *A*, and yet have no real competence. Caring-based leadership should strive for a notion of competence as a sense of *craft*, an idea that is vocationally fulfilling in a way that checking off the required boxes is not. If boxes need to be checked in order to earn accreditation or some other accolade, this can be acknowledged as necessary—but an activity such as that should never be confused with *excellence* fostered as an expression of love for the people we serve. We can hope for a day when official certification uses this language, but we should not wait for that day to clarify the value of caring as a motivating force in our practice.

In recent years a number of reports have been published about the rising sense of unhappiness among health care workers, including a sense of underaccomplishment, depression, and suicidal ideation. The caring-based approach to leadership can do much to address this. Perhaps one of the most surprising, and potentially helpful, summary ideas arising from this discussion is the idea of aesthetic knowing. There are many ways to characterize this, but one good way is just to say, "See the beauty in front of you." Here too the point I began with holds: If transformative leaders learn to see the beauty of the work their people do, that is a powerful lesson for the servants of the sick and dying. If we are going to care, whether as institutional leaders or clinicians, we must learn first to see. If we can learn to see, we have many beautiful surprises ahead of us that might even illuminate what is most needed in the health care reform debate we are going to have over the next decade.

Response to Chapter 7

Karen Olsen, MBA, BSN, RN
Vice President, Chief Nursing Officer
Mission Hospital

What is the value of a caring-based perspective in health care transformation?
Caring serves as an essential attribute for competent leadership in transformational health care. Without an authentic caring approach and attitude, a leader cannot convey a genuine mission, vision, or goals. When staff members do not feel cared for, it creates a challenge for personnel to provide compassionate care to patients or commit to overarching leadership objectives and initiatives. The lack of caring can result in staff members who may feel disengaged or disenfranchised from their work, the organization, and the patients or families they serve each day.

In today's health care environment, transformation demands flexible leadership structures and highly adaptable processes that are continually responsive to the ever-changing complexities. More traditional bureaucratic structures often fail in their efforts to innovate at the pace required by numerous demands on the health care system. Factors such as shrinking reimbursements, health care reform, and significant population health needs, in the context of the consumer's desire for patient-centered care, create opportunities for leaders who are risk takers and willing to innovate. A leader must care about the outcomes of his or her work as well as the individuals who strive to achieve those goals.

Highly effective leaders advance caring values in their everyday work through interactions, decision-making processes, and the way of being with individuals and teams. When each person is valued as a unique human being, the essence of caring can be infused within an organization and its work. This sense of belonging to and being part of something greater ensures that each member of the team and their contributions are valued and integral to the success of the organization. Caring must be hard-wired in the daily operations of an organization and the role of each leader.

In your experience, what would have to be in place in order to bring the ideas presented to fruition?
Nurses need supportive environments in which to create the lived experience of caring for each other and the patients and families they serve. Caring as a core element of nursing practice must be fully integrated in nursing educational programs and foundational

in hospital orientation programs for nurses. As nurses are oriented to their practice settings, they must learn and experience the dimensions of the caring environment. Through a careful and thoughtful socialization to the role as a member of a caring team, each nurse can actualize his or her potential. This socialization can begin prior to interviewing for a position. I have done this by inviting new graduates for a day-long education experience prior to interviewing for a position in the ED. This way, recent graduates have an opportunity to meet staff nurses and leaders without the pressure of an actual interview.

Caring must be core to the work of leaders so as to ensure that each patient and family receive care that matches their needs and expectations. Regardless of one's role, each member of the team serves as a leader in establishing and ensuring a caring environment. Each member of the leadership team has a moral imperative to care and create caring environments with a connectedness to each other, the work, and the organization. To support this work, I always hire for "attitude" as a primary qualification and create opportunities for staff nurses to connect regularly with leaders and other members of the team.

Specifically, nurse leaders must be chosen for their ability to lead and create caring environments. Dignity, respect, kindness, and empathy serve as essential leadership attributes in a caring organization. Nurse leaders must demonstrate commitment to and competency for creating caring environment and strive to continually advance relationship-based nursing practice. As a nurse leader, I always try to emulate the very characteristics that I expect from the leaders on my team as well as our staff nurses. The most important work I do each day is to recognize staff for their contributions and express my caring for them as an individual.

What ideas would you like to contribute to making the content even more practical?
Leaders must first and foremost commit to creating the time and space for caring. Strategies can include starting meetings with taking time for everyone to pause and "center." Leaders need to acknowledge the personhood of each member of the team, and take time to recognize each person as an individual. Making a personal connection with each member of the team can support an individual's sense of belonging and uniqueness. Knowing each member of the team helps a leader convey caring at both a personal and a professional level. When I first meet a staff member, I strive to learn more about him or her as a person and the things that are important in his or her life and work.

With the multitude of competing priorities, leaders can be at risk of shifting their focus away from the core value of caring. Placing patients and families as core to every decision and activity ensures that health care leaders' decisions are centered in caring. Such a value system must be shared and supported by every member of the team with an unwavering commitment. As a leader, I try to remain centered on this agenda and start every meeting with a moment for everyone to "center" and then focus on agenda items as our agenda for caring.

Caring does not mean offering employees and staff everything they want, but engaging them in the process when difficult decisions need to be made. Leaders need to listen and keep staff members informed about challenges, changes, and be open and transparent when difficult decisions are made. Listening requires one to be nonbiased and nonjudgmental; to be open to differences in ideas and perceptions. Creating a healthy work environment requires vision, unrelenting commitment, and the efforts of many individuals. Caring serves as core to the nursing profession and must be supported to its fullest. As a leader, I believe caring must be in the forefront of all aspects of my work whether it is answering an email, leading a meeting, or making difficult decisions—it is a moral imperative for nursing.

Chapter 8

Transforming Communication Processes

Communication is key to the transformation of health care. It is the intent of this chapter to address ideas that are believed to be necessary in creating health care systems grounded in the value of caring and acknowledging the importance of person. We have come to know that effective communication is vital not only in one's personal relationships, but also in one's organization. Especially in the health care organization, we believe the purpose of communication is meant to be the communication of caring.

In the health care setting, it is the role of leaders to set the tone for communication. How do beliefs and values of leaders influence communication? Organizational structure models communication expectations, whether the communication is formal or informal. The flow of communication is multidirectional. In hierarchical structures there is a chain of command one is expected to follow. Formal communication primarily occurs through a downward flow of information. The relationship in hierarchies is determined by the status of the employee. The nature of the hierarchy is communicated among members of the organization through the interactions of the members within a system.

The assumption with downward communicating is that the most important messages come from the *top*. Persons in these positions are considered to be an authoritative source. Generally, this way of sharing information ensures that a message is transmitted in a uniform way regarding things such as policies, organizational changes, and so on. In the downward mode, people are not engaged; there is no structure for feedback; information is often distorted; and there is no recipient design. Another vertical mode of formal communication is upward.

Examples of this are reports, surveys, or other information requested by managers in order to assist them in making decisions. The upward mode of communication may result in a poor quality of information if the purpose of the request is not clearly understood and therefore not properly valued. The issue with both forms of vertical communication is that there is often no, or little, dialogue, meaning-making, or shared understanding of the information (Jordan & Friends, 2006). Macknet (n.d.) asserts that communication is more than information transmission; communication requires dialogue to achieve shared understanding.

Tourish (2003) believes open, upward communication coupled with an open-door policy is key to organizational effectiveness. Inviting upward dialogue results in the promotion of shared leadership, increased willingness by managers to act on employee suggestions, increased tendency for employees to report positive changes in a manager's behavior, actual improvement in manager behavior due to feedback, decreased gap between the self-rating of the manager and employee, and the creation of new forums for gathering information, conflict resolution, and expressions of concerns. The success of upward communication is dependent on the openness of the managers and staff.

Communication can also flow horizontally. Horizontal communication is generally understood as that which occurs between employees who are at the same *level*. Because of the perceived equal status, communication is more open, free, and honest (McCroskey, 2006). The degree to which people communicate across the organization, problem solve with all employees and teams, and build accountability for superior outcomes is a manifestation of horizontal accountability (Ray & Elder, 2007). Relating in this way fosters trust and supports the growth of the organization.

The goals of communication tools are to convey information between human beings, which helps to bring people together to communicate/dialogue, to share meaning, and to generate new meaning. An organization is communication (Macknet, n.d.). The meaning in all forms of communication is co-constructed by the sender and receiver. Some communication, such as the following, may have mixed meanings:

> A manager requests a salaried employee keep a personal record of the time worked on a weekly basis to help demonstrate that person's value to the organization. The meaning of this request could be that the manager wanted to communicate that the employee was to put in the required hours or that the manager wanted to show the employer that the employee was consistently going above and beyond for the good of the organization and that the manager was aware of the employee's dedication.

The call today is for communication in all organizations to be open and continuous. In health care particularly, effective, open, and meaningful communication is critical. The importance of feedback from all levels of the health care system is vital for improving patient safety, improving care, and preventing medical errors (Institute of Medicine [IOM], 2004).

There must be no secrets. All information should flow freely and constantly so anyone in the system—including patients and families—can make well-informed health care decisions based on relevant facts (IOM, 2004, p. 79).

Despite the many reports on patient safety and the heightened need for effective communication, communication failures continue to be recognized as important latent factors affecting patient safety. Multiple reasons for the slow progress in this area include the complexity of the health care environment (multiple providers both in medicine and other health professionals), and "a tradition of professional fragmentation, of individualism, of a well-entrenched hierarchical authority structure, and of diffuse accountability" (Varpio, Hall, Lingard, & Schryer, 2008, p. S76).

A study by Sutcliffe, Lewtin, and Rosenthan (2004) found that communication failures are associated with vertical differences in the hierarchy, concerns with upward influence, role conflict and ambiguity, and struggles with interpersonal power and conflict. Studies of malpractice cases showed that physicians ignored important communication by nurses and that nurses withheld relevant information for diagnosis and treatment (Nembhard & Edmondson, 2006). The IOM report (2004) *Keeping Patients Safe* states "counterproductive hierarchical communication patterns that derive from status differences" (p. 361) are partly responsible for medical errors.

Transforming the pattern of communication is one of the greatest challenges facing those in health care systems. Many communication-based issues are directly linked to organizational structures and to the values and beliefs held by leaders and members of the organization. For reasons detailed in Porter-O'Grady's Foreword and Chapter 1 of this book, the traditional structure of health care systems cannot create the reform needed for effective communication and collaboration.

What is called for is the living of a caring-based value system, modeled in the Dance of Caring Persons, described in Chapter 2. This view unifies values, supports openness and honesty, and invites the voice of all members. It offers a new structure for being in relationship that honors the importance of each person's voice and his or her contribution to the health care system, recognizes the multiple ways of knowing that impact actions, and facilitates authentic communication.

HEARING THE VOICE

Employee comfort with expressing one's voice is necessary for the transformation of health care. Voice behavior is defined as "proactively challenging the status quo and making constructive suggestions" (Van Dyne, Cummings, & Parks, 1995, p. 266). Voicing is directional. It may be directed at peers (speaking out) or supervisors (speaking up). Liu, Zhu, and Yang (2010) found that social identity encourages speaking out and personal identity supports speaking up.

Those in leadership positions ought to be aware of the key role they play in developing a culture that supports hearing the voice of all employees. Transformational leadership supports hearing the employees' voice. It encourages employees to view issues from a new lens, to communicate views, and to challenge the status quo. A leader's motivational support of employees as individuals often results in an ongoing influence on their self-identity.

Employees respond to the role-modeling of leaders by understanding their values, beliefs, and behaviors. Engaged leadership may change the employee's relationship with the leader as well as their relationship with the organization. Strong personal relationships with leaders foster speaking up rather than maintaining silence (Liu et al., 2010).

The behavior of leaders communicates whether or not there is an openness to *hear* and influences whether or not speaking up is worth the risk. Deciding to voice means one is willing to address those in leadership positions. Employees decide to voice concerns by "reading the context for clues regarding context favorability" (Milliken, Morrison, & Hewlin, 2003, p. 1455). A favorable context is one in which the employee perceives that the leader will listen, the leader is open to change, the culture is supportive, and the fear of retaliation is small.

However, if the employee believes that speaking up could have significant risks, damage relationships, cause retaliation or labeling, or that it wouldn't make a difference, silence frequently ensues. As employees witness the consequences of speaking up, they too choose to be silent or to use their voice. Choosing silence has serious implications for organizations. These include that large amounts of significant important information are not shared with health care leaders, decisions are based on incomplete knowledge, the organizational ability to detect error and engage in learning is limited, and employees become dissatisfied and disengaged (Milliken et al., 2003).

A study of medical residents showed that silence began with voice (Sutcliffe, Lewton, & Rosenthal, 2004). When a person's voice wasn't heard and hoped-for actions didn't occur, they became silent. The experience taught them how to learn to express voice in different ways such as being more forceful or talking with someone else. The point of this study is that the voicing process—voice to silence—is iterative; learning is continuous (Blatt, Christianson, Sutcliffe, & Rosenthal, 2006).

Dyess, Boykin, and Bulfin (2013) describe hearing the voice of nurses in practice as a process of caring transformation. The process of *hearing* includes connecting and knowing, being and valuing, focusing and reflecting, and committing and dialoguing. They highlight the importance of the intention of leaders to the transformation of practice environments.

The following story of a nursing student reveals not only how using voice requires courage but also the importance of support to build confidence in voicing:

> In caring for a patient, the undergraduate student noticed what appeared to her to be an abnormal pulsation in the abdomen. After consulting with the faculty, the physician was called by the student (part of the learning to be colleague). The physician, angry that a student felt she could detect something like this, insisted that the student remain on the unit until he arrived. Shortly after the physician arrived, the patient was rushed to surgery with an aortic aneurysm. The physician never acknowledged the student's keen observational skills nor did he thank her for notifying him.

The student, initially fearful and regretting she had said anything, grew more confident in her knowledge base through this experience and the support of the faculty. Reflection on this experience and the importance of living courage in practice may influence her decision to voice concerns in the future.

Bunkers (2013) quotes Hannon et al. in noting that silence can be perceived as a betrayal of trust, as in this situation, and "violation of an implicit or explicit relationship-relevant norm" (p. 10) and thus an assault on human dignity. However, in the situation just described, the nursing student's expression of courageous caring helped her transform the potentially threatening experience into one of confidence-building.

In "Pizza Ship," a powerfully written narrative illustrating the power of communication in practice, Boyte (2004) made the point that "language counts" (p. 240). The story involved a hospitalized 10-year-old boy with cerebral palsy, neurological devastation, and pneumonia; an arrogant physician; and other caregivers who had been intimidated into silence. As the physician was making derogatory and heartless comments about the child and his parents, a nurse attempted to caution the physician that the child was awake and could most likely hear the conversation. Incensed at the nurse's attempt to silence her, the physician said, "What, him,...this POS can't understand anything" (p. 241). Another caregiver at the bedside inquired into the meaning of POS, and was derisively told in explicit terms that it meant "piece of sh*t." The procedure that was under way, drawing blood to determine whether the endotracheal tube could safely be removed, was concluded and the physician left. Sometime later, after the mother had returned to the room to learn that the child could be dismissed, the physician entered the room and the child's eyes lit up in recognition. "Pizza ship, pizza ship," he shouted excitedly. Brian's mother said, "Pizza Ship? Brian is a regular parrot...Did someone mention pizza around him?" (p. 241). On hearing the mother's question, the physician who had levied the original expletive "burned crimson [and] without a word, she turned around and quickly exited the room" (p. 241).

There are several communication lessons to be learned from Boyte's (2004) story—one is the power of language to hurt, and another is the power of silence to allow hurt to be inflicted. Many health care institutions are beginning to establish and enforce policies about bullying, intimidation, and verbal abuse (Samenow, Worley, Neufeld, Fishel, & Swiggert, 2013) in an effort to eliminate an outdated pattern of status-differential bullying communication. Although patterns aren't easily altered, a combination of an explicit caring-based culture and policies that are supported by specific correcting mechanisms can go a long way in eliminating the kind of situation described in "Pizza Ship" (Boyte, 2004).

Pross, Boykin, Hilton, and Gabuat (2010) studied knowing, patience, and courage as expressions of caring with practicing nurses. The results revealed that as knowing and patience scores increased, courage scores decreased. Although nurses expressed the importance of living courage in practice, it was almost invisible. As a result of this study, the nurse leader at this health care setting focused on supporting colleagues to live courage as follows:

> A nurse newly appointed to a nursing council was hesitant to participate verbally. Recognizing the scores for courage were in the low range for the staff, the nurse leader decided to mentor and support her colleagues in speaking her voice. As a result, the newly appointed nurse was able to take risks, make deliberate choices, and truly express what was important to her. (Pross et al., 2010, p. 146)

The nurse leader in this situation made explicit that there was no hierarchy, no center of power, and emphasized the importance of each person's voice to the organization. It is through a focus on knowing person as person and person as caring that each person comes to know self as caring and identifies with the significance of his or her voice to the organization.

One of the concepts of the theory Nursing as Caring, relevant to leaders and significant for enhancing communication, is *direct invitation* (Boykin & Schoenhofer, 2001). The original purpose of direct invitation was to make clear why one was in a nursing situation as a nurse and to create an openness—a special space—in which caring between the nurse and the patient is mutually lived. The nurse invites the one cared for to share that which matters most to them at that moment in time. Through this *caring between*, calls for nursing are heard and nurturing responses created. An exquisite, poetic description of a nursing situation shared by Chandra Sumlin-Brown reveals an experience in which direct invitation was used to hear the voice of the one nursed as follows:

> Seasons come and seasons go. There are seasons of emotions, confusion, denial, hope, despair, wellness, and sickness. As I experienced personal and professional seasons, I began to become a bigger and bigger part of the universe. The universe and I are becoming a whole. The sun shines brightly onto the white snow below. I am blind to everything in front of me. I cannot tell what might happen next. Anxiety consumed me as I saw a familiar face, in unusual circumstances. Although uncomfortable and frozen, I kept moving forward toward him. I am soon unthawed by his touch and highly warm conversation. His season was high in the galaxy with no direction. It would rain one minute and the sun would shine the next. My universe broadened with a mixture of hope and uncertainty. This perception of disbelief came in like a tornado.
>
> We are at opposite poles. I am patient, he is not. I am focused, he is unfocused. He is experiencing conflicting poles. He discusses how he feels his world is coming to an end and then in the same breath states how he is on top of the world. I am weary, but present in mind, body, and spirit. I distract him with communication of seasonal thoughts of past events and nourishment. With great apprehension, I welcome him into my universe realizing that no matter what his season, interaction and planning are needed. Interaction is often and brief. Communication is long, irrational, but eventually fruitful. He talked, talked, and talked. I listened, listened, and listened. He has high goals that are as untouchable as the sun. I reach for his finger tips and hold his hand bringing him once again back to earth. Finally, a reachable goal is set. Decisions were made together and implementation and transactions of the care plan began. However, I do not understand how he got to this state. Low to the ground, I plead with the universe for explanations and answers, for his galaxy to move toward stabilization. I pray that I would see a glimpse of the person I thought I knew. Time passed and communication, planning, and interactions were regular and becoming more rational. He is calmer, but yet not as clear as I remembered him prior to admission. I am more confident yet confused.

The restoration of the destruction of the galaxy is challenging, yet provides an opportunity to explore the rest of the galaxy. The potential of another storm is brewing. There are residual effects in his galaxy. He shares that he has had early warning signs, but did not take precautions. I call upon everyone asking for direction to prevent or slow down a likely undesirable season. The season was named and appropriate steps were taken to slow down a disastrous season. It was a global effort to improve his galaxy. His family was made aware of the discoveries in hopes to early identify and prevent a severe season in his future galaxy. My universe continues to expound with the awareness and knowledge that a nurse–patient relationship of communication, interaction, perception, and transaction attains mutually set goals. Feeling understood improves interpersonal, intrapersonal, and professional relationships. As nurses, when assessing patients, we must communicate verbally and nonverbally that we are present holistically to work with our patients. Patients' perception of nurses plays a major role in healing and nursing process as well as nurses' perception of patients. If a patient views a nurse as not listening, know it all, unsure or uncertain, impatient, inconsiderate, and so on, they are least likely to fully participate in the nursing process. Likewise, there is a potential for a nurse to be more passive with treatment planning if the patient is perceived as demanding, unreasonable, selfish, inconsiderate, loud, and so on. A necessary function of the nursing process consists of the nurse and patient communicating and interacting together, planning or making agreeable decisions or goals, and then acting to attain these goals.

In this nursing situation, the nurse through intentional presence lives courage and patience as she invites the patient into a common space where together they can come to know each other as caring; where the calls for nursing can be heard and responded to.

Direct invitation can also be used by leaders in health care organizations as a means to come to know employees as caring persons and to *invite* them to share honestly any issues or concerns. Through this invitation—either verbal or nonverbal—one communicates value and respect of person and appreciation of their ideas and what matters to them. The Dance of Caring Persons recognizes that each person brings commitment, knowledge, and expertise to the organization. It is the knowledge and expertise held by employees that is so critical to effective decision making by leaders. To create a culture where the flow of information is open, honest, and ongoing requires that leaders communicate respectfully and authentically. Direct invitation is a strategy that can be used to call forth the voice of all in the organization.

Strategies to Enhance the Voicing Process

Chief executive officers (CEOs) at award-winning health care institutions described strategies for increasing voicing in health care organizations (Adelman & Stokes, 2012). Some of their suggested strategies as well as other strategies are listed as follows:

- Establish personal knowing of employees by coming to know their names and stories. It is important for employees and leaders to come to know each other as a person in order to build trust
- Make oneself visible on a regular basis to promote trust, open avenues for communication, and instill the idea that one is approachable
- Extend to employees the invitation to communicate ideas and concerns and help them understand that it is only with all working together that the best and right decisions and actions occur
- Praise employees for living caring by risking to express their voice
- Conduct open forums to dialogue on issues and to answer questions
- Create an environment in which employees feel safe to share what matters to them

- Participate in rounding on units on a regular basis as a way to come to know concerns firsthand
- Create a culture for learning within cross-disciplinary teams

SENSE-MAKING

Voicing or remaining silent at critical points is part of the sense-making process. The process of deciding to voice begins when an issue is clear. The decision considers whether the issue is important enough to use voice and how confident one is in voicing the concern. Sense-making arises from dialogue when individuals share their perspective regarding a situation. The process emphasizes the importance of seeking different perspectives.

The process of sense-making occurs continuously in health care. Physicians and nurses "enact sensible environments (environments where sense-making can occur) by becoming more sensitive to all forms of communication, communicating their perspectives, and considering how each other's perceptual stance affects actions to be taken" (Manojlovich, 2010, p. 944). Leaders regularly reflect on organizational experiences and turn them into "words and salient categories that they can comprehend and then use as a springboard for action" (Blatt et al., 2006, p. 898). Whenever there is a change in the flow of events, sense-making results. Questions asked are, What is the story? What now? (Weick, Sutcliff, & Obstfeld, 2005). According to Weick, Sutcliff, and Obstfeld, the sense-making process includes the following:

- Noticing and bracketing
- Labeling
- Being retrospective
- Being presumptive
- Recognizing social and systemic factors
- Taking action
- Organizing through communication

Sense-making involves issues of identity. As mentioned earlier, the confidence of the provider in knowing self as caring determines whether or not voicing is used and whether or not one is comfortable in engaging others in dialogue on health situations. Being comfortable with colleagues points to the importance of various disciplines being clear on their unique disciplinary perspective. If nurses are not clear on their professional identity (Parse, 2013) or if they cannot clearly articulate their unique contributions to the health care team, their sense-making ability becomes limited as they may be hesitant to engage in a dialogue (Manojlovich, 2010).

The importance of the values and beliefs of the Dance of Caring Persons model is underscored by what we know of sense-making. In this model, rather than the usual unidirectionality between physicians and nurses, there is reciprocity. Each person's views are appreciated, shared, and respected. This openness eliminates the holding of information resulting in continuous learning of each person's unique contributions. Each person in the process of sense-making draws on his or her experiences and those of others to understand situations and create appropriate actions. Each person composes a story of what is happening so that action can be taken (Brown, 2006). Mayeroff (1971) refers to this expression of caring as alternating rhythms, moving from a broader perspective (experience) to a narrower perspective (a particular situation). In this process, "perceptions and experiences are transformed into words that all parties can comprehend, and which then serve as a springboard for action" (Manojlovich, 2010, p. 943). We propose that the common language of sense-making for health care systems is the language of caring. Caring is the lens through which one views the health situation—the experience—and comes to understand and respond.

All sense-making occurs through some mental model. From a caring perspective, one would ask, What is the caring in this situation? What actions would reflect the value of caring? In this nursing situation shared by Shelina Davis, the lens of caring guides sense-making:

This year, I met a young male who came to the emergency department with chest pain. We will just call him Bob. He underwent a cardiac catheterization and was found to have severe multivessel coronary artery disease and was referred to the cardiothoracic surgical team. I introduced myself to the small-framed gentleman and began to talk to him and ask him my usual questions. He rested on the recovery stretcher, very relaxed and very attentive to everything I explained. He asked questions along the way and seemed very accepting of (1) his newly diagnosed severe artery disease, (2) learning that he was a poor candidate for nonsurgical revascularization, and (3) being told that surgeons were prepared to take him for bypass grafting the next morning! I remember Bob coming to his decision rather quickly without any vacillation or discernible trepidation. The more I explained, the more eager he was to learn more.

After almost two hours of speaking with Bob and coming to know him, I learned he was a bit of a loner. He had never been married. His family lived in another state and he had not seen them in years. However, he had neighbors who were willing to help him at any time. I wrapped up the consult and began preparing him for the day's events. I remember thinking to myself how unusual this was for me because I normally would have to give patients and family members time to think and digest everything. Not Bob! By his verbal and nonverbal cues, I could tell he was ready for more. Every aspect of his hospital stay that I discussed, from preoperative testing to discharge home, he was open and accepting of things to come. I ended my extended visit with Bob, and I asked him if there was anything we had not covered that was important to him or any questions that I had not answered or needed clearing up. He smiled widely and replied, "Nope. I think I am ready!" He went off to surgery the next day.

Bob did very well postoperatively. I saw him every day through his recovery and continued to build a solid patient–provider relationship with him. He was discharged on postoperative day six with a follow-up scheduled in the office to see me. He presented for his first postoperative visit and had developed drainage, swelling, and pain at the distal end of his sternal incision. I opened the incision by sterile technique and realized the area of drainage was very large. I admitted him back into the hospital for incision and drainage of the entire area. Through it all, again, he was a trooper. A wound vacuum system was placed on the wound in the operating room and I saw him the next morning. I felt very good about his short stay and was even more excited that all had gone so well. Besides, I had more teaching to share about things to come. Just as I had done before, I explained to him everything to come. I explained that he would go home with the wound vacuum system and that nurses would come in every other day to change the foam packing. This time, he was very quiet. I continued on without missing a beat. Later that evening, I briefly thought about him, but I wasn't sure why. By the end of the week, postoperative day three, he was scheduled for discharge. As the nurse was preparing Bob for discharge, he began to have chest pains. Diagnostic testing was unrevealing and he was monitored for over the weekend. That Monday morning I made rounds and Bob seemed to be doing very well. I reviewed everything that happened over the weekend, and I began to recall my last encounter with Bob. Therefore, I decided to hang around for a couple of hours. Later, his nurse began to go over discharge information with him, and he began to complain of chest pain and dizziness. I entered the room and he looked terrified. He was pale, very fearful, and avoiding eye contact. He looked nothing like the Bob I had come to know. I asked the nurse to give us some time, and I sat down beside him and began to talk with him. Eventually, he began to reveal how he could not go home. He expressed how he felt no fear as he faced his own mortality being diagnosed with severe coronary disease and undergoing open heart surgery. He continued to tell me that everything had gone just as he had learned through teaching. He felt no fear until I told him that nurses would come into his home to do dressing changes. Turns out, Bob had two dogs that were deemed aggressive. He knew he could not have anyone in his home, but he didn't know how to tell me. He didn't know that he had options. He was afraid that his dogs would suffer as a result of his care needs. He feared that maybe they would be taken away. I realized then that I had missed something very special with Bob. His dogs were his close family. His dogs loved, comforted, and protected him. With them, he had no fear and felt he would be fine at home. Due to his special needs, I made arrangements for Bob to come into my office Monday, Wednesday, and Friday for dressing changes. He was very thankful, and so was I. He taught me a valuable lesson. Within half an hour, Bob was chasing the nurse down the hall for discharge information, asking questions, and being very attentive to his instructions for skin care and managing the wound vacuum system. He went home that afternoon and continued to eagerly learn, as he recovered from his surgical experiences. Nursing is learning and connecting to what matters to the patient and trying to make health care fit their needs; surely, the cares of the patient affect his or her experience in health, illness, and recovery.

In this lived experience, the nurse through her intentional and authentic presence entered Bob's world. She lived her caring with Bob as she expressed her knowing, patience, and hope. It is through her knowing Bob as caring person, that upon reflection, she became attuned to a specific call for caring. It is her knowing of and dialogue with Bob that allowed her to make sense out of what was happening to him. The nurse recognized Bob's call to be heard. She responded to his call by instilling hope as she presented alternatives to the nurses coming to his home for dressing changes. The nurse nurtured and supported Bob's living and growing in caring in ways that mattered to him.

Strategies for Sense-Making

Strategies for sense-making include the following:

- Seeing each health experience as an opportunity to learn
- Being concerned enough to ask your patients to repeat something you did not understand in their health story
- Costudying and dialoguing with colleagues on stories of practice
- Engaging in a process of understanding how to dialogue

NARRATIVE OR STORY

Perhaps a reflection on our own life will highlight the importance of story. There's something about us that wants to be heard—that wants to be told. We live to share, so to say, our lives. We can recall those early years—especially returning from school—when our parents wanted to know everything that happened each day and how eager we were to tell them the day's events. We recall how excited we became when we were praised by a teacher for knowing an answer and how special we felt when we met our first friends and anticipated being with them during lunch and recess, and if we were able, after school.

Those early experiences were so necessary and wonderful for us. Strangers came to know our names and wanted to know even more things about us. Gradually they became our friends. Not only did they *like* us but they were interested in us and what we did mattered to them—they listened to us and our stories.

Narratives or stories are the best way to communicate important experiences—especially those that have shaped us. Stories communicate values, teach, inspire, and motivate. They invite us to think, to reflect, and to come to understand complex situations. Stories are one way of conveying something of ourselves that often can begin only through this form. Starhawk reminds us that "to be valued we must first be seen, and that hearing another's story is a powerful way of valuing that person" (Nagai-Jacobson & Burkhardt, 1996, p. 57).

Throughout this book, stories have been used to communicate the human dimensions of health care. When a health care provider chooses to intentionally enter into the story of the one cared for, he or she creates the opportunity to affirm the worth of the person by listening caringly and carefully to what is being revealed (Charon, 2004). Entering into the stories of others calls for one to be vulnerable; to connect with the humanness of others, and to recognize the connectedness to oneself (Boykin & Schoenhofer, 1992). Being able to recognize, absorb, interpret, and be moved by stories requires a combination of textual skills (identifying the structure of the story), creative skills (imaging the many interpretations), and affective skills (tolerating uncertainty as the story unfolds; Charon, 2004).

Listening to the stories of those cared for has long been a strategy used by nurses. Today many physicians are beginning "to believe that narrative studies can provide the *basic science* of story-based medicine that can honor the patients who endure illness and nourish the physicians who care for them" (Charon, 2004, p. 863). We have seen earlier in this chapter ("Pizza Ship") and in a previous chapter ("Casey's Legacy") that physicians are using stories to understand and to teach (Boyte, 2001, 2004). Stories not only serve as a rich source for understanding patients but also a new way to understand diseases. They illustrate the power of listening and entering another's lived health experience, as we see in the following narrative shared by Barbara Edwards:

> My experience was with a patient that could easily be labeled "noncompliant." He routinely refused prescription medications and often left the hospital against medical advice. We met several days into his hospitalization. I was not the primary nurse but I entered his room to answer a call light.
>
> One morning I arrived on the unit to find several nurses standing in the hallway outside his room. Apparently he had been agitated on the night shift and was requesting a gun and threatening to kill himself. The nurses were frightened and not sure what to do. They had contacted the physician who ordered a sedative. After speaking with his nurse, I entered his room. He looked up at me and said "What are you doing here?" I responded by informing him that I was a nurse and concerned for him after hearing his threat of suicide. He told me I had no reason to be concerned; whether he lived or died was no concern of mine. I agreed in part. I told him that while I was not the nurse "assigned" to care for him that I still felt an obligation to him as a fellow human being. I shared that although I did not understand all of what he was going through, I was aware of his diagnosis of inoperable cancer. There was a long silence.
>
> After a few minutes, he told me to make myself useful and find him a gun. I did not respond for several minutes, as I didn't know what to say. Finally, I gathered the courage and spoke to him in a way that I had not spoken to a patient before. I told him that although he was upset with his current situation that suicide was not an option for him (I noticed in his chart that he was a practicing Catholic, had been visited by a priest, that he wore a crucifix, and had a tattoo of Jesus on his arm). Another long silence followed. Eventually he and I began to talk. He shared that as an ex-marine he didn't like being told what to do by nurses and doctors. He said he had been NPO for three mornings in a row and what he really wanted was a cup of coffee. We spoke for quite a while that day and over the next several days. He shared that his wife had died several years earlier and that when she died he lost touch with his son. I asked permission to contact the son. He said "no."
>
> The next day he asked for me to come to his room. When I got there he told me that if I still wanted to call his son, it would be fine with him and he handed me his number. I made the call and they were reunited.

This story retold serves as a reminder that listening is the most powerful way to connect with others. Through this connectedness there emerges a shared understanding.

When the nurse understood the patient's story, she could more accurately understand other information and data.

The story is the context for knowing and ought to become the source for determining individual outcomes in health situations. "The value of story begins with the insight and deepened understanding practicing nurses can gain into the meaning of their own practice" (Boykin & Schoenhofer, 1992, p. 248). Stories such as this one instill compassion and remind members of the health care organization that it is the person cared for who is the focus of one's work. Stories do indeed, as Langer and Riberich (2008) state, "strip away the details to get to the soul of a person or the issue at hand" (p. 57).

In health care, stories are also an effective way to communicate an organization's vision and values. In Chapter 7 on leadership, the story was told of how hospital employees, patients, families, and members of the community formed a circle of caring around the hospital to convey that living caring with those cared for, employees, and the community is what this health care organization valued. Their commitment to caring values was further communicated in numerous other ways. The vice president of nursing services, Nancy Hilton, created a process for storytelling that permeated the whole of the organization. This process, "huddling," began in the administrative suite with all leaders of the organization. She shares:

> We are in a big circle. Usually one of the executives starts with recognizing a department or an individual. All persons are invited to share a story of living caring or maybe a story that didn't start well but ended with service recovery. One morning I shared a story about a bedside shift report that did not go well for a particular patient. I was called to a nursing department because a patient wanted to complain to me. He listed a litany of reasons why bedside shift report was so important in making the connection with the patient. I was dumbfounded because he could have taught the class. He went on to explain also why the care boards were so valuable. I'm still nodding in full agreement. He then goes on to explain that the nurses did not offer him the direct invitation during bedside shift report this morning like they normally did. He heard the day shift nurse tell the night shift nurse that a report wasn't necessary because he was going home. He explained to me that it was extremely important because he needed to tell them that what mattered most to him this morning was to call his wife so she could pick him up before she went to work; otherwise, he would have to wait until 9 p.m. I was quickly able to orchestrate calling his wife and getting the discharge in order. Not only did I share this story in our "huddle" but I tell this story at every nursing orientation. Every nurse "gets it"—the value of bedside shift report focused on knowing the story of the person cared for.

Likewise, the director of the emergency department (ED), Jim Kruger, shared a story of a nurse living courage.

> We had a relatively young patient brought to the ED by ambulance. She was very ill. Her husband was at her bedside the entire time. After several hours, the woman died. The husband was very distraught. He said the worst part was he had to go home and tell their 15-year-old son that his mother had died. The ED nurse witnessing the husband's uncontrollable shaking and expression of deep anguish said he would drive this man home to tell his son and then drive them both back to the hospital to have some time and a little closure with the mom/wife.

These and other stories are told each day, Monday through Friday, at the beginning of the day. The expectation of the leaders is that all departments create a process for sharing stories in their departments on a regular basis. The sharing of stories makes it easier for one to hear stories. This process stimulates more stories and they become an important aspect of creating a sense of a community in which caring values are lived.

Aesthetic representations of stories of living caring may be communicated in different ways throughout an organization; on bulletin boards, in reports, through videos, and so on. Organizational stories teach many lessons. As in these stories, they teach us how to avoid making similar mistakes; they remind us of the values we hold dear; the importance of being present; and that how and what we say matters.

Strategies for Telling Stories

The use of stories in health care settings can be encouraged by the following:

- Listening to and sharing important stories of practice with colleagues
- Creating the space and time for stories to be shared regularly across disciplines and departments
- Bringing the language of caring to the core of all activities in health care

Communicating Through Technology

Unlike any other time in history, health care providers have the ability to be present to and with others wherever they may be. Although technology has rightly reaped its recognition especially in communication, can it take us only so far or bring us only so close to those cared for? The delivery of health care today and certainly that of tomorrow will expand well beyond the walls of any traditional health care settings. The point of care is where the person is residing. How will (or is) care delivered through cyberspace perceived as caring? Is health care technology at odds with human caring? How does one come to know a person as person? How does one establish presence and connect in ways that matter to the one cared for? How will outcomes of care be measured in the future? How does or will technology assist health care providers to achieve the goal of person-centered care?

The complexities of communication and establishing meaningful relationships deepen as one engages in the use of virtual communication. Although health care technologies for the delivery of care continue to advance, health care providers have been engaged in the use of information and communication technology for years. Examples of synchronous and asynchronous technologies include telephone, videoconferencing, e-mail, video-monitoring, telemetry, and telemedicine (especially in areas of radiology, pathology, dermatology, ophthalmology, and psychiatry). Data gathered through such technology adds to the empirical and personal knowing of person.

Poland, Lehoux, Holmes, and Andrews (2005) echo the view of Ihde, the classic philosopher of technology, that a person may relate to technology in one of two ways. It may serve as a "transparent mediator between oneself and the world" (p. 175). In this case there would be a smooth engagement of individuals within a world made possible via technology. On the other hand, technology may also act as an "opaque interference between oneself and the world, obfuscating the relationship between the individual, the technology, and the world" (p. 175). Although the proclaimed intent of health care technology is to empower the one seeking care by providing them with more information regarding their health, it can also have the effect of disempowerment and alienation.

The caring capabilities of technology that enhance communication have been described by Simpson (2008) as follows:

- *Efficiency*—because technology saves time, it allows nurses to spend more time with the patients
- *Audit trail*—technology supports the accountability and honesty necessary in communication
- *Data comprehensiveness*—technology allows for aggregation, evaluation, and dissemination of much data. Better decisions can be made regarding care

- *Data security*—there is better security with electronic data so a person's confidentiality is better maintained
- Anonymity—decreases biases; technology allows participants to collaborate from same or different places

Barnard and Sandelowski (2001) suggest that humane care and technology are a reflection of a "social construction rather than any essential difference between them" (p. 368). The view of technology at any point in time depends on the "eye of the beholder, the hand of the user, and the technological systems that influence integration and use" (p. 368). Sandelowski (2002) offers the following insight: The new virtual geography of nursing practice challenges traditional ideas, as it calls into question "how essential bodily presence is to being there" (p. 64) and to patients feeling that their nurse is there for them. How is presence communicated when the proximate body is no longer the channel of communication? Nursing is moving to cyberspace, a place "created and sustained by...computers and communication lines...a virtual world...entered equally from anywhere...where nothing is forgotten and yet everything changes" (p. 64). Sandelowski shares an illuminating quotation from Lombard and Ditton's work on presence and mediated communication:

> Telepresence...is successful when persons fail to perceive or acknowledge the existence of a medium in (their) communication environment and respond as (they) would if the medium were not there. (Sandelowski, 2002, p. 65)

How technology is viewed in health care depends on the lens of the health care provider. In a study by Varghese and Phillips (2009), advance practice nurses describe how they convey caring via telehealth. They stressed the importance of personhood and creating a way of being that fosters knowing person as person. They initiated this through empirical knowing—all available information was read prior to contact; and to begin to establish personal knowing, they sent to the person cared for information on who they were as nurse as well as information on their organization. Through telehealth, their presence was intentionally focused on listening, communicating, and staying connected. Some expressions of caring were identified as essential: honesty, dependability, competence, empowerment, and intentionality (Varghese & Phillips, 2009).

When practicing from the perspective of caring, technology is seen as an extension of self—an extension of one's senses—and an expression of living caring, of coming to know person as person, and person as whole in the moment. Technology in health situations is transformed in the aesthetics of practice. Living caring through technology requires knowing self as caring. The goal for the use of technology in health care must be on creating a caring, respectful relationship; on coming to know others; and on creating meaning through dialogue.

As always, being present and listening in health care situations are essential to the process of knowing other. Schneider (2001) quoted Issacs' perceptive injunction regarding listening: "Listening requires that we not only hear the words, but also embrace, accept, and gradually let go of our own inner clamoring. This means listening not only to others but also to ourselves and our own reactions" (Isaacs as cited in Schneider, 2001, p. 42). Schneider points out the advantages the virtual world offers for creating relationships. When the sender and receiver do not interact at the same time, there is more time to listen; and there is a sense of safety and trust. He specifically addresses the importance of establishing effective communication online and states that such communication requires:

> at least the same amount of energy used in listening as does real-world communication. It is about suspending judgment, speaking my own voice and inviting others to do the same,

and respecting myself and others. It is about creating the space or container where all this is possible. (p. 43)

Strategies for Communicating in the Virtual World

- Understand one's underlying intentions in using a particular technology
- Focus on coming to know person as whole who is living caring
- Listen attentively and respectfully
- Demonstrate competence in the technology used

SUMMARY

This chapter calls for leaders in health care to be reminded of the message from the introduction of Ralph Ellison's (1980) classic *Invisible Man*—a person who craves to be known but who is in effect invisible to those around him. Especially in a system that includes the terms "health" and "care" as descriptive of the nature of the system that thrives on its science and forward-looking technology, we need to be alert to the potential for any members being considered inferior because of their position or not being considered at all due to the large number of people who make up the particular health care organization. We must not lose sight of this primary responsibility, to "see," that is incumbent upon leaders who daily assume the task of caring for each of the members of their health care system.

In particular, from a perspective of caring, it is the responsibility of the leaders of health care to communicate openly, honestly, and authentically with those cared for as well as employees. It is the responsibility of the leader to ensure as best one can that all voices are heard, to know the stories of employees, and to live caring in responding to situations. It is the goal of leaders to humanize the health care environment by communicating the importance of each person.

The Dance of Caring Persons is a powerful symbol revealing an even greater meaning. We are—all of us—joined together in this movement called life, and each one of us finds our own identity by being aware of those journeying with us. The caring that is lived each moment in health care organizations communicates our connectedness to others and our commitment to live caring with them.

QUESTIONS TO CONSIDER

- Have you had experiences in which the lack of precise communication resulted in a detrimental effect?
- What situations have you encountered that caused you to remain silent rather than address issues that mattered? What was the experience like for you?
- Have you developed enough confidence to voice what matters to you?
- In what ways do your behaviors invite hearing the voice of others?
- How do you establish presence and connect in ways that matter to employees and those cared for?

REFERENCES

Adelman, K., & Stokes, C. (2012). Promoting employee voice and upward communication in healthcare: The CEO's influence. *Journal of Healthcare Management, 57*(2), 133–147.

Barnard, A., & Sandelowski, M. (2001). Technology and humane nursing care: (Ir)reconcilable or invented difference. *Journal of Advanced Nursing, 34*(3), 367–375.

Blatt, R., Christianson, M., Sutcliffe, K., & Rosenthal, M. (2006). A sensemaking lens on reliability. *Journal of Organizational Behavior, 27*, 897–917.

Boykin, A., & Schoenhofer, S. (2001). *Nursing as caring: A model for transforming practice.* Sudbury, MA: Jones & Bartlett.

Boykin, A., & Schoenhofer, S. O. (1992). Story as link between nursing's ontology, epistemology and practice. *Image: Journal of Nursing Scholarship, 23*(4), 245–248.

Boyte, W. R. (2004). Pizza ship. *Health Affairs, 23*(5), 240–241. doi:10.1377/hlthaff.23.5.240

Brown, A. (2006). A narrative approach to collective identities. *Journal of Management Studies, 43*(4), 731–753.

Bunkers, S. S. (2013). Theoretical concerns: Silence: A double-edged sword. *Nursing Science Quarterly, 26*(1), 7–11.

Charon, R. (2004). Narrative and medicine. *The New England Journal of Medicine, 350*(9), 862–864.

Dyess, S. M., Boykin, A., & Bulfin, M. J. (2013). Hearing the voice of nurses in caring theory-based practice. *Nursing Science Quarterly, 26*(2), 167–173.

Ellison, R. (1980). *Invisible man.* New York, NY: Vintage Books.

Institute of Medicine. (2004). *Keeping patients safe: Transforming the work environment of nurses.* Washington, DC: The National Academies Press.

Jordan, B., & Friends. (2006). *Communication in hierarchical organizations.* Unpublished manuscript. Retrieved from lifescapes.org

Langer, N., & Ribarich, M. (2008). Using narratives in healthcare communication. *Educational Gerontology, 35*(1), 55–62.

Liu, W., Zhu, R., & Yang, Y. (2010). I warn you because I like you: Voice behavior, employee identifications, and transformational leadership. *The Leadership Quarterly, 21*, 189–202.

Macknet, D. (n.d.). *Organizational communication. The role of humanity in organizations.* Retrieved from http://www.sonic.net/~davimack/OrgComm/OC_Final.htm

Manojlovich, M. (2010). Nurse/physician communication through a sensemaking lens. *Medical Care, 48*(11), 941–946.

Mayeroff, M. (1971). *On caring.* New York, NY: Harper & Row.

McCroskey, J. C. (2006). *An introduction to rhetorical communication* (9th ed.) Boston, MA: Allyn & Bacon.

Milliken, F., Morrison, E., & Hewlin, P. (2003). An exploratory study of employee silence: Issues that employees don't communicate upward and why. *Journal of Management Studies, 40*(6), 1453–1476.

Nagai-Jacobson, M., & Burkhardt, M. (1996). Viewing persons as stories: A perspective for holistic care. *Alternative Therapies in Health and Medicine, 2*(4), 54–58.

Nembhard, I., & Edmondson, A. (2006). Making it safe: The effects of leader inclusiveness and professional status on psychological safety and improvement efforts in health care teams. *Journal of Organizational Behavior, 27*, 941–966.

Parse, R. R. (2013). Editorial. "What we've got here is 'failure to communicate'": The meaning of the term *nursing perspective. Nursing Science Quarterly, 26*(1), 5.

Poland, B., Lehoux, P., Holmes, D., & Andrews, G. (2005). How place matters: Unpacking technology and power in health and social care. *Health and Social Care in the Community, 13*(2), 170–180. doi:10.1111/j.1365–2524.2005.00545.x

Pross, E., Boykin, A., Hilton, N., & Gabuat, J. (2010). A study of knowing nurses as caring. *Holistic Nursing Practice, 24*(3), 142–147.

Ray, D., & Elder, D. (2007). Managing horizontal accountability. *The Journal for Quality and Participation, 30*(4), 24–28.

Samenow, C., Worley, L., Neufeld, R., Fishel, T., & Swiggert, W. (2013). Transformative learning in a professional development course aimed at addressing disruptive physician behavior: A composite case study. *Academic Medicine, 88*(1), 117–123.

Sandelowski, M. (2002). Visible humans, vanishing bodies, and virtual nursing: Complications of life, presence, place, and identity. *Advances in Nursing Science, 24*(3), 58–70.

Schneider, F. (2001). Have you ever listened to your e-mail? A dialogic approach to online communication. *Reflections, 3*(2), 40–43.

Simpson, R. (2008). Caring communications: How technology enhances interpersonal relations. *Nursing Administration Quarterly, 32*(1), 70–73.

Sutcliffe, K., Lewton, E., & Rosenthal, M. (2004). Communication failures: An insidious contributor to medical mishaps. *Academic Medicine, 79*(2), 186–194.

Tourish, D. (2003). Critical upward feedback in organizations: Processes, problems and implications for communication management. *Journal of Communication Management, 8*(2), 150–167.

Van Dyne, L., Cummings, L. L., & Parks, J. M. (1995). Extra-role behaviors: In pursuit of construct and definitional clarity (A bridge over muddied waters). In L. L. Cummings & B. M. Staw (Eds.), *Research in organizational behavior* (Vol. 17, pp. 215–285). Greenwich, CT: JAI Press.

Varghese, S. B., & Phillips, C. A. (2009). Caring in telehealth. *Telemedicine and e-Health, 15*(10), 1005. doi:10.1089/tmj.2009.0070

Varpio, L., Hall, P., Lingard, L., & Schryer, C. (2008). Interprofessional communication and medical error: A reframing of research questions and approaches. *Academic Medicine, 83*(10), S76–S81.

Weick, K., Sutcliffe, K., & Obstfeld, D. (2005). Organizing and the process of sensemaking. *Organizational Science, 16*(4), 409–451.

Response to Chapter 8

Donna Linette, MS, RN, NEA-BC
Chief Nursing Officer
Atlantic Shores Hospital

Communication is foundational to the practice of nursing administration from a caring perspective. The most important aspect of my role is to support those providing direct care. In order to do this effectively, I must know each nurse as person, as caring. I want to know the story of each person so I know how to nurture and support their growth; know what matters to them; and know how their life might impact their work and ultimately patient care. Mostly, I need to listen and really hear what the nurse needs—to care exquisitely, to care for each other, and to care for self. More than ever I try to support the nurse in caring for self.

I am most grateful to a family who taught me the importance of listening to the voice of those cared for and their family.

> One of our patients had significant symptoms of his mental illness—the symptoms were severely interfering with his daily routine (volunteering at the mental health association drop-in center). He was hospitalized in an effort to develop a plan to curb these negative symptoms of schizophrenia. His treatment plan focused on all disciplines helping to relieve the effects of auditory hallucinations. One day as I was escorting his father to visit, I asked how he thought his son was doing—he stopped and said, "I wish that you (meaning all of the team) would focus on more than his symptoms. Does anyone here know that he graduated at the top of his class? Does anyone here know that he is a concert pianist?" This was a turning point for me, as I was beginning to change the philosophy of the department—this was a perfect example of how we were NOT treating the whole patient. Needless to say, we added his talents and have been working hard since to include strengths for all persons. Both our language of how we referred to this patient's needs, and our attention to the whole person, were an issue for communication within and among the team (including the person/patient and the family).

Leaders communicate caring through role modeling. This is a story of a situation in which I felt that the role modeling had been effective and the nurse "got it."

> Sometimes, caring for a person with a chronic mental illness means that you may see the same person come back to the hospital for treatment at another time. Unfortunately, this is

at times looked upon negatively and even the words I have heard some use to describe these persons—"frequent flyers," "problem patients," and so on—were so very objectifying and dehumanizing.

I went to one of the nursing units to meet with the team to let them know that patient MW was returning to their unit for further treatment. MW had previously presented with challenging symptoms, a family dynamic that also required extensive care, and not much interest in participating in his own course of treatment. The staff was frustrated with their inability to effectively treat him. The team members were quiet—not sure what to say exactly; and then the charge nurse asked the group, "I wonder how we can care for him differently this time?" I loved the question! To me it reflected that she was thinking about the whole person; the fact that a different approach to providing care was needed, and could be done; further, she led the team to welcome him back. At that moment, I thought—wow, she gets it.

Another example is continuing to use language that comes from a caring perspective. In residential treatment or correctional nursing, I was hearing "show of force" when help was called. It is amazing what a difference you can create by saying "show of support"—after all, isn't that what we are really trying to do?

The caring leader is one who encourages risk taking and allows each to follow his or her path; it is not always "popular" to be the nurse who speaks up; so we need to support courage while also drawing out the input from those who often do not speak up.

There must be understanding and support from all of the hospital leaders—nursing works collaboratively with other departments so we must share what we do, what the value of our work is, what the patient sees as important to care. We owe it to all to educate them on caring.

The nursing leader needs to create ways to hard-wire some of the concepts. Ongoing attention and education are needed to sustain a culture of caring. There are many ways to do this, such as:

- Creating an *Article of the Month* to share about caring
- Remembering that the nursing leader shares the lead in the Dance of Caring Persons
- Assuring that the nursing leaders speak the language of caring in all communications
- Establishing a nursing philosophy and plan—a working document—that firmly states caring is the essence of nursing
- Celebrating nursing stories that reflect caring
- Including caring on annual evaluations and in competency fairs
- Adding a "caring corner" to your nursing library
- Orienting each educational setting to the caring framework
- Adding *Caring* as a standing item to the monthly meeting agendas

Chapter 9

Prizing, Valuing, and Growing: Outcomes Reframed

The idea of outcomes—anticipated results of strategies deliberately designed to achieve clear purposes—depends on the idea of mission or purpose for a meaningful context. Porter O'Grady and Malloch (2012) have accurately pointed out that while responsibility was the watchword of the 20th century, the watchword for the 21st century is accountability. They have called for a new vision, one that encompasses both processes *and* outcomes, a "critical integration between means and ends, products and processes" (p. 261). In writing about reframing organizations, Bolman and Deal (2008) quoted DeGues, "They [organizations] need profits in the same way as any living organism needs oxygen. It is a necessity to stay alive but it is not the purpose of life" (p. 399). From that perspective, we would suggest that the new vision that is needed integrates not only processes and products, but also purpose. Further, we endorse the ultimate purpose of health care systems as a service purpose—systems intended to offer health services as an expression of human caring. Secondary purposes—professional and occupational satisfaction, employment, participation in commerce, and financial profit on monetary investments—important as they are to the lifeblood of health care systems, must reflect the ultimate purpose of the system. Clearly, outcomes as indicators of achievement of ultimate purpose should be recognized as means rather than as ends. Even the very concept of outcomes, as well as the processes of establishing and assessing outcomes, must align with the ultimate caring purpose of any health care system.

This chapter will be organized to address three integrated aspects related to the objective of reframing the idea of outcomes so that it reflects prizing, valuing, and growing. We will discuss strategies for evaluation and for acting on the results of evaluation, keeping in mind the nexus of purpose–process–product. Three central questions that will guide our discussion of this nexus are as follows:

How can we know that we are providing the care experience that each of us intends within our circle of influence?

How might we assure that this occurs and is sustained consistently, effectively, and meaningfully?

How might we intentionally build these expectations into the educational programs we offer across disciplines?

In addition to discussing and offering strategies for evaluation of outcomes, both institutional and clinical performance appraisal, we will also address the system functions in support of lifelong learning. We will begin by examining the idea of clinical performance evaluation, then move to system performance evaluation, and finally, coaching and formal learning system strategies.

Evaluation is an increasing concern of health care systems. In fact, in an era where the viability of all systems and institutions is being challenged, the evaluation process can and in many cases does become "the tail that wags the dog." This out-of-balance emphasis on the role of evaluation tends to produce a mentality of "token compliance," or as it is expressed in education, "teaching to the test." How can we understand evaluation in a new way that places it in the context of contributing to the mission of the health care system?

The answer we offer to that important question is the creation of a culture of caring, grounded in the philosophy of the Dance of Caring Persons. This chapter will provide examples and suggestions to stimulate creative thinking about the evaluation process and specific evaluation strategies. But first, let's examine two ideas basic to that cultural transformation: accountability and evaluation.

According to the *Oxford English Dictionary Online*, accountability has at its core the word *count;* the history of the word refers us back to its original meaning, which is to tell a story, to make known, to reveal or disclose, to relate. More readily recognizable uses of the idea of accountability refer to being answerable, or being called to render a reckoning, to explain, or to answer for—which takes us back to telling a story. Questions we might ask in relation to accountability include: Account for what? To whom? Key questions in evaluation include: "What counts?" and "How do we recognize what counts?" We will come back to this idea, but let's turn our attention to the idea of evaluation. Again, referring to the *Oxford English Dictionary Online* for the origins of this word, we find that it stems from the original meaning, *worth*. Evaluation is described as the act of appraising, to work out the value of something.

Stepping outside of the way we usually think about accountability and evaluation in health care systems offers an opportunity for a fresh look, a new understanding that draws on basic meanings of familiar concepts. We would like to introduce a new way of thinking about accountability and evaluation: prizing, valuing, and growing—dimensions of an evaluation process that acknowledge caring as the most fundamental service aim of health care systems (Schoenhofer & Coffman, 1994).

Prizing can be thought of as discovering, proclaiming, or imputing the worth of something. In our approach to this process, prizing is the establishment of mission, goals, and objectives—choosing that which is to be prized, that which "counts."

Valuing is recognizing the merits/worth of a representation of that which is chosen as prized in a way that tells a story about that which is valued. Translated into practical action, valuing is the process of weighing the evidence that describes a connection or relationship between that which is prized and the means selected to honor that which is prized, telling a story of the connection between means and ends. Valuing refers to that aspect of the evaluation process typically called planning and implementation.

Growing refers to specific expressions of the power of the valuing process to honor that which is prized—providing information that confirms the prizing, and sustains or enhances the valuing; growing refers to the coaching aspect of evaluation that offers recommendations for continuing development/support of implementation strategies.

The specific topic of retention can be used to illustrate the prizing, valuing, and growing process. Most health care systems have stated personnel policies that express staff retention as a prized objective. Retention of staff is prized for several reasons—reputation for excellence; nurturing recruitment and development investments; and avoiding unnecessary recruitment and retraining costs, including human systems costs.

A system of staff retention strategies is developed and implemented. Periodic measurements of indicators of staff retention are taken, and provide the basis for decisions about continuing, modifying, or discontinuing specific strategic plans related to staff retention, which can then become recommendations for sustaining and improving the means selected to ensure the viability of staff retention as a prized objective.

Central to this perspective on evaluation "is the assumption that the nature of being human is to be caring, free for choosing values, aspirations, and desires which give meaning to living" (Schoenhofer & Coffman, 1994, p. 127). Evaluation in health care organizations grounded in the Dance of Caring Persons needs to be conceptualized as more than the linear system of objectives—compliance, measurement, and outcome. Regardless of the aspect of a health care system being evaluated:

> it is necessary to live caring values such as honesty, humility, knowing, presence, and connectedness in the evaluation process. What this means in the context of the caring framework is that the human freedom to imagine, to hope, to choose, to be in authentic relationship, and to create meaning is what structures those activities traditionally termed evaluation (p. 128).

In this context, what we said in Chapter 3 about HCAHPS bears repeating: HCAHPS is only a sign, a representation, of what really matters, of the real value of that which is prized, and sought—that value is caring. Since the prized elements and characteristics of health care systems are numerous and diverse, a multidimensional approach to the valuing process is likely to yield the richest and ultimately most useful guidance to ensure the growth in viability and success of the organization.

Since evaluation involves all aspects of a health care system and all constituencies of that system, and as evaluation is integrally connected to each activity, components of prizing and valuing have been addressed in earlier chapters. In this chapter we will reintegrate those two dimensions of evaluation with the added dimension of growing—recommendations to sustain or modify strategies, for a full look at evaluation in a culture of caring—following the pattern in all constituencies of a health care system. Owen (2007), an educator, trainer, and author in the field of program evaluation, reminds us that evaluation has three phases: the planning phase, the data gathering/management phase, and the reporting phase. He also noted that negotiation is a skill that is important not only in the planning phase where value differences need to be reconciled, but also in the "disseminating" phase. Negotiating, more than directing, has key value implications for systems seeking to ground their activities in a framework of caring.

In a culture of caring, evaluation is understood as an expression of caring. What is it we care about, what is it that matters, that we prize, in health care systems? We care for each person involved in the enterprise—patients and their families, and direct and indirect caregivers, including all who contribute to the service we offer; we care for the service mission of the organization—effectiveness, efficiency, and equity in the performance of mission-directed activities; we care for the ethical and financial viability of the system; we care for the system itself which provides the infrastructure needed to achieve the service mission; and we care for persons—taxpayers, investors, benefactors, legislators, community leaders, and others—who underwrite the financial support essential to the viability of the implementation of the caring mission.

ASSESSING THE VALUE OF THE CARING EXPERIENCE

In the spirit of the Dance of Caring Persons, input into prizing, valuing, and growing is sought from persons belonging to the constituent groups comprising the health care system. The current widely employed HCAHPS measurements and other quantitative measurements are part of the picture that helps to tell a story in response to the questions "How are we doing?" and "Can we do better?" We have spoken previously about the value of using stories of nursing and other health care situations to illuminate understanding. Here is an example of combining numerical indicators with qualitative indicators derived from nurse and patient stories (Schoenhofer & Boykin, 1998). Although this example draws on a community nursing service, it does give an idea of the value of a broad approach to valuing:

> The patient had recently returned home after a period of hospitalization due to a mastectomy. She and her husband were retired and her husband was confined to the home because of severe cardiac problems. The wife, Mrs. H., was the primary caregiver for her husband, but needed assistance and support during her recuperation. This care was being provided by a local home health agency. Ms. Sue, the nurse practitioner (NP) caring for Mrs. H., was a member of the small, rural community in which the patient lived. Persons interviewed by the researcher included Mr. and Mrs. H., and the NP, Ms. Sue, with a focus on understanding the value of caring in the home nursing experience. Both qualitative and quantitative data were obtained from the nursing director and the chief executive officer of the home health agency. Additional data in the form of cost factors were obtained from the ambulance service, the hospital emergency department and the long-term care facility, community agencies that were included in considering the value of the experience of the NP caring in this specific instance. The cost analysis of having Ms. Sue as their nurse over this period of time versus having to seek care in the emergency department and in extended care demonstrated significant cost savings of $5,709 (1998 data) in this one-family care situation.

Table 9.1 illustrates the qualitative value of Ms. Sue's caring, from the perspective of Mrs. H., Ms. Sue, and the executives of the home health agency.

TABLE 9.1 Value Experiences in Nurse Caring Situations

Mrs. H.	Ms. Sue	CNO	CEO
Feels comfortable	Self-confidence	Staff retention	Minimal staff turnover
Complete nursing care	Commitment to honesty	Agency growth	Good reputation for the agency
Hopeful anticipation	Affirmation of commitment	Satisfaction that nursing goals are shared	Significant growth rate for agency
Personal sense of worth	Worthwhile collaboration	Affirmation of sense of nursing	Sense of assurance that agency is living up to its mission and goals "our presence is felt by the community in a family way"
Confidence	Confirmation of sense of who nursing is for	Sense of personal worth	Personal fulfilment "as if I'm doing a little bit of it too," "my living is not in vain"
Financial savings	Affirmation of self as loved, cared for		
Choice affirmed	Commitment to mutual goals supported		
Sense of connectedness			
Growing acceptance of interdependence			
Confirmation of self as caring person			

Findings from this study indicated that while caring in nursing must be paid for, in the words of Mrs. H, "it can't be bought"—but this study showed that an accounting of the value of caring in nursing can indeed be rendered, when qualitative descriptions and financial data are combined to present a complete picture. In hospital-based studies, Valentine (1989, 1997) found that there are direct correlations between effective nurse caring, patient satisfaction, and patient intention to return to the health care system as further need arises.

STRATEGIES FOR PRIZING, VALUING, AND GROWING

Individuals participate in the evaluation process in several ways, by focusing attention on personal commitment expressed to that which is prized in the health care system, by providing input to the process in relation to colleagues and processes, and by using information generated in the evaluation process. These structures support self-reflection and consideration of personal goals in relation to institutional goals, and they support strategies such as coaching and other authentic relationships and resources to assist with personal development, strategy development and implementation, along with valuing those activities.

The caring ingredients of Mayeroff, discussed in Chapter 2, offer an excellent framework for recommendations resulting from the prizing and valuing phases. Roach's 6 Cs of caring are helpful descriptors as well. Here is an example of how a corporate community hospital drew on these two sets of descriptors in their evaluation program:

> A hospital-based project was carried out to examine the assumption that a practice model grounded in caring would result in increased nurse and patient satisfaction as well as an increased reputation for the for-profit hospital (Boykin, Schoenhofer, Smith, St. Jean, & Aleman, 2003). The story of this project illustrates the necessity of relanguaging evaluation and traditional outcome statements. After nurses became immersed in this project, they recognized that the corporate appraisal system did not acknowledge their personal caring relationships of nursing practice nor did it reflect the values they held dear. As a result, they redesigned the system of evaluation of nursing practice to reflect caring values and renamed evaluation the "prizing system." The intent was to convey the importance of knowing each person as caring, and knowing and valuing how each person lived the value of caring in practice. The newly designed tool, based on Mayeroff's expressions of caring and Roach's 6 Cs, provided staff the opportunity to describe how they lived caring in their practice, and to discuss their hopes and dreams for growing in caring. In "evaluation" conferences, the nurse manager and employee discussed together how they might mutually support the other to live caring.

All constituencies of a health care system grounded in caring values will have a route to participation in evaluation of the effectiveness of aspects of the system in relation to that which matters and that which is prized, as expressed in the mission and objectives of the system. Selection and creation of these mechanisms would be guided by the essential values addressed in Chapter 2 and expanded upon in Chapter 3. All constituencies would have contributed to an expression of that which matters, that which is prized, and to the ongoing evolution of these understandings and strategies for accomplishing the mission, as discussed in Chapters 4 and 5.

STRATEGIES FOR VALUING THE PERFORMANCE OF CARING EFFECTIVENESS

Quantitative Surveys

Many survey instruments are available for evaluating the performance of caring effectiveness in nursing and health care. A number of them are collected in a book, *Assessing and Measuring Caring in Nursing and Health Science* (Watson, 2009). It should be noted that many of these tools were developed as research instruments, not as performance evaluation tools. In selecting research tools to use in performance evaluation, it is important to be certain that the question being asked in performance evaluation is the question being asked in the research instrument; otherwise, the tool will not make a reliable contribution to the story being told in prizing and valuing performance. Another aspect to be considered when choosing a research measurement tool as a performance measurement tool is the standard for reliability and for validity—those may be different in one use versus the other.

A set of "caring factor" surveys, developed by John Nelson (Nelson & Watson, 2011), consists of brief surveys of perception of caring experience in health care. The Caring Factor Survey can be a source of patients' or their family members' perceptions of the caring they experienced in the health care environment. It consists of 10 items scored on a 5-point scale, plus one open-ended question that asks for descriptions of caring behaviors experienced, and one demographic item. This basic survey is modified for use with several other groups involved in the caring process: care providers' perceptions of the care they are providing and another version on care that coworkers are providing. Another version is for use by employees to evaluate perceptions of their own self-caring, of the caring expressed by their unit or department managers, and of preceptors. The final version in this set assesses perceptions of patients or their family members regarding the caring they experienced from specific care providers. DiNapoli, Nelson, Turkel, and Watson (2010) used the tool to study caring in a clinical process.

The relational caring questionnaires were developed by Ray and Turkel (2009, 2012) from a synthesis of qualitative research data on the relationship among caring, economics, and outcomes. Quantitative research findings indicated that the hospitals with the highest mean scores related to organizational caring had the lowest number of patient falls and the lowest cost per adjusted patient day. These findings validated what registered nurses verbalized in the quantitative research, "Living the caring values in everyday practice makes a difference in nursing practice and patient outcomes."

Cheryl T. Beck, a recognized authority on nursing research, compared 11 survey instruments designed to measure caring (Beck, 1999). Beck sorted the instruments according to type, number of items, estimated time for completion, the variable measured, and the role category of intended respondents. Although Beck did not rank the instruments for quality, she did offer valuable information that could be used in deciding which one would be preferable under given circumstances.

The 43-item Caring Behaviors Inventory (Wolf, Giardino, Osborne, & Ambrose, 2007) has been widely used to assess nurse caring in a range of settings. Nkongho's (1990) Caring Ability Inventory, a 37-item survey based on Mayeroff's caring ingredients, designed to assess caring ability in relationships, has been used in nursing practice, nursing education, and pharmacy practice.

Duffy's Caring Assessment Tool (Duffy, Brewer, & Weaver, 2010) is an instrument that can be used to assess nurse–patient caring relationships from the perspective of Duffy's Quality-Caring Model. Valentine (1997, 1989) developed instruments to measure perceptions of caring effectiveness; studies demonstrated that when nurses and patients agreed that caring had occurred in a specific caring relationship, postoperative complications and length of stay were decreased. An instrument designed to assess peer evaluation of medical students' clinical competence, caring, and community service may have some utility for evaluating caring in physician practitioners in the health care system (McCormick, Lazarus, Small, & Stern, 2007).

The Jefferson Scale of Physician Empathy may be a helpful tool for self-evaluation, peer evaluation, and performance evaluation of physicians' caring, as empathy corresponds with an important aspect of caring—entering into the other's world and coming to know other as caring person (Lim et al., 2012).

It should be understood that because each person's experience of care is unique, the *predictability* of the outcomes is difficult to determine. Each situation holds its own values and complexities, calling for understanding and allowing the human perspective. Although in other areas of caring there are certain aspects that can be quantified, we must allow as part of our evaluation this significant personal experience. Unless the uniqueness of the experience is factored into the evaluation process, we lose sight of that most *prized factor.*

Evaluation processes that flow from and contribute to a culture of caring must have growing in caring as their ultimate aim. Summative evaluation—decisions to retain, promote, or terminate an individual's employment in a position or in the employing institution—must have growing in caring (formative evaluation) as the ultimate aim— formative for the person whose performance is being evaluated, as well as formative for the organization. Evaluation begins with prizing and valuing—with establishing the institutional vision and mission, and working out the strategies and tactics to actualize the mission in every facet of the health care system.

Designing an evaluation system capable of advancing the mission grounded in the Dance of Caring Persons requires considerable courage and creativity. Every element of the evaluation process needs to be selected or created to specifically reflect that framework. Commercially available evaluation systems will most likely need revision—sometimes involving minor tweaking and, in some cases, major reengineering. The evaluation system design team will need to be fully onboard with the framework so that all features of the evaluation system reflect the vision and contribution to actualization of the mission of the health care institution.

If the evaluation team is in-house, the team needs to be involved in the broad valuing processes that establish the institutional governing documents. If design of the evaluation system is to be outsourced, there will need to be a meaningful orientation and support process in place to ensure concordance with the institutional vision and mission. In effect, design team members become the practical champions of the caring framework by designing evaluation strategies and tactics that emerge from and support the framework.

We said earlier that even decisions for termination of employment must contribute to growing in caring, for the institution, yes, but also for the person whose employment is being terminated. Part of what this means in practical terms is that there are human resources programs in place that offer coaching in the position and counseling and other employee assistance programs.

A type of input into the valuing–prizing–growing process is the focused narrative— stories about caring. These stories could be invited from the person whose performance is being evaluated—stories that illustrate effectiveness of caring and stories that illustrate the areas for growing in caring effectiveness. Coworkers, patients and their families, and administrators could also be invited to offer stories that help paint the picture of both formative and summative performance evaluation.

PERFORMANCE APPRAISAL—INSTITUTIONAL

Strategies of benchmarking, report cards, dashboards, and other methods of systematization of data tracking and data analysis in the institutional performance appraisal process are a fact of life in the 21st century. Third-party reimbursement for health services are increasingly tied to these indicators. Although there is a significant role for policymakers in framing reimbursement policies to reflect caring values, the more immediate responsibility lies with providers and the health care systems that provide the infrastructure for their professional practice. It is the responsibility of leaders in a health care system—from the "C-Suite" through departments and even first-line leadership—to translate the language of external reimbursement policies into the language of caring, so that it becomes clear about what is being paid for. It was noted in the 2001 Institute of Medicine (IOM) report *Crossing the Quality Chasm* that outcomes of health care are not "encounters" but healing relationships. The relanguaging process is dynamic and reciprocal—as the language of what "counts" in policies changes, the language of what "counts" in practice changes, and vice versa, as the language of practice changes, the language of policy is influenced. In considering creating a culture of caring in a health care system, special attention needs to be given to these strategies and processes to ensure alignment with the institutional mission and core value of caring. When it gets down to practicality, it is these strategies that will determine what values are chosen and prized. In an article in the *Cambridge Journal of Economics*, Himmelweit (2007) analyzed caring from an economic theory perspective. She acknowledged that the primary thesis of her analysis was that "while caring is an economic activity, it has specific features that distinguish it from the economic activities involved in the provision of many other goods and services" (Himmelweit, 2007 p. 583). Those distinguishing features are as follows:

1. Care is the development of a relationship, not the production of an output that is separable from the person delivering it; this has implications for the extent to which productivity in caring can rise without affecting its quality.
2. Care needs, responsibilities for fulfilling them, and the resources to do so are unequally distributed and tend not to go together; this has implications for the extent to which public provision of care or support for carers will be needed if socially determined care needs are to be met.
3. Social and personal norms, which vary across societies, affect perceptions of who is seen to need care, who has responsibility for fulfilling their needs, and how that care should be delivered; this has implications for how family members are currently cared for in different countries and the political consensus about when and how the state should be involved in ensuring that different types of care needs are met (Himmelweit, 2007, p. 583).

It is the first of these features that most prominently aligns with the model for transformation we propose, the Dance of Caring Persons (Boykin & Schoenhofer, 2001). Perhaps the key idea in the first feature is that the production of care cannot be separated from the person—and we would add, "from the persons (plural) involved in the Dance." Bringing that perspective to institutional performance appraisal immediately changes the approach from a 1930s factory-model approach to a 21st-century human systems approach—one that takes into account the need for both creativity and predictability and integrates the humanizing need for both in a harmonious relationship.

We are very aware of a pattern of transformation promised but not delivered in health care systems—fidelity to the promise requires deliberate efforts to relanguage and redesign appraisal processes and materials to reflect a relanguaged and redesigned mission and vision for health care institutions. Commonly employed terminology must be examined for "fit." Listen to a conversation between colleagues in institutions—note that the language is dominated by terms from business to the exclusion of a language reflecting the ultimate purpose of the system—caring. Although it would be very naive to think that business interests could or even should be eliminated from health care, the weight carried by business interests regularly seems to outbalance the interests of caring.

Note too that while direct caregivers (physicians, nurses, allied health care providers in general) have agreed to learn the language of business, business interests in health care systems do not seem to have learned the language of caring. That state of affairs points to the responsibility of those in the caregiving professions to language their contributions as caring, and to teach through modeling that the "business" of the enterprise is caring. This imbalance can be corrected as a system genuinely creates a pervasive culture of caring. The language can change, but first, we must hear ourselves talking—we must pay attention to the language we are using to communicate about health care.

Often great efforts are made to relanguage an institution's core value statement, its mission statement, its vision, and even perhaps its strategic goals. But until that transformation is carried through to a relanguaging of the appraisal system, any change will be largely cosmetic, and will soon give way to the next "new wave" of marketing.

Health care organizations continue to formalize evaluation systems based on aggregate health conditions, which was started in the 1980s with Medicare's prospective payment organized around diagnosis-related groups (DRGs) and into the 21st century with the Agency for Healthcare Research and Quality's initiative to identify priority health issues around which to organize known best practices. Although the current focus on quality improvement in health care revolves around priority illnesses, the IOM and other groups do acknowledge that relationship outcomes have to be included in the set of evidence-based best practices for each illness condition.

What would a dashboard look like that was conveying appraisal of the effectiveness of direct care, and of the infrastructure in place to support that care? Take a moment to consider the language in the current institutional benchmarking/report carding/dashboarding system at your hospital or health care organization. To what extent is a culture of caring reflected in that language? How much information could be gleaned to answer the question: How effective are our system structures in supporting this institution as a caring environment, as an institution offering high-level caring services? What would we want to see in a "dashboard" or other device that gives us a quick reading on our institution as a service and culture of caring?

To a significant extent, that question has been answered in Chapter 6, with the discussion of relanguaging the mission, vision, and goals of the caring-based health care system. Part of the "dashboard" languaging lies in a willingness to design ways of valuing expressions of that mission, vision, and goal set—setting benchmarks that clearly convey the mission and vision of a culture of caring, designing infrastructure to enable the kind of worklife that makes those benchmarks feasible objectives, designing a variety of meaningful and credible ways of weighing the actual against the envisioned, and employing methods of encouraging desired outcomes that are congruent with the core value of caring. Just as planners and executives at all levels of the system will need to be supported in becoming acquainted with relevant aspects of caring science in order to plan and implement goals directed toward creating a culture of caring, designers of evaluation systems will need similar orientation.

In a resource book written by Peter Senge of Fifth Discipline fame, Senge, Kleiner, Roberts, Roth, and Smith (1999) addressed considerations regarding assessment of innovation, cautioning the "old" assessment measures are part of the "preinnovation" organizational culture and thus need to be addressed from that perspective. They identified two processes at work that tend to limit the effectiveness of appropriate assessment of results of innovations: short time horizons and traditional metrics inappropriately applied. As change leaders in health care systems plan and implement innovative strategies grounded in the principles of the Dance of Caring Persons, it will be important to accept that there are significant time delays between implementation of an innovation and realization of improvement from the innovation; Senge et al. (1999) noted "the 'results gap' between expected results and actual results drives negative assessments within the team" (p. 285). Another aspect that change leaders need to be aware of is the likelihood of "side effects," results that were not anticipated or at least not anticipated by persons not directly implementing the innovation. Senge et al. discussed several strategies to help counteract the potentially limiting effects of short time horizons and inappropriate metrics:

- Managing expectations in terms of helping people understand the sources of gestation periods between implementation and results
- Engagement of all leaders, at each level of the organization, in challenging the way traditional metrics are gathered, interpreted, and used; line managers do not have the authority to directly confront this issue, key executive leaders do have that authority, thus it is important to build executive partnerships around assessment processes
- "Learn to recognize and appreciate progress as it occurs" (Senge et al., 1999, p. 289); establish short-term targets and interim goals to help deal with the results lag; recognize unanticipated accomplishments and celebrate them; use data collection techniques to keep a record of the pattern of shifting views on measurement and assessment issues
- "Bring measurement and assessment into the service of learners, rather than having it feared as a tool for 'outside evaluators'" (Senge et al., 1999, p. 289); that is, using measurement and assessment for learning, rather than for control, engaging those immediately involved with particular innovations in the assessment process for learning purposes
- Building new capacity at all levels of the organization for measurement and assessment for learning (Senge et al., 1999).

STRATEGIES FOR PRIZING, VALUING, AND GROWING IN INSTITUTIONAL PERFORMANCE APPRAISAL

- Aligning broad guiding documents with the values of a culture of caring so that institutional language throughout the system supports those values
- Interpreting institutional benchmarks from the perspective of the Dance of Caring Persons, so that information is sought about that which matters in a culture of caring, integrating fiscal accountability as an expression of caring rather than placing it as a substitute for or in opposition to caring values
- Use Mayeroff's caring ingredients and Roach's 6 Cs of caring in the design of strategies to keep the ultimate value of caring front and center to all involved in appraising institutional effectiveness

Performance Appraisal: Staff

We turn now to appraising performance of clinical and ancillary staff, typically seen as a human resources departmental function that articulates with disciplinary-focused units, sometimes integrated as patient services departments. The design team for the evaluation subsystems for clinical staff performance needs to be based in part on professional standards for each of the participating professions.

> Nursing staff on a pilot unit in a corporate acute health care center designed a staff performance appraisal system grounded in the principles of the Dance of Caring Persons after realizing that the existing corporate appraisal system did not provide a satisfactory picture of nursing practice in that setting. Staff participated in designing a tool to assist in prizing and valuing their nursing practice. The tool asked that staff persons provide examples of how they live caring with patients; colleagues were asked to provide additional examples. Nurses

TABLE 9.2 Mean Press-Ganey Scores of Patient Satisfaction Pre and Post Initiation of a Professional Practice Model Based on the Dance of Caring Persons

ITEM EVALUATED	PREPILOT	POSTPILOT	+CHANGE
Friendliness/courtesy of nurse	86.4	93.3	6.9
Promptness response to call	77.5	90.0	12.5
Nurses' attitude toward requests	82.5	90.0	7.5
Attention to special/personal needs	82.5	86.7	4.2
Nurses keep you informed	77.5	83.3	5.8
Skill of the nurses	88.6	90.0	1.4

also provided a narrative describing self as living and growing in caring in specific ways during the evaluation period. The nurse manager reviewed these materials and then engaged the nurse in a valuing, prizing, and growing dialogue (Boykin, Schoenhofer, Smith, St. Jean, & Aleman, 2003). Broad objectives for this pilot project included improvement in patient satisfaction, using the metrics derived from the Press-Ganey questionnaire. The findings from this pilot, similar to findings from other similar pilots, indicate a significant improvement in patient satisfaction scores on the pilot unit, compared to similar units in the hospital and compared to preproject scores in the pilot unit (2003). Specific indicators of patient satisfaction before and following the initiation of a caring-based professional practice model in the pilot unit, are shown in Table 9.2.

STRATEGIES FOR PRIZING, VALUING, AND GROWING IN CLINICAL STAFF PERFORMANCE APPRAISAL

- Engage staff members in co-creating prizing processes
- Include executives in supporting measurement and assessment as processes for learning
- Use stories of practice to illustrate patterns of quality performance
- Invite stories from coworkers, patients and families, and supervisors as part of the staff evaluation process in which the staff member contributes stories of own caring practice—stories that illustrate expressions of caring and opportunities for learning and growing in caring
- Designate an area for communication of small successes and for unanticipated achievements to recognize growing in caring
- Consistently accompany metric and interpretations of metrics with stories of caring and stories that illustrate patterns of opportunities for valuing and growing in caring
- Use Mayeroff's caring ingredients and Roach's 6 Cs of caring to keep the ultimate value of caring front and center for all persons involved in appraising clinical effectiveness

GROWING IN CARING IN A LEARNING ORGANIZATION

The Dance of Caring Persons is grounded in the key assumptions that persons are caring by virtue of their humanness (Boykin & Schoenhofer, 2001). Caring is in the nature of human persons, and as with all intrinsic human characteristics, the effective and mature expression of caring can and should be developed through deliberate study and reflective practice. Health care systems are complex dynamic organizations, and to survive, they must be learning organizations. Health care systems that claim caring as a core value must incorporate the study of caring into their learning structures—structures that provide feedback into the system as well as formal education programs focused on orientation, in-service training, continuing professional development, and basic health-professional preparation. Infusion of learning about caring as an ongoing part of the feedback process—prizing, valuing, and growing—has been discussed, and in Chapter 6, we highlighted caring-based strategies for orientation programs. In this section we will focus on initiating and further developing an understanding of ways to live caring effectively in one's institutional role.

Health care skills acquisition and retraining programs in health care systems generally include topics such as patient and employee safety, ethics and legal rights and responsibilities, certification in lifesaving techniques, and other issues mandated by various external groups such as The Joint Commission and specific professional accreditation agencies. When an organization commits to a transformative framework grounded in caring, all of the standard training programs need to be enhanced by reframing them from the perspective of caring. This means that those who develop and deliver these programs need to have opportunities to study caring concepts and be supported in infusing each in-service topic with theoretical and practical knowledge of effective caring.

More than infusing each topic with knowledge of caring, the relevance of the topic needs to be framed in relation to its contribution to effective expressions of caring. For example, Locsin's middle range theory of technological competency might be adopted as the practical framework for all skills training and retraining. If every health-related technology training topic was presented from this perspective, all clinical staff could reconceptualize the use of specific skill sets as ways of expressing caring through their practice. This kind of deep reframing and reconfiguring of cognitive and psychomotor sets has the potential to embed the intentionality for caring as an active value.

Based on Locsin's (1995, 2005) work to clarify the caring potential of technological modes of health care, a growing body of information on the use of simulator-assisted learning is emerging. The work published by Eggenberger and Keller (2008), Eggenberger, Keller, and Locsin (2010), and Blum, Hickman, Parcells, and Locsin (2010) can help in-service educators and those responsible for continuing professional education programs design ways of using simulation labs to advance practical knowledge of caring.

Continuing professional education programs sponsored by a health care system that has adopted a caring framework also need to be reframed for a focus on topics in relation to caring. Some of the strategies for in-service education can be applied to continuing professional education programs. In addition, new topics will need to be introduced into the continuing education department's set of offerings. For example, theoretical concepts that have direct implications for practice applications grounded in caring might be useful additions to the curriculum. The body of health care research and caring is significant and growing, such that any clinical topic of interest can be presented in the context of caring. The two disciplines that have been most active in producing research on the topic of caring to date are nursing and education, although the study of caring as a dimension of other health care specialties is beginning to be recognized. Section IV provides a beginning guide to locating resources to promote growing in caring.

When health care systems that have adopted a values-based framework grounded in caring have contractual arrangements with training schools, colleges, and universities, specific strategies for growing in caring need to be designed for visiting students and faculty. When education programs in academic health science centers are also grounded in caring, students and faculty engaging in clinical learning experiences will be well versed in concepts of caring and specific effective caring practices, particularly when the entire clinical and educational programs of the academic health science center are integrated. However, when the "sending" academic programs are not grounded in the study of caring science, special attention will need to be given so that students and faculty can fully contribute to the Dance of Caring Persons that grounds the health care system.

Planning for effective clinical study in the health care setting grounded in caring should begin with an alignment between governing documents of the educational program and the health care system. Most educational program mission and objectives address the value of caring, if not explicitly, then implicitly, and these value expressions could be the cognitive and affective link between your health care system and the educational program seeking clinical placements. Once this connection is made explicit, plans can be made to orient faculty and students to the caring framework and the practices that flow from that framework. Most likely, the orientation could be similar to that provided to new clinical staff. Orientation materials that are available electronically could be shared with faculty and students prior to the initiation of the clinical learning experience; however, it will be important that there be an opportunity for dialogue between key health care system personnel and faculty and students to assure that faculty and students can truly engage in the Dance of Caring Persons that characterizes the clinical setting. Part of that dialogue would involve coming to know persons as caring, and developing shared meaning of key concepts of the caring framework through stories of personal and professional experience. Formal and informal evaluation of the clinical learning experience should reflect prizing, valuing, and growing patterns developed within the health care system.

In closing, reframing the appraisal/evaluation process in health care systems adopting the Dance of Caring Persons, as their expression of that which matters for the organization, is as crucial to the success of the transforming organization as designing governing documents, relationship and communication patterns, and work processes. The prizing, valuing, and growing process that has been the focal point of this chapter is a process that mirrors the complexity of today's health care systems and, as such, touches every function of the system. It offers the freedom for creativity so vital to the survival and success of complex learning organizations. Although temporary snapshot assessments are needed at points in time, the prizing, valuing, and growing process is not time-limited, but rather, it is a living part of the Dance of Caring Persons.

REFERENCES

Beck, C. T. (1999). Quantitative measurement of caring. *Journal of Advanced Nursing, 30,* 24–32.

Blum, C. A., Hickman, C., Parcells, D. A., & Locsin, R. (2010). Teaching caring nursing to RN-BSN students using simulation technology. *International Journal for Human Caring, 14*(2), 41–50.

Bolman, L. G., & Deal, T. E. (2008). *Reframing organizations: Artistry, choice and leadership* (4th ed.). San Francisco, CA: Jossey-Bass.

Boykin, A., & Schoenhofer, S. O. (2001). *Nursing as caring: A model for transforming practice.* Sudbury, MA: Jones & Bartlett.

Boykin, A., Schoenhofer, S. O., Smith, N., St. Jean, J., & Aleman, D. (2003). Transforming practice using a caring-based model. *Nursing Administration Quarterly, 27*(3), 223–230.

DiNapoli, P., Nelson, J., Turkel, M., & Watson, J. (2010). Measuring the caritas process: Caring factor survey. *International Journal for Human Caring, 14*(3), 15–20.

Duffy, J. R., Brewer, B. B., & Weaver, M. T. (2010). Revision and psychometric properties of the Caring Assessment Tool. *Clinical Nursing Research.* doi:10.1177/1054773810369827

Eggenberger, T., Keller, K., & Locsin, R. C. (2010). Valuing caring behaviors within simulated emergent nursing situations. *International Journal for Human Caring, 14*(4), 23–29.

Eggenberger, T. L., & Keller, K. B. (2008). Grounding nursing simulations in caring: An innovative approach. *International Journal for Human Caring, 12*(2), 42–47.

Himmelweit, S. (2007). The prospects for caring: Economic theory and policy analysis. *Cambridge Journal of Economics, 31*(4), 581–599. doi:10.1093/cje/bem011

Institute of Medicine. (2001). *Crossing the quality chasm: A new health system for the 21st century.* Washington, DC: The National Academies Press.

Lim, B. T., Moriarty, H., Huthwaite, M., Gray, L., Pullon, S., & Gallegher, P. (2012). How well do medical students rate and communicate clinical empathy. *Medical Teacher.* doi:10.3109/01421 59X.2012.715783. Retrieved from http://informahealthcare.com/doi/pdfplus/10.3109/0142 159X.2012.715783

Locsin, R. C. (1995). Machine technologies and caring in nursing. *Image: Journal for Nursing Scholarship, 27*(3), 201–203.

Locsin, R. C. (2005). *Technological competency as caring in nursing: A model for practice.* Indianapolis, IN: Sigma Theta Tau International.

McCormick, W. T., Lazarus, C., Stern, D., & Small, P. A., Jr. (2007). Peer nomination: A tool for identifying medical student exemplars in clinical competence and caring, evaluated at three medical schools. *Academic Medicine, 82*(11), 1033–1039.

Nelson, J., & Watson, J. (2011). *Measuring caring: International research on caritas as healing.* New York, NY: Springer Publishing Company.

Nkongho, N. (1990). The caring ability inventory. In O. Strickland & C. Waltz (Eds.), *Measurement of nursing outcomes* (pp. 3–16). New York, NY: Springer Publishing Company.

Owen, J. M. (2007). *Program evaluation: Forms and approaches* (3rd ed.). New York, NY: The Guilford Press.

Porter-O'Grady, T., & Malloch, K. (2012). *Leadership in nursing practice.* Sudbury, MA: Jones & Bartlett Learning.

Ray, M., & Turkel, M. (2009). Relational caring questionnaires. In J. Watson (Ed.), *Assessing and measuring caring in nursing and health sciences* (2nd ed.). New York, NY: Springer Publishing Company.

Ray, M. A., & Turkel, M. C. (2012). Transtheoretical evolution of caring science in complex systems. *International Journal for Human Caring, 16*(2), 28–49.

Schoenhofer, S., & Coffman, S. (1994). Prizing, valuing, and growing in a caring-based program. In A. Boykin (Ed.), *Living a caring-based program* (pp. 127–165). New York, NY: National League for Nursing.

Schoenhofer, S. O., & Boykin, A. (1998). The value of caring experienced in caring. *International Journal for Human Caring, 2,* 9–15.

Senge, P., Kleiner, A., Roberts, C., Roth, G., & Smith, B. (1999). *The dance of change: Mastering the twelve challenges to change in a learning organization.* New York, NY: Doubleday.

Watson, J. (2009). *Assessing and measuring caring in nursing and health science* (2nd ed.). New York, NY: Springer Publishing Company.

Wolf, Z. R., Giardino, E. R., Osborne, P. A., & Ambrose, M. S. (2007). Dimensions of nurse caring. *Journal of Nursing Scholarship, 26*(2), 107–112.

Valentine, K. (1989). Caring is more than kindness: Modeling its complexities. *Journal of Nursing Administration, 19*(11), 28–35.

Valentine, K. (1997). Exploration of the relationship between caring and cost. *Holistic Nursing Practice, 11*(4), 71–81.

Response to Chapter 9

Marian C. Turkel, PhD, RN, NEA-BC, FAAN
Director, Professional Nursing Practice and Research
Einstein Healthcare Network

I want to acknowledge the richness, depth, and beauty of the caring scholarship that has been shared from the perspectives of Dr. Boykin, Dr. Schoenhofer, Dr. Valentine, and other scholars throughout this book. The integration of theory, research, and practice exemplars validate the value of caring not only as a substantive area of research and study within the discipline, but as the essence of professional nursing practice and core focus of organizational transformation.

In this time of uncertain health care transformation in our country with a focus on economics, costs, and reimbursements, having organizational culture grounded in caring is more important than ever. For the first time since the inception of value-based purchasing, one third of hospital reimbursement will be linked to patient satisfaction data and two thirds to patient quality/safety data. As discussed and referenced throughout this book, caring has been studied, researched, measured, and shown to make a difference in patient outcomes. The use of stories to come to know self and others as caring person and to understand the meaning of caring within the nursing situation has been part of the curriculum at Christine E. Lynn College of Nursing for over 20 years and is central to the Dance of Caring Persons. Only recently, the Institute for Healthcare Improvement has recognized the use of story as a way to demonstrate quality patient experiences.

Within the health care industry, words such as "customer satisfaction" and "patient satisfaction" are being replaced with words such as the "patient experience" or the "patient journey." Mission and vision statements are being revised to include words such as "caring," "compassion," "love," and "humanistic values." The time is now for the nursing profession to make caring explicit in professional models of care delivery, organizational transformation, and research.

Nursing leaders need to value and conduct role model caring before sustainable organizational cultural transformation can occur. As leaders, we need to make caring explicit through creativity and innovation within the professional model of care and reframing the language within the organization. Using a caring theory guided approach to practice is very different than a "customer service scripted" or "fix it" approach to "rapidly improve" patient scores. Philosophy, values, stories, and ethics are foundational to professional practice framed in caring theory.

Customer service approaches may provide direction, new approaches, or restructuring of processes within organizations, but they are not grounded in the tenets and values of caring. A colleague of mine reframed the language in a subtle yet meaningful way. The organization was using a customer service approach and one of the words used in describing the model of care as part of rounding was the word "potty." Recognizing that this did not promote human dignity or enhance personhood, the language was reframed to personal needs by the organization. Another colleague "tweaked" a scripted customer service phrase requiring the registered nurses (RNs) to end each patient visit with the statement "Is there anything else I can do for you? I have the time" to "Is there anything else I can do for you? I will take the time." The intent of the scripted approach is to anticipate needs and improve communication, but the nurses felt it was not authentic because in reality they often do not have the time.

Working in collaboration with non-nursing leaders to provide education on caring and having other professionals and paraprofessionals identify tangible examples of how caring values can be become part of their practice is essential. I am reminded of Sister Roach's belief that caring is not unique to nursing but unique in nursing. Non-nursing leaders/employees may not connect with caring as a substantive area of study or think of it as foundational to the discipline, but they can begin to identify ways to express caring in interactions with colleagues and patients. A medical clerk shared this example with me, "I know on Sunday many visitors come after church and they get mixed-up about what section of the 6th floor their family member is on. Instead of just pointing them in the right direction, I walk with them, you know some are using crutches or a cane and I don't want them to walk alone or get lost."

As nurse leaders, we need also to remember to practice self-care. To compassionately care for others we need to care for self. It is important to appreciate self as a caring person and realize that if we do not care for ourselves it is impossible to compassionately care for others. Einstein Healthcare Network nursing employees have education related to self-care including research on the value of self-care and strategies for self-care while at work and after work. Part of the yearly evaluation for all nursing employees including RNs, patient care associates, and medical clerks is identifying a personal plan for self-care. One of the nurse managers does hand massages for the staff when they feel stressed or overwhelmed and other managers have created small self-care lounges on the unit where employees can meditate, rest, or simply reflect on their thoughts.

As I moved from academia to practice, I became involved with integrating caring theory into practice in various organizations. In some it was only to have a theory for the purposes of the Magnet Recognition Program® documents; in others it became interconnected with the mission, vision, and values of the organization. What was most helpful to me when I started the process at Einstein Healthcare Network was to relate caring theory to the values of the organization, *Einstein Brilliance and Compassion In All We Touch:* humanity, humility, honor, affinity, integrity, empathy, responsibility, and respect. The practice reality within most organizations is multiple competing organizational priorities and it is important for transformation to a culture grounded in caring values to be viewed as interconnected and providing a foundation to our care beliefs and values instead of "one more thing we have to do." I also knew for the transformation to be authentic it needed to take time and that some nursing units would be more open to innovation and creativity than others, so I started on the units where I was welcomed and as we made changes, I linked them to outcomes, some traditional, others nontraditional. Traditional outcomes included improvement in patient satisfaction, RN satisfaction, and quality/safety data. To me, the nontraditional outcomes were the most surprising and meaningful. Examples of these included "finding joy and meaning at work" through creation of caring story boards on the unit; caring hands to help the novice nurse; staying after work to pray and sing with a patient who was afraid and lonely; "experiencing love and humility" through buying warm clothes and clothes for children at a local school; and having bake sales on the unit to buy personal hygiene items and underwear for patients. In nursing, we need to honor and reframe that language of nontraditional outcomes and remember the quote by Einstein: "Not everything that can be measured counts, and not everything that counts can be measured."

Some of the early initiatives included nursing employees focusing on caring for colleagues, replacing asking patients "What is your goal for the day?" with asking "What matters most to you today?" and avoiding the labeling of patients as mean, aggressive, or difficult.

Language was reframed to say the challenging nursing situation or expression of noncaring behaviors. Meetings started with sharing of caring stories and a centering experience. I started small and kept moving forward. On the majority of the nursing units the caring is authentic and truly valued by the manager and the nursing employees, caring is integrated into nursing orientation and the nursing education classes. Peer review was grounded in caring theory language, the "charge nurse" worship was reframed with caring science language and received the highest evaluations ever after the change was made. Caring theory serves as the framework for evidence-based projects and nursing research and many of these initiatives have been published and/or presented at national conferences.

In terms of valuing, prizing, and growing related to outcomes, nurse managers identified some very tangible yet innovative ways to recognize caring as part of the traditional performance evaluation. Starting 3 years ago, all nursing services employees were invited to write a caring story as part of their self-evaluation; the stories are growing in terms of the depth, reflection, and understanding of the meaning of caring.

One story was recently published in the *International Journal for Human Caring* and I have collected so many more that we are now considering publishing a book on our stories as a way to inform others how caring has reframed not only our practice of nursing, but also how we view the outcomes of care. This year for the annual performance evaluation, one of the nurse managers wrote all of the employee feedback grounded in the language of caring; this was done on over 90 evaluations. This is reflected in the following narrative:

> Denise is thorough in assessing and reassessing her patients and their response to nursing initiatives and revises the plan of care according to their needs. Her patients value her authenticity and the time she takes to listen to them. Her approach is invaluable in developing and sustaining helping-trusting authentic caring relationships.

Inspirational and reflective wisdom guides my personal journey on coming to know and understand the meaning of caring; all of which came from my mentors at Florida Atlantic University. Their collective values and ideas shaped my thinking related to caring and ground me as a person when I am integrating caring theory into practice, or helping others on their journey. I am honored to share them and invite you to reflect on the following:

> Trust the process and be open to all possibilities.
>
> Dr. Marilyn Parker

Look for the caring underneath the uncaring expressions.

Dr. Savina Schoenhofer

All nursing occurs within the context of the nursing situation and nursing leaders need to draw upon multiple ways of knowing (empirical, aesthetics, ethical, and personal) to inform and guide their practice.

Dr. Anne Boykin

Resources

Resources by Chapter

CHAPTER 1

1. Features in Affordable Care Act (ACA) that support seven initiatives proposed by Halvorson and Isham
   a. Aspects of the ACA that support patient safety and quality:
   Include efforts for quality improvement through establishing an interagency work group to improve collaboration across federal, private, and public initiatives. Payment reductions to hospitals for readmissions determined to be preventable, eventually the rate for preventable readmissions would be posted for public review. The legislation empowers Medicare to promote programs that form accountable care organizations. If organizations choose to do that and save money, they will share in the savings, and they will be rewarded for higher quality and better patient outcomes. Understanding that health disparities affect overall health, data about race and ethnicity and preferred language must be collected so that care can be personalized to that person's risks and needs and trend data can be compared across states.
   b. Aspects of the ACA that support promotion of consumer choice and market models:
   The ACA has several aspects that affect access to the market for different segments of the population: students, employees in small businesses, seniors, and currently uninsured or financially challenged citizens. This broadens the marketplace for covered lives. The multiple ways to enter the market preserve consumer choice. In addition, there are requirements about having coverage for preventive services and a definition of required benefits. This allows consumers to choose less extensive coverage at a lower cost while at the same time establishing a threshold for covered services. Information for consumers to choose insurance products based on quality will also be available to aid in consumer choice.
   c. Affordable Care Act aspects that reflect population health:
   These aspects of the ACA help to develop processes for transformation in

pilot projects so that lessons can be learned and adapted, adopted, or abandoned and inform the spread of accountable care organizations. In addition, the fee for service for Medicaid patients will be increased to the Medicare level with the hope of motivating providers to accept the increased number of Medicaid patients.

d. Prevent monopolistic and competitive behavior:
This is not overtly addressed in the ACA, as it relates to other aspects of law.

e. Aspects of the ACA that address the uninsured:
Children and adults will not be able to be refused insurance coverage for a pre-existing condition, nor will they be able to have existing insurance terminated when the person becomes ill. Annual and lifetime coverage limits will be phased out by 2014. Medicare part D related to prescriptions will be changed to close the "doughnut hole" requiring personal payment for medications that reach a specified threshold. Safety net services such as those provided by community health centers will receive funding to care for the uninsured. Taxes imposed on employees and self-employed persons for Medicare will be increased as well as a fee for the insurance industry to cover the cost of the uninsured and health care reform. Insurance premiums will be offered on a sliding scale and will be able to be purchased in either federal or state health care exchanges, which will promote greater transparency related to comparative rates and coverage options.

f. Affordable Care Act provisions related to workforce:
More loans for students in all fields related to primary care will be available to encourage students to choose health care careers that focus on prevention and chronic condition management.

g. Affordable Care Act related to technology:
All health insurers must participate in efforts to simplify the administrative processes related to claims submission and payment in an effort to reduce the administrative overhead costs associated with the current system.

Sources for references to the ACA are as follows:

The Patient Protection and ACA, available at http://frwebgate.access.gpo.gov/cgi-bin/getdoc.cgi?dbname=111_cong_bills&docid=f:h3590eas.txt.pdf

The Health Care and Education Affordability Reconciliation Act of 2010, available at http://docs.house.gov/rules/hr4872/111_hr4872_amndsub.pdf; Summary and other supporting documents available at http://www.rules.house.gov/111_hr4872_secbysec.html.

2. An example of moving from volume-based to value-based care, using care of a person with diabetes as the focus of the example.
An example may help to illustrate the dynamic tension that exists between a curative, diagnosis-related health care focus and carative personalized health care. Let us take diabetes as a case study. Diabetes is the sixth leading cause of death in the United States. Of the children born in the year 2000, one of three will develop diabetes in their lifetime and one of two will develop it if they are Hispanic or African American. The increased prevalence of obesity in the past three decades has affected health outcomes, quality of life, and health costs in the United States and is becoming one of the most pressing public health issues in the United States today (p. 1). Two thirds of American adults and one third of American youth are overweight or obese. If trends continue, 75% of the Americans will be overweight or obese by 2018. Higher rates of obesity are

linked with greater prevalence of chronic conditions as well as cancer, heart disease, depression, and other conditions. (Public Health Law Center, Access to Healthy Food: Challenges and Opportunities, 2012, St. Paul, Minnesota: William Mitchell College of Law.)

3. The American Diabetes Association (ADA) has developed a basic set of care standards for physicians and practitioners to follow with their diabetic patients, which if adopted, have the potential to reduce complications early and reduce major complications such as amputation, blindness, and kidney failure by more than 50% (Halvorson & Isham, 2003, p. 162). The effect of using these guidelines in practice would have health benefits and reduce unnecessary variation in care. Yet, they are not widely adopted. In fact many hospitals that used to have ADA diabetes programs have ceased programs because the reimbursement rate for services does not cover program costs. In sum, payment incentives for prevention have not been aligned with the population health needs.

4. This may be changing as payment from Medicare is based on performance measures that, when collected, would report key health outcomes. Health technology support is required for such data collection and reporting and though available in larger health systems, it is not widespread in smaller practices, thus affecting widespread adoption.

5. Despite the trend to move toward pay for prevention and performance, the reimbursement systems are still largely focused on high-technology treatments such as bariatric surgery that is employed to prevent progression of diabetes and its complications, rather than prevention of the condition itself. The treatment requires specialized teams, and pre- and post-surgical preparation and monitoring. When successful, complications related to diabetes such as heart disease, kidney failure, blindness, and amputation can be averted. Yet in our current health care system we have specialized centers that pay for end-stage renal disease (ESRD) and have low reimbursement for services that prevent diabetes at its earlier stages of risk. Slowly this is changing, for example, Medicare will now pay for office visits to treat obesity, allowing for treatment of risk factors before complications of diabetes are evident. Medicare is one of the few payers that will cover for certified diabetes education by certified diabetes education programs, though these programs have been shown to have measurable benefits to patients.

6. For hospitals, investing in diabetes prevention programs aimed at keeping patients out of the hospital is counter to the incentives associated with reimbursement. Hospitals are paid on the volume of patient days, procedures, and emergency room (ER) visits. Though incentives are beginning to change (e.g., denial of payment if there is a return to the hospital within 30 days for same diagnosis, or complications from procedures), hospitals themselves are not incentivized to prevent admissions. This misalignment of incentives is beginning to change as hospital and physician groups begin to consider becoming accountable care organizations as a way to integrate care of patients across settings.

7. Diabetes represents just one example of the challenges of realigning the reimbursement systems from a procedural and volume-based model to a prevention and value-based model aligned with measured outcomes and accountability for patient health across the continuum of care. The Patient Protection and ACA provides some mechanisms for realigning payment incentives toward this goal, continuum of care. A shift toward a value- versus volume-based model is one of

the major challenges facing health care today and will require transformational changes in order to achieve. Our goal is to have the Dance of Caring Persons model assist in such transformation.

CHAPTER 2

Electronic Media (Websites, Videos, etc.)

Nursing As Caring website (http://www.nursingascaring.com)

Boykin, A., & Schoenhofer, S., (2001). *Nursing as caring: A model for transforming practice* [eBook]. Free download from Nursing As Caring website and from http://www.gutenberg.org/ebooks/42988

Website of Anne Boykin Institute for Advancement of Caring Knowledge (http://fau.edu/AnneBoykinInstitute)

Books and Journals

International Journal for Human Caring (http://www.humancaring.org/journal/index.htm)

Journal of Art and Aesthetics in Nursing and Health Sciences (http://nursing.fau.edu/index.php?main=1&nav=879)

Smith, M. C., Turkel, M. C., & Wolf, Z. (Eds.). (2012). *Caring in nursing classics: An essential resource.* New York, NY: Springer Publishing Company.

CHAPTER 4

Electronic Media (Websites, Videos, etc.)

Nightingale Songs, a publication of aesthetic expressions of nursing (http://nursing.fau.edu/index.php?main=1&nav=475)

Journal of Art and Aesthetics in Nursing and Health Sciences (http://nursing.fau.edu/index.php?main=1&nav=879)

Consultants

Anne Boykin Institute for the Advancement of Caring in Nursing (http://nursing.fau.edu/AnneBoykinInstitute)

American Nurses Credentialing Center (ANCC). (2011). *Forces of magnetism.* Retrieved from http://nursecredentialing.org/Magnet/ProgramOverview/ForcesofMagnetism.aspx

http://nursecredentialing.org/Magnet

Paul Plsek (www.directedcreativity.com)

Implementation Management Associates (www.imaworldwide.com)

Institute for Healthcare Improvement (www.ihi.org)

Interaction Associates Return on Involvement™. (www.interactionassociates.com)

The Advisory Board (www.advisory.com)

Robert Wood Johnson Foundation: Transforming Care at the Bedside (TCAB; www.rwjf.org)

Watson Caring Science Institute (http://www.watsoncaringscience.org)

Elsevier CPM Resource Center (www.cpmrc.com)

Creative Health Care Management (http://chcm.com)

Professional Organizations

International Association for Human Caring (IAHC; http://humancaring.org)

Mission

The IAHC provides the forum for discovery and dissemination of caring science. The IAHC hosts an international research conference each year and publishes the *International Journal for Human Caring*, now in its 16th year of publication. Dr. Valentine was the founding managing editor of the journal and Drs. Boykin and Valentine were the first team of editors for the journal. In the journal's first year in print, published scholarship increased by 160%. Dr. Zane Wolf is now the editor of the journal and it serves as a forum for publishing scholarly works on caring.

CHAPTER 7

Corley, M., Elswick, R. K., Gorman, M., & Clor, T. (2001). Development and evaluation of a moral distress scale. *Journal of Advanced Nursing, 33*, 250–256.
Lake, E. (2002). Development of the practice environment scale of the nursing work index. *Research in Nursing and Health, 25*, 176–188.
Kramer, M., & Schmalenberg, C. (2004). Development and evaluation of essentials of magnetism tool. *JONA, 34*(7/8), 365–378.

The concept of transformational leadership was first described by Burns (1978) in a book called *Leadership* (New York, NY: Harper and Row).

The IHI's implementation (2010) guide for medical home initiatives also highlights engaged leadership as a key strategy along with "continuous and team-based healing relationships, patient-centered interactions, quality, access, care coordination, and evidence-based care." Subject: Implementation Guide/Engaged Leadership: Strategies for Guiding PCMH Transformation from Within. Retrieved from IHI website June 29, 2013, http://www.improvingchroniccare.org/downloads/engaged_leadership.pdf

Transformational leadership is characterized by synthesizing, intuitive, qualitative thinking (J. M. Skelton-Green, *Canadian Journal of Nursing Administration*, Sept.–Oct. 1995).

Bennis and Nanus, 1985, in their seminal work *Leaders*, list four core activities for transformational leaders.

Streater, M. L. (2009). *What drives your leadership? Leadership advance online*. Issue 18. Retrieved June 29, 2013, from http://www.regent.edu/acad/global/publications/lao/issue_18/Streater_leadership_drive_1.pdf

Reading List

BASIC BOOKS ON CARING

Boykin, A., & Schoenhofer, S. O. (2001). *Nursing as caring: A model for transforming practice.* Sudbury, MA: Jones & Bartlett.

Leininger, M. M. (1988a). *Caring: An essential human need.* Detroit, MI: Wayne State University Press.

Leininger, M. M. (1988b). *Care, the essence of health and nursing.* Detroit, MI: Wayne State University.

Mayeroff, M. (1971). *On caring.* New York, NY: Harper & Row.

Roach, S. M. (2002). *Caring, the human mode of being* (2nd ed.). Ottawa, ON: CHA Press.

Smith, M. C., Turkel, M. C., & Wolf, Z. R. (2012). *Caring in nursing classics: An essential resource.* New York, NY: Springer Publishing Company.

Watson, J. (2008). *The philosophy and science of caring* (Rev ed.). Boulder, CO: University Press of Colorado.

SELECTED BOOKS AND JOURNAL ARTICLES ON CARING

Almerad, S., Alapack, R. J., Fridllund, B., & Ekebergh, M. (2008). Beleaguered by technology. *Nursing Philosophy, 9*(1), 55–61.

Alpers, R. R., Jarrell, K., & Wotring, R. (2011). The Tapestry of Influence project: Cultivating caring in the caring profession. *Teaching and Learning in Nursing, 6,* 144–145.

Bailey, D. N. (2009). Caring defined: A comparison and analysis. *International Journal for Human Caring, 13*(1), 16–31.

Bailey, D. N. (2011). Framing client care using Halldorsdottir's theory of caring and uncaring behaviors within nursing and healthcare. *International Journal for Human Caring, 15*(4), 54–66.

Barnard, A. (2003). Philosophy of technology and nursing. In P. G. Reed, N. C. Shearer, & L. H. Nicoll (Eds.), *Perspectives on nursing theory* (4th ed., pp. 613–625). Philadelphia, PA: Lippincott Williams and Wilkins (Reprinted from *Nursing Philosophy, 3*[1] [2002], 15–26).

Barry, C. D., & Purnell, M. (2008). Uncovering meaning through the aesthetic turn: A pedagogy of caring. *International Journal for Human Caring, 12*(2), 19–23.

Beckerman, A., Boykin A., Folden S., & Winland-Brown J. (1994). The experience of being a student in a caring-based program. In A. Boykin (Ed.), *Living a caring-based program* (pp. 79–92). New York, NY: National League for Nursing.

Bent, K. N. (1999). The ecologies of community caring. *Advances in Nursing Science, 21,* 29–36.

Bevis, E. O., & Watson, J. (1989).*Toward a caring curriculum: A new pedagogy for nursing*. New York, NY: National League for Nursing.

Boykin, A. (1990). Creating a caring environment: Moral obligations in the role of dean. In M. Leininger & J. Watson (Eds.), *The caring imperative in education* (pp. 247–254). New York, NY: National League for Nursing.

Boykin, A. (1994). Creating a caring environment for nursing education. In A. Boykin (Ed.), *Living a caring-based program* (pp. 11–25). New York, NY: National League for Nursing.

Boykin, A. (Ed.). (1994). *Living a caring-based program*. New York, NY: National League for Nursing.

Boykin, A., Bulfin, J., Baldwin, S., & Southern, R. (2004). Transforming care in the emergency department. *Topics in Emergency Medicine, 26*(4), 331–336.

Boykin, A., & Schoenhofer, S. (1990). Caring in nursing: Analysis of extant theory. *Nursing Science Quarterly, 3*(14), 149–155.

Boykin, A., & Schoenhofer, S. O. (1991). Story as link between nursing practice, ontology, and epistemology. *Image, 23*(4), 245–248.

Boykin, A., & Schoenhofer, S. (1997). Reframing nursing outcomes: Enhancing personhood. *Advanced Practice Nursing Quarterly, 1*(3), 60–65.

Boykin, A., & Schoenhofer, S. O. (2001). The role of nursing leadership in creating caring environments in health care delivery systems. *Nursing Administration Quarterly, 25*(3), 1–7.

Boykin, A., & Schoenhofer, S. O. (2011). Caring and the advanced practice nurse. In L. M. Dunphy & J. E. Winland-Brown (Eds.), *Primary care: Art and science of primary care nursing* (3rd ed., pp. 19–24). Philadelphia, PA: F. A. Davis.

Boykin, A., Schoenhofer, S. O., & Linden, D. (2010). Anne Boykin and Savina O. Schoenhofer's theory of nursing as caring. In M. E. Parker & M. C. Smith (Eds.), *Nursing theories and nursing practice* (3rd ed., pp. 370–386). Philadelphia, PA: F. A. Davis.

Boykin, A., Schoenhofer, S., Smith, N., St. Jean, J., & Aleman, D. (2003). Transforming practice using a caring-based model. *Nursing Administration Quarterly, 27*(3), 223–250.

Brown, C. J. (2009). Self-renewal in nursing leadership: The lived experience of caring for self. *Journal of Holistic Nursing, 27*(2), 75–84.

Buber, M. (reprinting 1996). *I and Thou*. New York, NY: Simon & Schuster.

Carper, B. (2011). Fundamental patterns of knowing in nursing. In P. G. Reed & N. C. Shearer (Eds.), *Perspectives on nursing theory* (5th ed., pp. 377–384). Philadelphia, PA: Lippincott Williams and Wilkins (Reprinted from *Advances in Nursing Science, 1*[1] [1978], 13–23).

Carter, L. C., Nelson, J. L., Sievers, B. A., Dubek, S. L., & Pipe, T. B. (2008). Exploring a culture of caring. *Nursing Administration Quarterly, 32*(1), 57–63.

Chinn, P., & Watson, J. (Eds.). (1994). *Art and aesthetics of nursing*. New York, NY: National League for Nursing.

Chinn, P. L. (1999). Scholarship: The paradoxes of the 14 C's. *Advances in Nursing Science* (Handout provided in class).

Cooper, M. C. (1988). Covenantal relationships: Grounding for the nursing ethic. *Advances in Nursing Science, 10*(4), 48–59.

Cossette, S., & Forbes, C. (2012). Psychometric evaluation of the Caring Nurse Observation Tool: Scale development. *International Journal for Human Caring, 16*(1), 16–25.

Cowling, W. R., Smith, M. C., & Watson, J. (2008). The power of wholeness, consciousness & caring: A dialogue on nursing science, art and healing. *Advances in Nursing Science, 31*(1), E41–E51.

Davidson, A., Ray, M., & Turkel, M. (2011). *Nursing, caring, and complexity science: For human environment well-being*. New York, NY: Springer Publishing Company.

Donaldson, S. K., & Crowley, D. (1978). The discipline of nursing. *Nursing Outlook, 26*(2), 113–120.

Duffy, J. R. (2003). Caring relationships and evidence-based practice: Can they coexist? *International Journal for Human Caring, 7*(3), 45–50.

Duffy, J. R., Baldwin, J., & Mastorovich, M. J. (2008). Using the quality-caring model to organize patient care delivery. *Journal of Nursing Administration, 37*(12), 546–551.

Duffy, J. R., & Hoskins, L. M. (2003). The quality-caring model: A blending of dual paradigms. *Advances in Nursing Science, 26*(1), 77–88.

Dunn, D. J. (2009). The intentionality of compassion energy. *Holistic Nursing Practice, 23*(4), 222–229.

Eggenberger, T. L., & Keller, K. B. (2008). Grounding nursing simulations in caring: An innovative approach. *International Journal for Human Caring, 12*(2), 42–46.

Erdmann, A. L., deAndrade, S. R., Ferreira deMello, A. L., Klock, P., Nascimento, K. C., Koerich, M. S., & Backes, D. S. (2011). Practices for caring: Brazilian research groups. *International Nursing Review, 58*, 379–385.

Ericksson, K. (2001). Caring science in a new key. *Nursing Science Quarterly, 15*(1), 61–65.

Falk Rafael, A. (2000). Watson's philosophy, science, and theory of human caring as a conceptual framework for guiding community health nursing practice. *Advances in Nursing Science, 23*(2), 34–49.

Finch, L. P., Thomas, J. D., Schoenhofer, S. O., & Green, A. (2006). Research as praxis: A model of inquiry into caring in nursing. *International Journal for Human Caring, 10*(1), 28–31.

Finfgeld-Connett, D. (2008). Metasynthesis of caring in nursing. *Journal of Clinical Nursing, 7*(20), 196–204.

Finfgeld-Connett, D. (2008). Qualitative convergence of three nursing concepts: Art of nursing, presence and caring. *Journal of Advanced Nursing, 63*(5), 527–534.

Flanagan, J. (2009). Patient and nurse experiences of theory-based care. *Nursing Science Quarterly, 22*(2), 160–172.

Freshwater, D. (2004). Aesthetics and evidence-based practice in nursing: An oxymoron? *International Journal for Human Caring, 8*(2), 8–12.

Fridh, I., Forsberg, A., & Bergbom, I. (2009). Close relatives' experiences of caring and of the physical environment when a loved one dies in an ICU. *Intensive and Critical Care Nursing, 25*(3), 111–119.

Gadow, S. (1980). Existential advocacy: Philosophical foundations in nursing. In S. Spicker & S. Gadow (Eds.), *Nursing images and ideals*. New York, NY: Springer Publishing Company.

Gadow, S. (1993). Covenant without cure: Letting go and holding on in chronic illness. In J. Watson & M. Ray (Eds.), *The ethics of care and cure: Synthesis in chronicity* (pp. 5–14). New York, NY: National League for Nursing.

Gadow, S. (2009). Relational narrative: The postmodern turn in nursing ethics. In Reed & Shearer (Eds.), *Perspectives on nursing theory* (5th ed., pp. 571–580). Philadelphia, PA: Lippincott Williams and Wilkins (Reprinted from *Research and Theory for Nursing Practice, 13*[1] [1999], 57–70).

Gaut, D. (1983). Development of a theoretically adequate description of caring. *Western Journal of Nursing Research, 5*, 313–324.

Gramling, K., & Smith, M. (2001). What you need to know: Artful caring pedagogy in health assessment. *International Journal for Human Caring, 6*(1), 7–11.

Haldorsdottir, S. (1991). Five basic modes of being with another. In D. A. Gaut & M. Leininger (Eds.), *Caring: The compassionate healer*. New York, NY: National League for Nursing.

Hills, M., & Watson, J. (2011). *Creating a caring science curriculum: An emancipatory pedagogy for nursing*. New York, NY: Springer Publishing Company.

Iranmanesh, S., Axelsson, K., Savenstedt, S., & Haggstrom, T. (2009). A caring relationship with people who have cancer. *Journal of Advanced Nursing, 65*(6), 1300–1308.

Johns, C., & Freshwater, D. (2005). *Transforming nursing through reflective practice*. Oxford, England: Blackwell.

Jones, M., Hendricks, J. M., & Cope, V. (2012). Toward an understanding of caring in the context of telenursing. *International Journal for Human Caring, 16*(1), 7–13.

Koerner, J. (2007). *Healing presence: The essence of nursing*. New York, NY: Springer Publishing Company.

Krysl, M. (1988). *Midwives and other poems*. New York, NY: National League for Nursing.

Krysl, M., & Watson, J. (1988). Poetry on caring and addendum on center for human caring. *Advances in Nursing Science, 12*–17.

Lavore, M., DeKonick, T., & Blondener, D. (2006). The nature of care in light of Emmanuel Levinas. *Nursing Philosophy, 7*(4), 225–34.

Leininger, M., & McFarland, M. (2006). *Culture care diversity and universality: A worldwide nursing theory* (2nd ed.). Sudbury, MA: Jones & Bartlett.

Leners, D. W., & Sitzman, K. (2006). Graduate students' perceptions: Feeling the passion of caring online. *Nursing Education Perspectives, 27*(6), 315–319.

Levy-Malmberg, R., Eriksson, K., & Lindholm, L. (2008). Caritas: Caring as an ethical conduct. *Scandinavian Journal of Caring Sciences, 22*(4), 662–667.

Locsin, R. (2001). *Advancing technology, caring and nursing.* Westport, CT: Auburn House Press.

Locsin, R., & Purnell, M. (2008). Rapture and suffering with technology in nursing. *International Journal for Human Caring, 11*(1), 38–43.

Locsin, R. C., & Purnell, M. (2009). *A contemporary nursing process: The (un)bearable weight of knowing in nursing.* New York, NY: Springer Publishing Company.

Longo, J. (2009). The relationships between manager and peer caring to registered nurses' job satisfaction and intent to stay. *International Journal for Human Caring, 13*(2), 26–33.

Lundqvist, A., & Nilstun, T. (2009). Noddings' caring ethics theory applied in a pediatric setting. *Nursing Philosophy, 10*(2), 113–123.

McCance,T. V., McKenna, H. P., & Boore, J. M. P. (1999). Caring: Theoretical perspectives relevant to nursing. *Journal of Advanced Nursing, 30*, 1388–1395.

Meng, M., Xiuwei, Z., & Anli, J. (2011), A theoretical framework of caring in the Chinese context: A grounded theory study. *Journal of Advanced Nursing, 67*, 1523–1536. doi:10.1111/j.1365–2648.2010.05573.x

Mitchell, G. (1997). Questioning evidence-based practice for nursing. *Nursing Science Quarterly, 10*(4), 154–155.

Morse, J. M., Bottorff, J., Anderson, G., O'Brien, B., & Solberg, S. (2006). Beyond empathy: Expanding expressions of caring. *Journal of Advanced Nursing, 53*(1), 75–87.

Morse, J. M., Bottorff, J., Neander, W., & Solberg, S. (1991). Comparative analysis of conceptualization and theories of caring. *Image: Journal of Nursing Scholarship, 23*(2), 119–126.

Morse, J. M., Solberg, S. M., Neander, W. L., Bottorff, J. L., & Johnson, J. L. (1990). Concepts of caring and caring as a concept. *Advances in Nursing Science, 13*(1), 1–14.

Munhall, P. L. (2004). Unknowing: Toward another pattern of knowing in nursing. In P. G. Reed, N. C. Shearer, & L. H. Nicoll (Eds.), *Perspectives on nursing theory* (pp. 368–374). Philadelphia, PA: Lippincott Williams and Wilkins (Reprinted from *Nursing Outlook, 41*[3] [1993], 125–128).

Nelms, T. (1996). Living a caring presence in nursing: A Heideggerian hermeneutical analysis. *Journal of Advanced Nursing, 24*, 368–374.

Nelson, J., & Watson, J. (2011). *Measuring caring: International research on caritas as healing.* New York, NY: Springer Publishing Company.

Newman, M. (2008). *Transforming practice: The difference that nursing makes.* Philadelphia, PA: F. A. Davis.

Newman, M. A., Simes, A. M., & Corcoran-Perry, S. A. (2009). The focus of the discipline of nursing. In P. G. Reed, N. G. Shearer, & L. H. Nicoll (Eds.), *Perspectives on nursing theory* (5th ed., pp. 601–606). Philadelphia, PA: Lippincott Williams and Wilkins (Reprinted from *Advances in Nursing Science, 14*[1] [1991], 1–6).

Newman, M. A., Smith, M. C., Dexheimer Pharris, M., & Jones, D. (2008). The focus of the discipline revisited. *Advances in Nursing Science, 31*(1), E16–E27.

Noddings, N. (2010). Moral education in an age of globalization. *Educational Philosophy and Theory, 42*, 390–396. doi:10.1111/j.1469–5812.2008.00487.x

Norman, V., Rutledge, D. N., Keefer-Lynch, A. M., & Albeg, G. (2008). Uncovering and recognizing nurse caring from clinical narratives. *Holistic Nursing Practice, 22*(6), 324–335.

Nyberg, J. (1990). The effects of care and economics on nursing practice. *Journal of Nursing Administration, 20*(5), 13–18.

O'Connell, E., & Landers, M. (2008). The importance of critical care nurses' caring behaviours as perceived by nurses and relatives. *Intensive and Critical Care Nursing, 24*(6), 349–358.

O'Connor, M. (2008). The dimensions of leadership: A foundation for caring competency. *Nursing Administration Quarterly, 32*(1), 21–26.

Paley, J. (2001). An archeology of caring knowledge. *Journal of Advanced Nursing, 36*, 188–198.

Papastavrou, E., Efstathiou, G., & Charalambous, A. (2011). Nurses' and patients' perspectives of caring behaviours: Quantitative systematic review of quantitative studies. *Journal of Advanced Nursing, 67*, 1191–1205. doi:10.1111/j.1365–2648.2010.05580.x

Papastavrou, E., et al. (2011). A cross-cultural study of caring through behaviours: Patients' and nurses' perspectives in six different EU countries. *Journal of Advanced Nursing.* doi:10.1111/j.135–2648.201.05807.x

Parcells, D. A., & Locsin, R. (2011). Development and psychometric testing of the technological competency as caring in nursing instrument. *International Journal for Human Caring, 15*(4), 8–13.

Paterson, J., & Zderad, L. (1988). *Humanistic nursing.* New York, NY: National League for Nursing.

Persky, G. J., Nelson, J. W., Watson, J., & Bent, K. (2008). Creating a profile of a nurse effective in caring. *Nursing Administration Quarterly, 32*(1), 15–20.

Powers-Jarvis, R. S. (2012). Between nursing, caring and technology: Being alive is more than having a beating heart. *International Journal for Human Caring, 16*(1), 48–53.

Purnell, M. J. (2009). Gleaning wisdom in the research on caring. *Nursing Science Quarterly, 22*(2), 109–115.

Quinn, J. (1992). Holding sacred space. The nurse as healing environment. *Holistic Nursing Practice, 6*(4), 26–36.

Quinn, J. F., Smith, M., Ritenbaugh, C., Swanson, K., & Watson, M. J. (2003). Research guidelines for assessing the impact of the healing relationship in clinical nursing. *Alternative Therapies in Health and Medicine, 9*(3, Suppl.), A65–A79.

Ray, L. (1999). Evidence and outcomes: Agendas, presuppositions and power. *Journal of Advanced Nursing, 30*(5), 1017–1026.

Ray, M. A. (1997). Consciousness and the moral ideal: A transcultural analysis of Watson's theory of transpersonal caring. *Advanced Practice Nursing Quarterly, 3,* 25–31.

Ray, M. A. (1997). The ethical theory of existential authenticity: The lived experience of the art of caring in nursing administration. *Canadian Journal of Nursing Research, 29*(1), 111–126.

Reed, P. G. (2009). Nursing: The ontology of the discipline. In P. G. Reed & N. C. Shearer (Eds.), *Perspectives on nursing theory* (5th ed., pp. 614–620). Philadelphia, PA: Lippincott Williams and Wilkins (Reprinted from *Nursing Science Quarterly, 10*[2] [1997], 76–79).

Reed, P. G., & Shearer, N. C. (Eds.). (2011). *Perspectives on nursing theory* (6th ed.). Philadelphia, PA: Lippincott Williams & Wilkins.

Roach, S. (2002). *Caring, the human mode of being: A blueprint for the health professions* (2nd ed.). Ottawa, CA: Canadian Hospital Association Press.

Roach, S. (2002). *Caring from the heart: The convergence of caring and spirituality.* New York, NY: Paulist Press.

Rykkje, L., Eriksson, K., & Raholm, M.-B. (2011). A qualitative metasynthesis of spirituality from a caring science perspective. *International Journal for Human Caring, 15*(4), 40–53.

Schoenhofer, S. O. (1994). Transforming visions for nursing in the timeworld of *Einstein's Dreams. Advances in Nursing Science, 16*(4), 1–8.

Schoenhofer, S. O. (2001). Infusing the curriculum with literature on caring: An idea whose time has come. *International Journal for Human Caring, 5*(2), 7–14.

Schoenhofer, S. O. (2001). A framework for caring in a technological dependent nursing practice environment. In R. C. Locsin (Ed.), *Advancing technology, caring and nursing* (pp. 13–11). Santa Barbara, CA: Praeger.

Schoenhofer, S. O. (2001). Outcomes of caring in high technology practice environments. In R. C. Locsin (Ed.), *Advancing technology, caring and nursing* (pp. 79–87). Santa Barbara, CA: Praeger.

Schoenhofer, S. O. (2002a). Choosing personhood: Intentionality and the theory of Nursing As Caring. *Holistic Nursing Practice, 16*(4), 36–40.

Schoenhofer, S. O. (2002b). Philosophical underpinnings of an emergent methodology for nursing as caring inquiry. *Nursing Science Quarterly, 15,* 275–280.

Schoenhofer, S. O., Bingham, V., & Hutchins, G. C. (1998). Giving of oneself on another's behalf: The phenomenology of everyday caring. *International Journal for Human Caring, 2*(2), 23–29.

Schoenhofer, S. O., & Boykin, A. (1998). Discovering the value of nursing in high-technology environments: Outcomes revisited. *Holistic Nursing Practice, 12*(4), 31–39.

Schoenhofer, S. O., & Boykin, A. (1999). The value of caring experienced in nursing. *International Journal for Human Caring, 2*(4), 9–15.

Schroeder, C. (1993). Cost effectiveness of a theory-based nurse-managed center for persons living with HIV/AIDS. In M. E. Parker (Ed.), *Patterns of nursing theories in practice* (pp. 159–179). New York, NY: National League for Nursing.

Schroeder, C., & Astorino, G. (1996). The Denver Nursing Education Project: Promoting the health of persons living with HIV/AIDS. In E. L. Cohen (Ed.), *Nurse case management in the 21st century* (pp. 63–67). St. Louis, MO: Mosby-Year Book.

Schroeder, C., & Maeve, M. K. (1992). Nursing care partnerships at the Denver Nursing Project in Human Caring: An application and extension of caring theory in practice. *Advances in Nursing Science, 15*(2), 25–38.

Sherwood, G. D. (1997). Metasynthesis of qualitative analysis of caring. *Advanced Practice Nursing Quarterly, 3*, 32–42.

Silva, M. C., Sorrell, J. M., & Sorrell, C. D. (1995). From Carper's patterns of knowing to ways of being: An ontological philosophical shift in nursing. *Advances in Nursing Science, 18*(1), 1–13.

Smith, M. C. (1992). Is all knowing personal knowing? *Nursing Science Quarterly, 5*(l), 2–3.

Smith, M. C. (1997). Nursing theory-guided practice: Practice guided by Watson's theory. The Denver Nursing Project in Human Caring. *Nursing Science Quarterly, 10*, 56–58.

Smith, M. C. (1999). Caring and the science of unitary human beings. *Advances in Nursing Science, 3*, 32–42.

Smith, M. (2004). Review of research related to Watson's Theory of Caring. *Nursing Science Quarterly, 17*(1), 13–25.

Soderlund, M., & Eriksson, K. (2006). The role of interpretation in caring science. *International Journal for Human Caring, 10*(3), 30–37.

Swanson, K. M. (1991). Empirical development of a middle range theory of caring. *Nursing Research, 40*, 161–166.

Swanson, K. M. (1999). What's known about caring in nursing: A literary meta-analysis. In A. S. Hinshaw, J. Shaver, & S. Feetham (Eds.), *Handbook of clinical nursing research* (pp. 31–60). Thousand Oaks, CA: Sage.

Thorkildsen, K. M., Eriksson, K., & Raholm, M.-B. (2012, July 27). The substance of love when encountering suffering: An interpretative research synthesis with an abductive approach. *Scandinavian Journal of Caring Sciences, Early View.*

Thornberg, P., Schim, S. M., Paige, V., & Grunbauch, K. (2008). Nurses' experiences of caring while letting go. *Journal of Hospice & Palliative Care Nursing, 10*(6), 382–391.

Thornton, L. (2005). The model of whole-person caring: Creating and sustaining a healing environment. *Holistic Nursing Practice, 10*(3), 106–115.

Touhy, T., & Boykin, A. (2008). Caring as the central domain in nursing education. *International Journal for Human Caring, 12*(2), 8–15.

Turkel, M. C. (2007). Dr. Marilyn Ray's theory of bureaucratic caring. *International Journal for Human Caring, 11*(4), 57–70.

Valentine, K. (1988). History, analysis and application of the carative tradition in health and nursing. *Journal of the New York State Nursing Association, 19*(4), 2–8.

Valentine, K. (1989). Caring is more than kindness: Modeling its complexities. *Journal of Nursing Administration, 19*(11), 28–35.

Valentine, K. (1991a). Nurse/patient caring: Challenging our conventional wisdom. In D. A. Gaut (Ed.), *Caring: The compassionate healer* (pp. 99–113). New York, NY: National League for Nursing.

Valentine, K. (1991b). A comprehensive assessment of caring and its relationship to health outcomes. *Journal of Nursing Quality Assurance, 5*(2), 59–68.

Valentine, K. (1992). Strategic planning for professional practice. *Journal of Nursing Care Quality, 6*(3), 1–12.

Valentine, K. (1993). Utilization of research on caring in the development of a nurse compensation system. In D. Gaut (Ed.), *Caring: A global agenda*. New York, NY: National League for Nursing.

Valentine, K. (1995). Values, vision, and action: Creating a care-focused nursing practice environment. In M. Leininger (Ed.), *Power, politics, public policy: A matter of caring* (pp. 99–115). New York, NY: National League for Nursing.

Watson, J. (1988). *Human science, human care*. New York, NY: National League for Nursing.

Watson, J. (1990a). The moral failure of the patriarchy. *Nursing Outlook, 28*(2), 62–66.

Watson, J. (1990b). Caring knowledge and informed moral passion. *Advances in Nursing Science,* 13(1), 15–24.

Watson, J. (1999). *Postmodern nursing and beyond.* New York, NY: Churchill-Livingstone.

Watson, J. (2000). Leading via caring-healing: The four-fold way toward transformative leadership [25th Anniversary Edition]. *Nursing Administration Quarterly, 25*(1), 1–6.

Watson, J. (2002a). Caring in nursing science: Contemporary discourse. In J. Watson (Ed.), *Assessing and measuring caring in nursing and health science.* New York, NY: Springer Publishing Company.

Watson, J. (2002b). Intentionality and caring-healing consciousness: A theory of transpersonal nursing. *Holistic Nursing Practice, 16*(4), 12–19.

Watson, J. (2003). Love and caring: Ethics of face and hand. *Nursing Administration Quarterly, 27*(3), 197–202.

Watson, J. (2005a). Metaphysics of virtual caring communities. *International Journal for Human Caring, 6*(1), 41–45.

Watson, J. (2005b). *Caring science as sacred science.* Philadelphia, PA: F. A. Davis.

Watson, J. (2006). Caring theory as ethical guide to administrative and clinical practices. *Nursing Administration Quarterly, 30*(1), 48–55.

Watson, J. (2008a). *Assessing and measuring caring in nursing and health sciences* (2nd ed.). New York, NY: Springer Publishing Company.

Watson, J. (2008b). *The philosophy and science of caring* (Rev ed.). Boulder, CO: University Press of Colorado.

Watson, J., & Foster, R. (2003). The Attending Nurse Caring Model: Integrating theory, evidence and advanced caring-healing therapeutics for transforming professional practice. *Journal of Clinical Nursing, 12,* 360–365.

Watson, J., & Smith, M. C. (2003). Caring science and the Science of Unitary Human Beings: A trans-theoretical discourse for nursing knowledge development. In P. G. Reed, N. B. Shearer, & L. H. Nicoll (Eds.), *Perspectives on nursing theory* (4th ed.). Philadelphia, PA: Lippincott Williams and Wilkins (Reprinted from *Journal of Advanced Nursing, 37*[5] [2002], 452–461).

White, J. (1995). Patterns of knowing: Review, critique and update. In P. G. Reed, N. C. Shearer, & L. H. Nicoll (Eds.), *Perspectives on nursing theory* (4th ed., pp. 247–257). Philadelphia, PA: Lippincott Williams and Wilkins.

Wolf, Z. (2013). *Exploring rituals in nursing: Joining art and science.* New York, NY: Springer Publishing Company.

Wolf, Z., Zuzelo, P., Goldberg, E., Crothers, R., & Jacobson, N. (2006). The caring behaviors inventory for elders: Development and psychometric characteristics. *International Journal for Human Caring, 10*(1), 49–59.

Index